THE BRITISH SCHOOL OF OSTEOPATHY
1-4 SUFFOLK ST., LONDON SW1Y 4HG
TEL: 01-930 9254-8

MEASURING HEALTH:
A Guide to Rating Scales and Questionnaires

KU-245-041

IAN McDOWELL
and
CLAIRE NEWELL

University of Ottawa

New York   Oxford
OXFORD UNIVERSITY PRESS
1987

Oxford University Press

Oxford   New York   Toronto
Delhi   Bombay   Calcutta   Madras   Karachi
Petaling Jaya   Singapore   Hong Kong   Tokyo
Nairobi   Dar es Salaam   Cape Town
Melbourne   Auckland

and associated companies in
Beirut   Berlin   Ibadan   Nicosia

Copyright © 1987 by Oxford University Press, Inc.

Published by Oxford University Press, Inc.,
200 Madison Avenue, New York, New York 10016

Oxford is a registered trademark of Oxford University Press

All rights reserved. No part of this publication may be reproduced,
stored in a retrieval system, or transmitted, in any form or by any means,
electronic, mechanical, photocopying, recording, or otherwise,
without the prior permission of Oxford University Press.

Library of Congress Cataloging-in-Publication Data
McDowell, Ian.
    Measuring health.
    Includes bibliographies and index.
    1. Health surveys. 2. Social surveys.
I. Newell, Claire. II. Title. [DNLM: 1. Health Surveys.
2. Questionnaires. WA 900.1.M478m]
RA408.5.M38   1987   362.1′0723   86-8556
ISBN 0-19-504101-1

1 2 3 4 5 6 7 8 9
Printed in the United States of America
on acid-free paper

The British School of Osteopathy

* 7 9 5 *

This book is to be returned on or before
the last date stamped below.

13 JUN 1988
3 OCT 1988
13 OCT 1988
-7 DEC 1990
12/11/90
10 DEC 1990
10 JAN 1991
13 FEB 1991

26 JUN 1992
-4 JUL 1993
29 SEP 1994
14 MAY 1996
11 DEC 1996

14 FEB 1997
11 JUL 1997
5 OCT 1998
18 FEB 1999
16 OCT 2007
22 SEP 2010

McDOWELL, Ian

MEASURING HEALTH

Preface

A major problem for epidemiological and health care researchers has been the lack of a concise source of information on health measurement methods. Many health measurements have been developed for use in health and social surveys, in epidemiological studies and in clinical trials. Descriptions of these methods, however, have been widely scattered in social science, medical, management and methodological journals, so that keeping abreast of the field is a formidable task. Furthermore, there are few summaries that compare one method with another and few that indicate which is the most valid for a particular application. The present reference book is intended to fill this gap. These methods have been termed "sociomedical" measurements, and they cover a variety of topics, including physical disability, emotional and social well-being, pain, life satisfaction, and quality of life.

We have written this book with two main purposes. First, we review the current status of health measurement, describing its theoretical and methodological bases and indicating areas in which further development is required. Second, and more important, we describe the leading health measurement methods, and comment on the current state of the field. These two themes will clearly appeal to different audiences—to the users and to the developers of measurement scales. Our experience as research consultants has repeatedly shown us that the greatest problem lies in persuading researchers not to invent their own unique measurement scale until they have carefully reviewed the numerous measurement methods that are already available. Our primary focus is therefore on the first theme: the provision of a guide to existing health measurement methods. The methods we review all use subjective judgments obtained from questionnaires or rating scales; they do not include laboratory measurements of the functioning of body systems or processes. We give full descriptions, including copies of the instruments, of 50 measurement methods; we summarize the reliability and validity of each and provide all the information necessary for readers to select the most appropriate measurement for their purposes, and then to apply and score the method chosen. As an introduction to the available health measurements, this book is intended principally as a reference work for social scientists, epidemiologists and other health care researchers, for health planners and evaluators: in short, for all who need to measure health status in research studies. It should also be of value to clinicians who wish to select a way to record the progress of their patients.

This seems to be an appropriate time to produce this book because we have recently seen the completion of the testing of several important measurement methods; at the same time there is a growing awareness among granting agencies and researchers of the importance of applying measurements that have proven reliability and validity.

Ottawa, Canada   I. McD.
May 1986   C. N.

Acknowledgments

This book was written while the principal author was supported by a Career Health Scientist Award from the Ministry of Health in Ontario, Canada. We gratefully acknowledge the support of the Ministry of Health, and also of the University of Ottawa; of the various people who have helped us, particular thanks are due to Monica Prince, who kept the word processor to heel with consummate skill.

I. McD.
C. N.

Contents

List of Exhibits

MEASURING HEALTH

1

Introduction

BACKGROUND

Our experience as research consultants has shown us that researchers and clinicians are often unaware of the wide variety of measurement techniques that are available for use in health services research. This has been detrimental in several ways. Research funds are wasted when studies do not use the best available techniques, and unless comparable measurement methods are used in different studies, the accumulation of scientific evidence is seriously delayed. The development of health measurements has so far been an uneven process with deficiencies in some areas of measurement, while others show a proliferation of methods which vary only in minor detail. In general, the developments that have been made in health measurement techniques are slow to filter down to those who might wish to use them. It often seems easier to create a new index than to search out and use an existing one, as illustrated by the many researchers who have reinvented the Activities of Daily Living scale (several of the largely minor variants on the ADL theme are summarized in Chapter 3).

In the chapters that follow we review a selection of the leading health measurement methods. Our descriptions are intended to be sufficiently detailed to permit readers to choose, and then apply, the most suitable instrument. We have included several sections that give critical comparisons between the methods examined, and throughout the book we have paid careful attention to the accuracy of the information provided.

SELECTION OF INDICES FOR REVIEW

Because there are too many indices to review in a single book, we have had to be selective in the scales we present. This was especially the case in areas such as the Activities of Daily Living indices and scales of social functioning. We narrowed our selection in several ways. First, we omitted whole areas of measurement from consideration such as indices of child health, which have been well summarized by Johnson (1). We have also omitted indices designed to assess very specific forms of impairment (scales of hand function, functional indices for quadriplegics, etc). Psychological measurements with a clinical focus, such as anxiety and depression scales, were excluded in part because they have already been described (2, 3), but also because they are so numerous that they would fill a volume of their own. We have, however, compromised in the area of psychological health indicators by including more general indices of "psychological well-being" as these are frequently used in health surveys and in outcome evaluation studies. We excluded measurements that are still in the preliminary stages of development, as any description would rapidly become outdated. We do not include complete survey questionnaires, nor do we cover questions on risk factors such as smoking or alcohol consumption. The scales that we do discuss all measure a specific aspect of health; they may be incorporated within a broader survey questionnaire. They cover the following topics: functional disability and handicap, psychological well-being, social health, quality of life, pain and general health measurements that assess the physical, emotional and social aspects of health.

Within each of these fields we have been highly selective, attempting to review the best methods available. Our definition of "best" relied principally on the evidence for the validity and reliability of each measurement. We considered only measurements for which published information is available, including evidence of reliability and validity. Unpublished scales have been reviewed elsewhere, by Ward and Lindeman (4) and by Bolton (5). As we made our selection, it became clear that the evidence for the validity of many scales is remarkably thin, so we were able to base our selection almost exclusively on the measurement properties of the scale. The few exceptions to this are scales that hold particular conceptual or methodological interest in the development of the field. We recognize, of course, that a different selection could have been made, but the scope for choice applies mainly to the less important methods, and in each chapter there are instruments that are clearly superior and whose inclusion cannot reasonably be disputed.

STRUCTURE OF THE BOOK

As we are writing for a broad audience, including those not familiar with the methodological bases for health measurement, Chapter 2 provides a brief historical review of the origins and development of the field, giving an outline of the theoretical and technical foundations of health measurement methods. This discussion provides the reader with an appreciation of the general quality of the methods available, with an introduction to the central themes of validity and reliability, and with an explanation of the various approaches to assessing the validity and reliability of measurement methods. The explanations provided are sufficient to permit the reader to understand our descriptions of the measurement methods, but it should be made clear that this book is not intended to serve as a text on how to develop a measurement scale.

Chapters 3 to 8 are the heart of the book, presenting our reviews of measurement instruments. They cover indices of functional disability, emotional well-being, social health, quality of life and pain, as well as general indices that span more than one of these themes. Each chapter opens with an introductory discussion of measurement techniques in that field, followed by a summary of the measurements we review, comparing their scope and quality. These "consumer's reports" take the form of tables that will assist the reader in selecting the most suitable scale for his purpose. Following these tables, we present the reviews of the measurement methods, ordered from the simpler to the more complex within each chapter. This is intended to reflect the general evolution of the methods, and also to aid the reader in selecting a method of appropriate length and complexity. To ensure the accuracy and completeness of our reviews, each was checked by the person who originally developed the method or by an acknowledged expert.

From our experience in writing these reviews, it has become clear that many methods lack information on relevant issues such as precisely for whom the measurement is intended, how valid it is and exactly how it is to be administered. For the leading instruments, however (see, for example, Goldberg's General Health Questionnaire), detailed information is available on all such points; in this respect the contrast between the more and the less adequate scales is very noticeable. Some general guidelines that could be followed by those who develop and publish descriptions of health measurement methods are given in Chapter 9, the concluding chapter.

STYLE AND CONTENT OF THE REVIEWS

Several general points must be made concerning our reviews. First, we found it necessary to do more than merely reproduce existing descriptions of the various methods, for it is remarkable how often there are discrepancies between the various published descriptions of a given method. Where we have found discrepancies, such as between different versions of a questionnaire, we have sought the guidance of the original author concerning the correct version to use. Second, wherever possible we have avoided technical terms and the jargon that is at times used in the original sources. We have frequently clarified obscure statements in the original publications. At the same time, we provide a factually accurate review of each method, and restrict comments and statements of our own opinions to the Commentary section of each review. Inevitably, however, some technical terms have to be used, especially in the sections on reliability and validity. We have defined these in a Glossary of Technical Terms at the end of the book. In the same vein, we have avoided repeating the interpretations of authors concerning the validity of their scales; virtually every author claims his method to be valid and so we have preferred to let the statistics speak for themselves.

FORMAT FOR THE REVIEWS

A standard format is followed in reviewing each measurement. It should be stressed that while we have written the reviews, each was checked for accuracy and completeness (in 1983–1985) by the person who originally developed the method, or by an acknowledged expert, to ensure that we are providing author-itative descriptions of the measurement methods. The following information is given for each measurement.

Title

The title of each method is that given by the original author of the instrument.

Author

The attribution of each method to an author is primarily for convenience; we recognize that most methods are developed by team effort. In certain cases additional authors are cited where they had a continuing involvement in the development of the method.

Year

This is the year the method was first published, followed by that of any major revisions.

Purpose

The purpose of the measurement is summarized in our own words, based as far as possible on those used by the original author. We have indicated the types of person the method is intended for (specifying age, diagnostic group) where this was stated. Frequently the precise purpose of the method is not made clear by the test developer; occasionally it is restated differently in dif-ferent publications and we have tried to resolve such inconsistencies.

Conceptual Basis

Where specified by the original author, this indicates what theoretical approach was taken to measuring the topics described in the Purpose.

Description

The description indicates the origins and development of the instrument, and shows the questionnaire or rating scale where space permits. Details of admin-istration and scoring are given. If the method is too long to reproduce, we show typical questions. Where there are several versions of the instrument, we have sought the advice of the original author of the method, and in general have reproduced the most recent version.

Exhibits

Within the Description section, we have reproduced a copy of the question-naire or rating scale. Occasionally, where space does not permit us to show the entire instrument, we have included only one or two sections of it. We have followed the format of the original method as closely as possible, and as all use a slightly different layout, this explains the apparent inconsistencies between the exhibits.

Reliability and Validity

For most instruments we have summarized all of the information that was available when our book was being prepared. For a few scales (notably in Chapter 4 on psychological well-being) there is such extensive data on validity that we have been selective. We have taken the majority of the information from published sources, but at times this has been supplemented or corrected following correspondence with the original author.

Alternative Forms

This outlines alterations that have been made to the questionnaire, including abbreviations and translations. We have only listed versions that could be considered authoritative, and do not include minor variants.

Reference Standards

Where available, these provide a valuable source of information against which the user can compare the results of his own study.

Commentary

Our descriptions of each measurement are as objective as possible; our own comments have been restricted to this section. Here we summarize the strengths and weaknesses of the method and outline how it compares to others with a similar focus. This is intended to help the reader choose between alternative measurements and to suggest where further developmental work may be carried out. Read in conjunction with the summary tables at the beginning of each chapter, the Commentary should guide the reader in his choice of a measurement.

Address

Most of our reviews were examined by the original test developer, who often provided us with additional information. This is also the person from whom materials such as users' manuals or copies of the questionnaire may be obtained. The address we give was correct as of 1985.

References

We do not list all available references to the measurements, but cite those that we found to provide useful information on the instrument and on its validity or reliability. For most instruments we reviewed additional references to studies that used the method but unless data on its quality were reported, such references have not been listed. The interested reader will be able to locate further references through the Science Citation Index.

Each chapter is introduced by a brief, historical overview of the measurement methods it contains; this is followed by a summary table comparing the salient characteristics of the measurements reviewed in that chapter. This is intended as a "consumer's guide" to the various methods and gives the following information:

1. The numerical characteristics of the scale: nominal, ordinal, interval or ratio.
2. The length of the test, as indicated by the number of items in contains.
3. The applications of the method: clinical, research or survey.
4. The method of administering the scale: self-administered, by an interviewer, or requiring an expert rater (e.g., physician or physiotherapist). Where a scale may be administered in several ways we have recorded the simpler method: self- rather than interviewer-administered. Where the length of time needed to administer the scale was given, this is indicated.
5. We have made a rating that indicates how widely the method has been used because, other things being equal, it will be advantageous to select a commonly used measurement technique. Our rating refers to the number of separate studies in which the method has been used, rather than to the number of publications that describe the method, for one study can often give rise to a large number of reports. Three categories indicate how widely the scale has been used: a few (1 to 4) published studies have used the method, several (5 to 8) studies by different groups, or many studies (9 or more different studies).
6. Four ratings summarize evidence of reliability and validity. The first and third summarize the *thoroughness* of reliability and validity testing:

> 0 = no reported evidence of reliability or validity
> + = very basic information only
> + + = several types of test, or several studies have reported reliability/validity
> + + + = all major forms of reliability/validity testing reported.

Because the thoroughness of testing may be independent of the results obtained, two other ratings summarize the *results* of the reliability and validity testing:

> 0 = no numerical results reported
> ? = results uninterpretable
> + = weak reliability/validity
> + + = adequate reliability/validity
> + + + = excellent reliability/validity.

Because of the large numbers of indices reviewed, and the range of topics they include, Chapters 3 and 8 also contain summary tables comparing the scope of each of the measurements reviewed.

The introduction to each chapter reviews the historical evolution of the methods and is intended to illustrate the common themes that link the individual measurement methods, for they are seldom developed in isolation from each other. The conclusion to each chapter gives a brief summary of the current state of the art in that area of measurement and suggests directions for further developmental work. The concluding section also mentions other measurements we consider to have merit but which we did not include as formal reviews because of lack of space or insufficient evidence on their quality.

EVALUATING A HEALTH MEASUREMENT: THE USER'S PERSPECTIVE

Finally, we recognize that everyone would like a guide book to make recommendations about the "best buy." This, of course, is a difficult judgment to make without knowing about the study in which the reader intends to use the method. We give several indications of the relative merits of the scales, but all of the methods we review have different strengths, so we can only make suggestions to the reader on how to use the information in this book to choose an appropriate measurement.

The user must decide exactly what he requires of the measurement. For example, will it be used to evaluate a program of care, or to study individual patients? What type of person will be assessed (what diagnosis, age group, level of disability)? What time-frame must the assessment cover: acute or long-term conditions? How broad-ranging an assessment must be made, and how detailed does the information need to be? For example, would a single rating of pain level suffice, or is a more extensive description of the type as well as the intensity of the pain needed? Bear in mind that this may require 15 minutes of the patient's time and that a person in pain will be unenthusiastic about answering a lengthy questionnaire. The user must decide, in short, on the appropriate balance to strike between the detail and accuracy required, and the effort of collecting it. This information can be gleaned from the "consumer's report" tables at the beginning of each chapter.

Turning to how the user evaluates the published information on a measurement method, the following characteristics should be considered:

1. Is the purpose of the method fully explained and is it appropriate for the intended use? Make certain that the method has been tested on the types of person to whom the user is intending to apply it.
2. Is the method broad enough for the application, neither asking too many, nor too few questions? Is it capable of identifying levels of positive health where this is relevant?
3. What conceptual approach to the measurement topic does it use? For example, which theory of pain does it reflect, and is this approach consonant with the orientation of the study? Is the theory well-established

(e.g., Maslow's hierarchy of needs) or is it an idiosyncratic notion that may not correspond to a broader body of knowledge?

4. How feasible is the method to administer and how long does this take? Can it be self-administered? Is professional expertise required to apply or interpret the instrument? Does it use readily available data (e.g., information already contained in medical records) and will it be readily acceptable to respondents? What response rates have been achieved using the method? Is the questionnaire readily available and is there a cost involved? Above all, is there a clear instruction manual that specifies how the questions should be asked?

5. Is it clear how the method is scored? Is the numerical quality of the scores suited to the type of statistical analyses planned? If the method uses an overall score, how is this to be interpreted?

6. What degree of change can be detected by the method, and is this adequate for the purposes? Does the method detect qualitative changes only, or does it provide quantitative data? Might it produce a false negative result due to insensitivity to change (e.g., in a study comparing two types of therapy)? Is it suitable as a screening test only, or can it provide sufficiently detailed information to indicate diagnoses?

7. How strong is the available evidence for reliability and validity? How many different forms of quality testing have been carried out? How many other indices has it been compared with? How many different users have tested the method, and did they obtain similar results? How do these compare to the quality of other scales?

A difficulty is commonly encountered in comparing two indices, one of which has excellent validity results in one or two studies, while the other may have been more widely tested but shows somewhat less adequate validity. We advise the reader to pay attention to the size of the validation studies: frequently, apparently excellent results obtained from initial, small samples are not repeated in larger studies. Ultimately the selection of a measurement contains an element of art and perhaps even luck; it is often prudent to apply more than one measurement wherever possible. This has the advantage of reinforcing the conclusions of the study when the results from ostensibly similar methods are in agreement, and it also serves to increase our general understanding of the comparability of the measurements we use.

The chapter that follows describes the methodological bases for health measurements; it provides sufficient information to permit readers to interpret the reviews in Chapters 3 to 8 and to answer the questions raised above. The chapter is intended primarily as an introduction for those who do not have a grounding in the theory of measurement; those who do may prefer to proceed to Chapter 3.

References

(1) Johnson OG. Tests and measurements in child development: handbook II. San Francisco: Jossey-Bass, 1976.

(2) Mittler P, ed. The psychological assessment of mental and physical handicaps. London: Tavistock, 1974.

(3) Sweetland RC, Keyser DJ. Tests: a comprehensive reference for assessments in psychology, education and business. Kansas City, Missouri: Test Corporation of America, 1983.

(4) Ward MJ, Lindeman CA. Instruments for measuring nursing practice and other health care variables. Vol. 2. Washington, DC: Department of Health, Education and Welfare, 1978. (DHEW Publication No. HRA 78–54).

(5) Bolton B. Measurement in rehabilitation. In: Pan EL, Newman SS, Backer TE, Vash CL, eds. Annual review of rehabilitation. Vol. 4. New York: Springer, 1985:115–144.

2

The Theoretical and Technical Foundations
of Health Measurement

For over a hundred years, most Western nations have collected statistical data characterizing social conditions. The data, describing birth and death rates, education, crime, housing, employment and economic output, reflect issues of public concern and often become the focal point for social reform movements. Measurements of health have always formed a central component in such public accounting, and are used to indicate the major health problems confronting society, to contribute to the process of setting policy goals and to monitor the effectiveness of medical and health care.

Social indicators of this kind are based on aggregated data expressed as regional or national rates; they are intended to give a picture of the health of populations rather than of individual people. Indicators of the health of individuals have also been developed and are principally used to evaluate the outcomes of care or in detailed epidemiological studies of the causes and consequences of differences in health (1). While both population and individual health indices are necessary and both will continue to be developed, this book deals only with indicators at the individual level. Population measurements such as rates of morbidity and mortality, or the mathematical indicators developed by Chen, by Chiang and others, are not considered here.*

There will probably always be a debate over how best to measure health, and one reason for the debate lies in the complexity and abstract nature of health itself. Like attitude or motivation, health cannot be measured directly, but the process of measurement requires several steps. Measurement is the process of applying a standard scale to a variable, but there is no standard scale for health; rather, its measurement relies on assembling a number of health *indicators,* each of which more or less adequately represents an element of the overall concept. Numerical scores are then assigned to the indicators, following which these may be assembled into an overall score. Reflecting this indirect approach,

*Information on such methods is contained in the winter 1976 issue of Health Services Research, pp442–463.

an often-quoted definition of measurement is "the assignment of numbers to objects or events to represent quantities of attributes according to rules" (2). The "objects or events" that may be used to indicate a person's health are of many types, ranging from a tumor analyzed in a laboratory to a movement of a limb observed by a physiotherapist, from estimates of working capacity to expressions of personal feelings. Of particular interest to us is a recent evolution in the range of indicators that have been used to measure health, and this trend will be reviewed below. Following that, we will review the methods that may be used to assign numbers to indicators of health.

THE EVOLUTION OF HEALTH INDICATORS

The earliest population health indices used readily available numerical indicators such as mortality rates. Mortality is unambiguous and, because death must be recorded by law, the data are generally complete. But as societies evolve, health problems alter in salience and new health indicators must be chosen to reflect changing health issues. The resolution of one type of health problem serves to reveal a new layer of concerns, a process that Morris has called "the onion principle" (3). As an example, the infant mortality rate is often used as an indicator of health levels in preindustrial societies, where rates are high and where reductions can be relatively easily achieved. As infant mortality declines, however, several things happen. First, a law of diminishing returns begins to apply, so that further reductions require increasingly large expenditures of resources. Second, as the infant mortality rate declines, the numerator becomes so small that it provides a less representative indicator of the health of the broader population. This is especially true if growing numbers of those who survive exhibit health problems associated with low birth weight or prematurity, problems rarely encountered when infant mortality is high. In a similar way, the currently increasing life expectancy in industrial countries may raise the prevalence of disability in the population (4, 5). In each case, the resolution of one health problem casts new issues into prominence and reduces the usefulness of the prevailing health indicator, necessitating its replacement by others. It may also increase pressure to modify the prevailing definition of health.

It should be recognized, however, that the selection of a particular health indicator has several important consequences. Indicators are deliberately chosen to reflect problems of social concern and ones for which improvement is sought. Because of this, a given indicator does not serve merely as a passive marker of health, but may come to be a rallying point for programs of social reform: to reduce infant mortality or rates of alcoholism, for example. Social reforms are based on the information that is available to us, so the selection and publication of indicators of health are choices that reflect, but in turn come to influence, social and political goals. The very choice of indicators therefore tends to affect the health of the population; reference to an indicator focuses attention on that problem, such as infant mortality, and the resulting interventions (if successful) will tend to reduce the prevalence of the problem, in turn reducing the value of the measurement. The identification of new concerns tends to raise a demand for new indices of health to monitor progress towards the new goals, and so the cycle begins again.†

The rising expectations of the past 150 years have led to a shift away from viewing health in terms of survival, through a phase of defining it in terms of freedom from disease, thence to an emphasis on the individual's ability to perform his daily activities, and now to the current emphasis on positive themes of happiness, social and emotional well-being, and quality of life. Only where problems of high premature mortality are no longer a pressing social concern does it become relevant to think of health in the World Health Organization's terms of "physical, mental, and social well-being, and not merely the absence of disease and infirmity" (7, p459). But here, again, measurements interact with progress. Just as language molds the way we think, our health measurements influence (and are influenced by) the way we define and think about health. When it was introduced in the 1950s, the WHO definition of health was criticized as unmeasurable, but the subsequent development of techniques to measure the concepts it includes, such as "well-being," contributed to the current wide acceptance of the definition. Goldsmith has reviewed a number of definitions of health and has discussed the implications of these for measuring health (8, 9).

This book is concerned with the adequacy of health indices: do the available methods successfully reflect an explicit and accepted definition of health? This is the theme of validity, the assessment of what a measurement measures, and of how it can be interpreted. A valid health index provides information about health status, not about some other variable, such as personality (1). Historically, it was concern over the validity of measurement that led to questions over the interpretation of many of the population health indices and that fostered the development of indicators of the health of individuals. For example, population indices such as the rates of consultations with physicians can only be interpreted as indicators of health if we can determine how the numbers of services provided are related to health status. Do more consultations imply better health in a population, or that there is more illness to be treated? Consultation rates may form more valid indicators of health expenditures than of health. Similar problems arise in interpreting indicators such as rates of bed days or work-loss days: these can reflect both health and the provision of care, for improved access to care may result in activity restrictions ordered by physicians. Without the care there might have been less activity restriction but a greater risk of long-term damage to the individual's health (10). Studies have, indeed, shown increases in disability days as the availability of medical services grows (11). One way out of the dilemmas in interpreting population indicators is to ask questions of individuals, providing a more direct reflection of health, rather than of the availability of care.

Measurements of individual health may be based on laboratory or diagnostic tests, or they may rely on indicators in which a person (the patient or a clinician) makes a judgment that forms the indicator of health. The latter are often

†A good general discussion of these issues is given by Moriyama (6).

termed "subjective" measurements, and we use the term in this sense here. Unfortunately, "subjective" is also used in other ways, for example to indicate whether the variable to be measured is observable or not (1). In this definition of subjective, the ability to climb stairs is considered an objective indicator because it can be observed, whereas pain or feelings are subjective because they are unobservable. For reasons of simplicity and cost, most health measurements use self-report rather than observation, so that even though stair-climbing ability could be observed, it is normally measured by self-report and so we have included it and similar indicators under the rubric of subjective measurements.

Subjective health measurements may be grouped into three main categories: those that record general feelings of well-being, those that record symptoms of illness, and those that focus on the adequacy of a person's functioning (12). Subjective measurements of each of these types hold several advantages. They amplify the data obtainable from morbidity and mortality statistics by describing the quality rather than merely the quantity of survival. They give insights into matters of human concern such as pain, suffering or depression that could never be inferred solely from physical measurements or laboratory tests. They give information about individuals whether they seek care or not, they can reflect the positive aspects of good health, and they do not require invasive procedures or expensive laboratory analyses. They may also offer a systematic way to record and present "the small, frantic voice of the patient" (13). Subjective measurements are, of course, little different from the data collected for centuries by physicians when taking a medical history. The important difference lies in the standardization of these approaches and the addition of numerical scoring systems.

Despite these potential advantages of subjective indicators, several problems delayed their acceptance. Contrasting sharply with the inherent reliability of mortality rates as a source of data, asking questions of a patient seemed to be abundantly susceptible to bias. There was also the question of completeness: population health indicators apply to the whole population rather than only to a limited number of individuals. Applying individual health measurements to whole populations is prohibitively expensive, although questions on health were asked in the Irish census as far back as 1851 (14).

Gradually, however, indices of personal health that relied on subjective judgments came to be accepted. The reasons for this included several methodological advances in survey sampling and data analysis made at the time of World War II. The war brought with it the need to assess the physical and mental fitness of large numbers of recruits for military service. Evidently, indicators showing rates of disease or disability were of no use for this; indicators of the health of individuals applicable on a large scale were accordingly developed and standardized. Wartime screening tests of physical capacity later influenced the design of post-war questionnaires (14, 15), while the psychological assessment techniques developed by Lazarsfeld, Guttman, Suchman and others during the war formed the basis for the first generation of psychological well-being measurements in the post-war years (see Chapter 4).

A major contribution of this wartime work concerned the application of numerical scaling techniques to health indices. Because subjective reports of health are not inherently quantitative, some form of rating method was required to translate statements such as "severe pain" into a form suitable for statistical analysis. The scaling techniques originally developed by social psychologists to scale attitudes soon found application in health indices. The use of these (and later of more sophisticated) rating methods permitted subjective health measurements to rival the quantitative strengths of the traditional indicators. After the war survey sampling techniques were refined by political scientists concerned with predicting voting behavior. This gave the basis for using individual measurements to provide data that were representative of the larger population. Coming somewhat later, technical advances in data processing had a profound effect on the range of statistical analyses that could be applied to data. This encouraged the refinement of questionnaires through techniques such as factor analysis and also simplified the analysis and presentation of the voluminous information collected in health questionnaires.

In more recent years the scope of subjective indices has been extended to cover virtually every aspect of daily functioning: physical, emotional, and social. Elinson termed these new methods "sociomedical" indicators of health (13). By assessing the whole person in his environment, these complement more traditional laboratory measurements that focus on parts of people, or elements of physical functioning. It is with sociomedical health measurements that this book is concerned.

THEORETICAL BASES FOR MEASUREMENT: PSYCHOPHYSICS AND PSYCHOMETRICS

Before we review the procedures for evaluating the accuracy of health measurements, a more fundamental question needs to be addressed: what evidence is there that subjective judgments form a sound basis for making measurements of health at all? Set against the Western tradition of mathematics and the exact sciences, it is by no means self-evident that such "soft" data can be considered as anything more than a crude approximation to measurement. Indeed, many health measurements *are* exceedingly crude and merely affix numbers to subjective judgments that are qualitative rather than quantitative. This, however, need not be so, as will be seen from some of the more sophisticated instruments reviewed in this book. To introduce the scientific basis for health measurement, we will begin with a brief introduction to psychophysics and psychometrics, describing the procedures used to assign numerical scores to subjective judgments. The following sections presume a familiarity with some basic statistical terms that are, however, defined in the "Glossary of Technical Terms."

The arguments for considering subjective judgments as a valid approach to measurement derive ultimately from the field of psychophysics. Psychophysical principles were later incorporated into psychometrics, from which most of the techniques used to develop subjective measurements of health were derived. Psychophysics is concerned with the way in which people perceive and make judgments about physical phenomena such as the length of a line, the loudness of a sound, or the intensity of a pain: psychophysics investigates the characteristics of the human being as a measuring instrument.

> If you shine a faint light in your eye, you have a sensation of brightness—a weak sensation, to be sure. If you turn on a stronger light, the sensation becomes greater. Clearly, then, there is a relation between perceived brightness and the amount of light you put in the eye. . . . But how, precisely, does the output of the system (sensation) vary with the input (stimulus)? Suppose you double the stimulus, does it then look twice as bright?
>
> The answer to this question happens to be no. It takes about nine times as much light to double the apparent brightness, but this specific question, interesting as it may be, is only one instance of a wider problem: what are the input-output characteristics of sensory systems in general? Is there a single, simple, pervasive psychophysical law? (16, p29).

In 1960, Stevens's answer to this question was that psychophysics had apparently discovered such a law that was becoming well substantiated by empirical evidence. Before describing this law, we should briefly establish a context for Stevens's claim by outlining the earlier history of psychophysics. This will then shed light on the way in which we can interpret subjective judgments of more abstract qualities such as pain, disability or depression.

The search for a mathematical relationship between the intensity of a stimulus and its perception began with the work of Gustav Fechner, whose major text was published in 1860. Subjective judgments of any stimulus, Fechner discovered, are not simple mirrorlike reflections of the event. For example, it is easy for us to feel the four-ounce difference between a one- and a five-ounce weight, but distinguishing a 100-pound weight from one four ounces heavier is much less certain. To discern the mathematical form of the link between the level of a physical stimulus and our perception of it, Fechner proposed a method of scaling sensations based on "just noticeable differences," and then recording the objective magnitude of just noticeable differences at different levels of the stimulus. A difference of one ounce may be noticeable when dealing with small weights, whereas with larger weights a just noticeable difference would be much larger. In this case our perceptions are more attuned to detecting small differences at lower levels of a stimulus than they are at higher levels. Fechner concluded that a geometric increase in brain activity (i.e., the stimulus as received by the senses) is accompanied by an arithmetic increase in conscious sensation. This relationship is conveniently expressed as a natural logarithm, and details of the derivation of Fechner's law are given, for example, by Baird and Noma (17).

Fechner's approach agreed with empirical data, it was intuitively appealing and it also incorporated Weber's law of 1846, which proposed that the magnitude of just noticeable differences was proportional to the absolute level of the stimulus. Fechner's law became accepted, and psychophysics turned its attention to other issues for over 70 years. During this time, however, considerable evidence had accumulated from various sources that the logarithmic relationship did not fit all types of stimuli. Experimental investigations of how people judge the loudness of sounds, the intensity of an electric shock or the saltiness of food, for example, showed that the logarithmic relationship between stimulus and response did not always apply, but it proved hard to find a more adequate mathematical formulation. Eventually, in the mid-1950s, the logarithmic approach was replaced by the more generally applicable power law proposed by Stevens (16). Like Fechner's law, the power law recognized that humans can make consistent, numerical estimates of sensory stimuli; it agreed, also, that the relationship between stimulus and subjective response was not linear, but it differed from Fechner's law by stating that the exact form of the relationship varied from one sensation to another. This was described by an equation with a different power function exponent for each type of stimulus, of the following general form:

$$R = kS^b,$$

where R is the response, S the level of the stimulus, and b an exponent that typically falls in the range 0.3 to 1.7 (17, p83; 18, p25). The exponent for force of handgrip is 1.7, while that for sound pressure is 0.67. The varying exponents imply that subjective responses to different types of stimulus grow at different, but characteristic, rates. The size of the exponent is an indicator of psychological sensitivity to the stimulus. The exponent of 0.67 for loudness means that a doubling of decibels will typically be judged as only two thirds louder. Sensitivity to electrical stimulation is much greater, with an exponent of 3.5; this holds implications for describing responses to pain. When the exponent b is unity, the relationship between stimulus and response is linear, as proposed by Weber's law. This is the case for judging line lengths, so that a line of 2 inches is judged to be twice as long as one of 1 inch. This convenient result underlies the interpretation of visual analogue response scales used in several health indices. Other aspects of psychophysical research that have a bearing on health measurement come from work done to validate the power law.

Considerable attention has been paid to validating the power law, and some of the most convincing evidence comes from a technique known as cross-modality matching. In the research to establish the power law, judgments were made by rating responses on numerical scales, so of course these judgments could be influenced by the way in which people perceive and use the numerical rating scale itself (17, p82). Since the power law response exponents are known (in terms of numerical judgments) for many different stimuli (line length, loudness, brightness, pressure and so on) arithmetical manipulation of these exponents should indicate how a person would judge one stimulus by analogy to another. Thus, in theory, a certain loudness of sound should be judged equivalent to a predictable brightness of light or pressure of handgrip. Experimental testing of the predicted match would test the internal consistency of the power law: if A equals B and A equals C, then B should equal C. Equally important, it would also show whether the use of numerical scales confounds the measurement process. As it turns out, the experimental fit between observed and predicted values was remarkably close, often within a 2% margin of error (18, pp27–31). This holds important ramifications for health measurement: people can make subjective judgments in a remarkably internally consistent manner, even when asked to make abstract comparisons—comparisons of the type that are frequently incorporated in subjective health measurements. Furthermore, visual analogue judgments of pain and ratings of functional disability on a 1 to 10 scale become more plausible on the basis of the evidence of the cross-modality matching experiments. Finally, the validation studies of the power law suggested that people can make accurate judgments of stimuli on a ratio, rather than merely on an ordinal scale of measurement: that is, people can judge in a consistent manner how many times stronger one stimulus is than another. The application of this more sophisticated "magnitude estimation" rating procedure to health measurement represents a plausible direction for future work; a review of the practical procedures for deriving ratio scale values for measurement instruments is given by Lodge (18).

Traditionally, psychophysics studied subjective judgments of stimuli that may be measured on physical scales such as decibels, millimeters of mercury, and so on. The very purpose of using subjective judgments in the social sciences or in the health field, however, was because there exist no objective, physical ways to measure the phenomena under consideration. Various books provide extended discussions of the way that the psychophysical methods have been adapted for use in measuring qualities for which there is no physical scale (19–21). This is the field of psychometrics, and the work done by psychologists in this area is now beginning to be applied in developing health measurement methods. Preliminary results suggest that a similar internal consistency of judgment holds for ratings of health as for other psychological measurements.

The following sections introduce two further issues involved in making subjective estimates of health levels. How are numerical values assigned to statements describing levels of health, and how far are subjective judgments influenced by the personal bias of the rater, instead of giving an accurate reflection of the actual level of health?

NUMERICAL ESTIMATES OF HEALTH: SCALING METHODS

Most of the health indices described in this book record responses in the form of descriptive statements: "severe pain," "I am unable to work," "I feel downhearted and blue." Many scaling methods exist for translating these indicators into numerical estimates of severity (19–22), and once this is done they may be combined into an overall score, termed a "health index." Scaling methods vary in complexity. Ideally, we want the most adequate numerical scale possible, but this requires a great deal of work in constructing the measurement. It may also place additional demands on the respondent, as seen in scales such as Tursky's pain rating scale.

A distinction between four ways of using numbers in measurement is fundamental to all scaling methods, and these lie in a hierarchy of mathematical adequacy. The lowest level is not a measurement, but a classification: nominal or categorical scales use numbers simply as labels for categories (such as males and females). No inferences can be drawn from the relative size of the numbers used: whether males are coded 1 or 2 is arbitrary. The only mathematical expression that can be used is that $A = B$ or $A \neq B$. For the second type, ordinal scales, numbers are again used as labels for response categories, but the numbers reflect the increasing order of the characteristic being measured, such as "mild," "moderate" and "severe" disability: $A > B$ or $B > A$. The actual value of the numbers, and the numerical distance between each category, hold no intrinsic meaning: a change from scale point 3 to point 2 is not necessarily equivalent to a change from 2 to 1. This is where considerable debate begins among methodologists. Strictly speaking, it is not appropriate to calculate differences between ordinal scores by subtraction, or to combine them by addition, because the resulting scores cannot be meaningfully compared: differences of a certain number of points between scores may not represent equivalent contrasts at different points on the scale. This is not to say that adding ordinal scales to make an overall score cannot be done—it is frequently done. While purists may criticize (23), pragmatists argue that the errors produced are small (19, pp12–33). Although many health indices do calculate overall scores on the basis of adding ordinal scales, the reader should be aware that this may lead to incorrect conclusions.

Adding scores is, however, permissible with the third type of scale. An interval scale is one in which numbers are assigned to the response categories in such a way that a unit change in scale values represents a constant change across the range of the scale. Temperature in degrees Celsius is an example. Because $A - B = C - D$, it is possible to interpret differences in scores: to add and subtract them and calculate averages. It is not, however, possible to state how many times greater one score is than another, which is the distinguishing feature of the fourth type of scale, the ratio scale. This may be expressed as $A \times B = C$ and $C / B = A$. This improves on the interval scale by including a zero point, making it possible to state that one score is, for example, twice another; the measurement of pressure is an illustration.

Psychometric texts distinguish between two main categories of scaling task used to convert responses to scale values: direct subjective estimates versus discriminant models that use Thurstone's law of comparative judgment (19, pp50–66). Both approaches have been used in developing health indices, and are very briefly introduced below.

The crudest (but most commonly used) approach to scaling is to rank order the responses in terms of severity and then to assign a numerical code to each response category. A critical review of this practice, which entails translating verbal labels such as "frequently" or "strongly agree" into largely arbitrary numerical equivalents, is given by Bradburn and Miles (24). Because people use the same adjectives in different ways we cannot assume that "frequently" implies the same thing to different people, nor that it implies the same frequency when referring to common as to rare health problems.

The first refinement to this approach is to use one of several category scaling procedures. Several of the measurements described in this book have used the equal-appearing interval scaling method to produce what is assumed to be an interval scale. In this approach a sample of people are asked to judge the relative severity (or "utility" in the economic term) of each of the items used in the health index. Verbal descriptions of the response categories, such as "severe pain," "moderate pain" and "mild pain," are sorted by each person into ten to fifteen ordered categories to reflect the relative severity of the problem implied by each statement. For each description a score is derived from the median of the category numbers to which the statement is assigned by the raters. Transformations may be applied, and the resulting score is used as a numerical indicator of the judged severity of that response. This approach has been used in scales such as the Sickness Impact Profile.

Objections to category scaling derive from the use of a fixed number of categories in the scaling task. People are capable of making much more accurate judgments of the relative magnitude of stimuli than such scales permit. A more sophisticated approach to scaling statements about health therefore has people judge the relative severity implied by each statement on scales with no limits placed on the values. This technique is known as magnitude estimation, and its proponents argue that it produces a true ratio scale estimate of the absolute value of the stimulus. At present, magnitude estimation has been used in very few health indices, and the simpler categorical rating methods are still the most commonly used, despite their technical inferiority. Objections have been raised against magnitude estimation, and both magnitude estimation and category scaling will probably continue to be used as their appeal is different: accuracy and theoretical sophistication versus simplicity (17).

As well as providing scale values for a single question, there are procedures for analyzing the scale properties of sets of questions. A method sometimes used in measuring functional abilities is the Guttman approach to scalogram analysis (see "Glossary"). This procedure identifies groups of questions which stand in a hierarchy of severity. In a Guttman scale an affirmative reply to a question high on the severity scale will imply an affirmative reply to each question lower on the scale. This gives some evidence that the items measure varying levels of a single aspect of health such as functional disability or depression. On such a scale a person's status can be described by noting the question at which his or her replies switch from being affirmative to negative. Indices that use Guttman scaling include Meenan's Arthritis Impact Measurement Scale and Lawton and Brody's Physical Self-Maintenance Scale. Guttman scaling is less well suited to the measurement of psychological attributes, which seldom form cumulative scales (19, p75). These various scaling methods are described in more detail in many sources (17–20, 22, 25, 26).

IDENTIFYING AND CONTROLLING BIASES IN SUBJECTIVE JUDGMENTS

Psychophysical experiments have shown that people can make accurate and internally consistent judgments of phenomena. This is the case, at least, when the individual is making objective judgments in a setting designed to emphasize that the task is an experimental one. Consistency in judgment may hold true for laboratory experiments concerning the length of lines or brightness of lights, but judgments of health may not be as dispassionate: in real life people have a personal stake in the estimation of their health. One person may exaggerate symptoms in order to be classified as sick and to qualify for a pension, while another may show the opposite bias and minimize ailments in the hope of returning to work. Judgments of psychological qualities may be even more susceptible to bias in self-report, and perhaps this is why so much attention is paid to validating psychological measurements. Goldberg cites the example of a person who is regarded by outside observers as fanatically tidy but who may judge himself untidy. Thus, subjective ratings of health combine an estimate of the severity of the health problem with a personal tendency to exaggerate or hide the problem—a bias that varies among people and over time. Several studies have examined how question phrasing and the respondent's personal attitudes may influence response bias—see, for example, reports from the National Opinion Research Center in Chicago (27).

Many types of bias have been identified in subjective measurements. Some reflect personality traits of the respondent: defensiveness, hypochondriasis, or a tendency to portray oneself in a good light by giving socially desirable responses. Other biases reflect the way people interpret questionnaire response scales: some prefer to use the end-position on response scales, while others prefer the middle (see 28, pp26–34). Two approaches have been used to deal with bias in health measurement. The first bypasses the problem, and argues that health care should consider the problem as perceived by the patient, including possible exaggeration, for this forms an integral part of his overall complaint: consideration of "the whole patient" is a hallmark of good care. From this viewpoint it can be argued that the biases inherent in subjective judgments do not threaten the validity of the measurement process: health is as the patient perceives it. The counter-argument is that this is a convenient simplification, and that the interests of correct diagnosis and appropriate patient management demand that health measurements should disentangle the objective estimate from any personal response bias. As an example, different forms of treatment are appropriate for the person who complains of a pain of organic origin from one whose report of pain is exaggerated by psychological distress.

Most health indices do not disentangle the subjective and objective components in the measurement and thereby seem to assume that the admixture of subjective and objective data is inevitable. Three approaches are seen among the relatively few indices that do try to separate subjective and objective components. First, the questionnaire may be completed by someone other than the patient, but who is very familiar with the patient. This approach is used in Katz's rating of social adjustment, and in Pfeffer's rating of functional disability. The second way of handling response bias is seen in scales that make an explicit assessment of the patient's emotional response to his condition. This approach is seen in the pain measurements of Pilowsky, Leavitt and Zung. The third approach is a statistical method of analyzing responses that provides two scores: one indicating the patient's ability to distinguish low levels of the stimulus (a notion akin to estimating the size of just noticeable differences), and the other an indication of the patient's personal response bias. This statistical approach, known as signal detection theory or sensory decision theory, is applied in a few health indices such as Tursky's pain measurement and so deserves a brief mention here; fuller discussions are available (17, 29–31).

Signal detection theory originated from the question of how people distinguish signals from background noise in radio and radar applications. In an experimental situation, two types of stimulus are presented in random order—noise alone or noise plus low levels of signal—and the ability of an individual to identify the presence of a signal against the noise is recorded. Applied to pain research, the stimulus is usually an electric shock and the "noise" is a low level of current. For each trial the respondent judges whether or not the stimulus was present and from the resulting pattern of true and false positive responses two indices are calculated: discriminal ability and response bias. In pain research, this technique has been used to study whether the use of analgesics influences pain by altering discriminability (i.e., by making the stimulus feel less noxious), or by shifting the response bias (making the respondent less willing to call the stimuls "painful"). Studies of this type are further described in Chapter 7. Signal detection analyses represent some of the most complex methods currently being applied to analyze subjective judgments of health. The field is relatively new, and although there is some disagreement over the interpretation of the results (31), the method may become more widely used in future.

From the signal detection analyses, characteristic graphs known as receiver operating characteristic (or ROC) curves may be drawn (29, 32). These illustrate changes in response patterns as a function of the strength of the stimulus, the likelihood of there being a stimulus, and the implications of the presence of the stimulus for the individual. Although developed as a way to examine the influences that bias individual judgments, the approach has been applied by epidemiologists in summarizing the validity of screening tests. Before we discuss validity, however, we must review the conceptual definitions that have been used to describe "health," and against which the validity of a measurement is checked.

CONCEPTUAL BASES FOR HEALTH MEASUREMENTS

It may appear obvious that a health measurement must be based on a specific conceptual approach: if we are measuring health, what do we mean by "health"? And yet by no means do all of the methods we review in this book offer a clear conceptual explanation of what they measure or of the value judgments they incorporate. In our descriptions we distinguish between the purpose of each index and its conceptual basis. The first provides a brief description of what the measurement is meant to do, such as to assess functioning in the elderly, while the conceptual basis specifies what approach is used to make this assessment and why. The conceptual definition of an index relates it to a broader body of theory and shows how the results obtained may be interpreted in the light of that theory.

A basic issue in constructing a health index is how to choose among the virtually unlimited number of questions that could potentially be included. There are two ways of approaching this problem: questions may be chosen from an empirical, or from a theoretical, standpoint. The two approaches are roughly equally represented in the methods we review.

The empirical approach to index development is typically used when the measurement has a practical purpose, for example to predict which patients are most likely to be discharged home following a rehabilitation program. After testing a large number of questions, statistical procedures based on correlation methods are used to select those that predict the eventual outcome. These item analysis statistics are described in the next section. This approach has frequently been used, and has a practical appeal. It does, however, suffer the weakness that the user cannot necessarily interpret why those who answered a certain question in a certain manner tended to have better outcomes: the questions were not selected so as to relate to any particular theory of rehabilitation. Many illustrations exist; the questions in the Health Opinion Survey were selected because they distinguished between mental patients and normal people, and while they succeed in doing this, the debates over what exactly they measure have continued for 25 years. A more recent example is Leavitt's Back Pain Classification Scale, which was developed empirically to distinguish between pain of an organic origin and pain related to emotional disorders. It succeeds well, but Leavitt himself comments: "Why this particular set [of questions] works as discriminators and others do not is unclear from research to date" (see Chapter 7). Accordingly, the method may have clinical value, but does not advance our understanding of the phenomenon of pain as a response to emotional disorders and how this operates.

The alternative approach to developing a health measurement is to choose questions that are considered relevant from the standpoint of a specific theory of health. Science advances mainly by developing and testing theories, so some indices have been explicitly developed to represent particular theoretical approaches to health, and their use in turn permits the theory to be tested. Melzack's McGill Pain Questionnnaire was based on his theory of pain; Bush's Quality of Well-Being Scale is based on an explicit conceptual approach to disability. Basing a measurement on a particular conceptual approach holds important advantages. By linking the measurement with a body of theory, it enables the method to be used analytically, rather than simply descriptively: studies using these methods may be able to explain, rather than merely to describe, the patient's condition in terms of that theory. The conceptual description also provides a guide to the appropriate procedures to be used in testing the validity of the method. The conceptual approaches used in many indices share common elements that will be introduced here, while finer details of the conceptual basis for each method are given in the reviews of the individual indices.

The majority of indices of physical health, and some psychological indices, build their operational definitions of health on the concept of functioning: how far is the individual able to function normally and to carry on his typical daily activities? In this view, someone is healthy if he is physically and mentally able to do the things he wishes and needs to do. The phrase "activities of daily living" epitomizes this approach. There are many discussions of the concept of functional disability, including those by Gallin and Given (33) and Slater (34). As Katz pointed out, functional level may be used as a marker of the existence, severity and impact of a disease even though knowledge about its etiology and pathogenesis is not advanced enough to permit measurement in these terms (14, p49). Measuring functional level offers a convenient way to compare the impact of different types of disease on different populations at different times. Stating that an index of disability will assess functioning, however, does not indicate what questions should be included. At this more detailed level, indices diverge in their conceptual basis; approaches that have been used include psychological theories such as Maslow's hierarchy of human needs, biological models of human development (as in Katz's ADL scale), or sociological theories such as Mechanic's concept of illness behavior.

Alterations in function are commonly assessed at three sequential stages: impairment, disability and handicap (35–38). "Impairment" refers to a reduction in physical or mental capacities. Impairments are generally disturbances at the organ level; they need not be visible and may not have adverse consequences for the individual: impaired vision can normally be corrected by wearing glasses. Where the effects of an impairment are not corrected, a "disability" may result. Disability refers to restriction in a person's ability to perform a function in a manner considered normal for a human being (to walk, to have full use of one's senses, and so forth). In its turn, disability may or may not limit the individual's ability to fulfil a normal social role, depending on the severity of disability and on what the person wishes to do. "Handicap" refers to the social disadvantage (e.g., loss of earnings) that may arise from disability. A minor injury can handicap an athlete but may not noticeably restrict someone else; a condition producing mild vertigo may prove handicapping to a construction worker but not to a writer. Although medical care generally concentrates on treating impairment, the patient's "problem" is usually expressed in terms of disability or handicap, and the outcome of treatment may therefore best be assessed using disability or handicap indicators, rather than measures of impairment. The term "disablement" has been proposed to refer to both disability and handicap: a field normally covered by subjective health indices. A thorough discussion of these terms and of alternative conceptual approaches that have been made to the same topics is given by Duckworth (36).

The positive aspect of health is increasingly often mentioned and is linked to resilience and resistance to disease. Here health implies not only current well-being but also the likelihood of future disease. This is relevant because planning health services requires an estimate of what the burden of sickness is likely to be in the future. Nor is it appropriate to consider as equally healthy two people at equal levels of functional capacity, if one has a presymptomatic disease that will very seriously affect future functional levels. For this reason, some indices (such as the Functional Assessment Inventory or the Quality of Well-Being Scale) include assessments of prognosis alongside the assessment of current health status. This prognosis is, of course, only related to health, for there are other reasons, such as an accident, which could drastically alter future health levels, but which are not an aspect of a person's health.

The conceptual basis for a health index narrows the range of questions that could possibly be asked, but a relatively broad choice remains among, for example, the many questions that could be asked to measure "functional disability." Whether the index reflects a conceptual approach to health or whether it is developed on a purely empirical basis, procedures of item selection and item analysis are used to guide the final stages of selecting and validating the questions to be included in the measurement.

THE QUALITY OF A MEASUREMENT: VALIDITY AND RELIABILITY

Someone learning archery must first learn to hit the center of the target, and then to do this consistently. This is analogous to the difference between two characteristics of a measurement: validity and reliability (39). The validity of measurement would be represented by the aim of the shooting—how close, on average, the shots come to the center of the target. The reliability (or consistency) of a measurement would be represented by how close successive shots fall to each other, wherever they land on the target. Ideally, a close grouping of shots should lie around the center of the target (reliable and valid), but a close grouping of shots may consistently fall away from the center of the target, representing a test that is reliable but not valid, perhaps due to some bias in the measurement. Other characteristics of a measurement may also be enumerated, but have so far received little attention in the field of sociomedical measurement. For example, precision may be important: a concept analogous to the number of decimal places to which a measurement is expressed.

Anyone who reviews discussions of validity and reliability will be struck by the diversity of ways in which writers approach these concepts. There are clear differences, for example, in the level of abstraction of definitions of the terms. Thus, validity is often defined as the extent to which a test measures what it is intended to measure, a definition used by many epidemiologists. Some psychologists would note, however, that uses may be found for tests that go beyond the purpose originally intended. Mortality rates may be intended to indicate levels of health or need for care, but the infant mortality rate may also serve as an indicator of socioeconomic development. This commends a broader definition of validity: the range of interpretations that may be placed on a test; what do the results mean? This approach recognizes that valid applications of a test may go beyond the purpose for which the method was originally designed. In this view, it is not the measurement itself that is valid or invalid, but the use to which it is put. There are objections to this definition, however: it may encourage an excessively empirical approach in developing measurements, for rather than beginning from a clear statement of the purpose of the scale, methods may be created whose precise intent (and therefore interpretation) is unclear. There are many examples of these, especially in the field of functional disability measurement. The result of using such scales is that we do not know how to interpret their results in terms of a broader body of theory, so that general understanding is not advanced. This can only be rectified by closely linking the validation process to a conceptual expression of the aims of the measurement. To avoid this problem, we argue that health indices should measure a specific and defined aspect of health, generally described in terms of a particular concept or theory. This approach then corresponds to the narrower definition of validity: does the instrument measure what it is supposed to? In keeping with this emphasis on specifying the precise aims of the method, we report the concept that each measurement is intended to reflect, whenever this was explained by the original authors. The provision of a conceptual description of a health index indicates how it relates to a body of theory; it also serves as a guide to the validation process which takes the form of testing how closely it meets its purpose as specified in the conceptual formulation.

The practical concern then becomes how we tell if a measurement is striking close to the center of the target and measuring what it is supposed to. There are many ways of testing validity, the choice depending on the purpose of the method (e.g., screening test or outcome measurement) and on the level of abstraction of the topic to be measured. The following section gives a brief review, introducing the methods that will be mentioned in the reviews. More extensive discussions are given in many sources (see, for example, references 19, 21, 40–42).

ASSESSING VALIDITY

Most validation studies begin by referring to content validity. Each health measurement represents a sampling of questions from a larger number that could have been chosen. Similarly, the measurement instrument that is selected is one of a number of instruments that could have been used, and the score obtained at the end of this multi-stage sampling process is of interest to the extent that it is representative of the universe of questions that could have been asked: the theme of content validity. Content validity refers to how adequately the sampling of questions reflects the aims of the index, as specified in the conceptual definition of its scope. For example, in a patient satisfaction scale, do all the items appear relevant to the concept being measured, and are all aspects of satisfaction covered? Often, content validity is not tested formally: it may be impossible to prove conclusively that the items chosen are representative of all possible items (see 43). A common procedure to establish content validity is to ask experts to comment on the clarity and completeness of the questionnaire. Occasionally, formal tests of linguistic clarity are used to test whether the phrasing of the questions is clear.

Following content validation, more formal, statistical procedures are used to assess the level of validity of a measurement. These procedures will either review the validity of the complete measurement, or of each individual question. The latter procedures are known as "item analysis." The term "item" is used to refer to the questions asked in a health index, simply because not all indices use actual questions: some use rating scales and others use statements with which the respondent agrees or disagrees. If the complete questionnaire is shown to lack validity, individual questions are normally examined and those that are weakest are deleted or altered with the aim of improving the overall validity results. Several statistical procedures may be used in testing validity.

In the simplest case there is already an accepted way to measure the concept in question, a criterion or "gold standard" against which the new measurement may be compared. This typically occurs when the new instrument is being developed as a simpler, more convenient alternative to a standard measurement. The new and the established tests are applied to a suitable sample of people and the results are compared using an appropriate correlation statistic. This procedure is variously known as correlational, concurrent or criterion validation. As an example, a questionnaire on hearing difficulties may be compared with the results of audiometric testing. Typically, the correlation of each question with the criterion score is used to select the best questions and thereby refine draft versions of the questionnaire. A variant of this approach is known as predictive validation, used when a test is intended to predict an aspect of future health status. Predictive validity is tested in a prospective study in which patient outcomes are compared to the measurements made at the start of the study. Since this may demand a long and expensive investigation it is rarely used; there are also logical problems with the approach. It is likely that during the course of a prospective study (and perhaps as a result of the prediction) interventions will be applied to selectively treat the individuals at highest risk. If successful, the treatment will alter the predicted outcome and wrongly make the test appear invalid. To avoid this problem, predictive validity is more commonly tested over a very brief time-interval, making it equivalent to concurrent validity.

Our chapter on psychological measurements describes several screening tests, and their validation illustrates the next level of complexity in the validation process. Here there is a criterion score, normally in the form of a diagnosis made independently by a clinician. The task is to show how well the test agrees with this classification, and also to identify the threshold score on the test that most clearly distinguishes between well and sick respondents. The test is applied to the contrasting groups of respondents and the patterns of their responses are compared. Two main types of potential error are recognized: a test may fail to identify people who have the disease, or it may falsely classify people without the disease as being sick. The "sensitivity" of a test refers to the proportion of persons with a disease who are correctly classified by the test as having the disease, whereas "specificity" refers to the proportion of truly nondiseased persons who are so classified by the test. Several extensions to these analyses exist, some of which will be encountered in this book. For example, Goldberg illustrates various ways of combining sensitivity and specificity estimates to give a single estimate of the adequacy of the test. He also gives formulae for calculating the prevalence of a disease using a screening test of imperfect, but known, sensitivity and specificity, correcting for the imperfections in the test (28, p93). Sensitivity and specificity analyses require that the score obtained using the test be divided into two categories, indicating presumed sick and presumed well. Changing the cutting point will alter the proportions of well and sick people correctly classified by the test such that an increase in sensitivity is associated with a decrease in specificity. Accordingly, the two parameters may be plotted graphically at different cutting points for the test in a further application of the ROC analyses described earlier. The true positive ratio (sensitivity) is plotted against the false positive ratio (1 − specificity) for various cutting points. The curve produced illustrates the trade-off between sensitivity and specificity, and the area under the curve provides an indicator of the usefulness of the test (32, 44).

For most of the measurements covered in this book, however, gold standards do not exist. This is especially the case where a measurement is designed to reflect an abstract, conceptual definition of health. In this situation, evidence from several validation procedures must be assembled, a process known as "construct validation." None of the construct validation procedures alone offers definitive proof of validity, and as will be shown below, all suffer from logical and practical limitations. The reviews in this book illustrate most of the types of evidence used to indicate construct validity, and these are briefly described here.

Correlational Evidence

Hypotheses are formulated which state that the measurement will correlate with other methods that measure the same concept; the hypotheses are tested in the normal way. The method is sometimes compared with several other indices using a multivariate procedure such as multiple regression. Hypotheses may also state that the test will *not* correlate with tests which measure different themes. For example, a test of "Type A behavior patterns" may be expected to measure something distinct from neurotic behavior. Accordingly, a low correlation would be hypothesized between the Type A scale and a neuroticism index and, if obtained, would lend reassurance that the test was not simply measuring neurotic behavior. Naturally, this provides little information on what it *does* measure.

Correlating one method with another would seem straightforward, but there are logical problems. Because a new measurement is often not designed to replicate precisely the existing method against which it is being compared, the expected correlation is often not high. But how high should it be, given that the two indices are inexact measurements of similar, but not identical, concepts? Here lies a common weakness in reports of construct validation: few studies declare what levels of correlation are to be taken as demonstrating adequate validity. All too often an author reports whatever correlation he obtains and then concludes that the test is thereby shown to be valid! A reasoned statement on the expected strength of correlation coefficients should precede the empirical test of validity.

Several comments may be made to assist the reader in interpreting reported validity correlations. First, because in practice there is always some error of measurement, the maximum attainable correlation between two health indices is never perfect but is limited by the unreliability of each of the measurements being compared. The maximum correlation that could be obtained is the product of the square roots of the reliabilities of each index (41, p84). If reliability coefficients are known, therefore, it is possible to compare the observed correlation to the maximum theoretically obtainable. Second, there are several ways of translating a correlation coefficient into terms that are more interpretable for the user. These are all based on the assumption that the measurement is being used to predict a criterion, and the purpose is to assess how much the accuracy of prediction is increased by knowing the score on the measurement. The simplest approach is to square the correlation coefficient, showing the reduction in error of prediction that would be achieved by using the measurement compared to not using it. As an example, if a health measurement correlates 0.70 with a criterion, using the test will provide an almost 50% reduction in error compared with simply guessing. Note that the value of a measurement in these terms declines increasingly steeply below a validity coefficient of roughly 0.50. The derivation of this approach is given by Helmstadter (41, p119); he also describes other ways of interpreting validity coefficients. The coefficient of alienation, for example, is an inverse measure of the effectiveness with which a prediction can be made, and uses the formula

$$\sqrt{1 - r_{xy}^2}.$$

The adequacy of validity (and reliability) coefficients may also be interpreted in the light of the values typically observed. The concurrent validity correlations between the tests reviewed in this book are low, typically falling between 0.20 and 0.60, with only occasional correlations between very similar instruments (such as the Barthel and PULSES scales) falling above 0.70.

Factorial Validity

This is an empirical way of establishing content validity using a statistical technique known as factor analysis. This examines how far the various items in an index accord in measuring one or more common themes. It is appropriate to use this method when a measurement contains separate components, each reflecting a different aspect of health. Using the pattern of intercorrelations among replies to questions, the analysis forms the questions into groups (or factors) that appear to measure common themes, each factor being distinct from the others. As an example, Bradburn selected questions to measure two aspects of psychological well-being, positive and negative affect. Factor analyses of the questions confirmed that they fall clearly into two distinct groups, which were homogeneous and unrelated to each other, and which by inspection appeared to represent positive and negative feelings. Where factor analysis is used to examine only the internal structure of a test, rather than its correlation with other tests, this is logically very similar to testing the internal consistency of the measurement, an aspect normally considered under reliability testing and discussed in a later section.

Factor analysis is widely used (and all too frequently misused), in the studies reported in this book; several principles guide its appropriate use (45). The variables analyzed should be measured at the interval scale level, the response distributions should be approximately normal and there should be at least five times more respondents in the sample than there are variables to be analyzed. Because so many health indices use categorical response scales (such as "frequently," "sometimes," "rarely" and "never") the first and second of these principles are very often contravened.

Group Differences or Discriminant Evidence

An index that is intended to distinguish between different categories of respondent (e.g., well and sick) may be tested by applying it to samples of each group, and by analyzing the scores for significant differences. Significant differences on index scores would disprove the null hypothesis that the method fails to differentiate between them. This approach is very frequently used, but like all other validation procedures is not free of logical limitations. At times we cannot be certain about people's health status. For example, screening tests for emotional disorder may compare psychiatric patients with the general population, but there is likely to be a proportion of the general population who suffer from undiagnosed emotional disorders. Furthermore, even though patients with a given diagnosis may show a high score on an index, this does not necessarily prove that high scores obtained on the index in a community survey imply that diagnosis (43).

In summary, construct validation of a health measurement is part science, but to a large extent an art form. There is seldom a definitive way to prove validity, and the choice of validation approaches is always open to debate. Some general principles exist, however. Good validation studies proceed by stating clear hypotheses and testing them, having explained why those hypotheses were considered the most relevant. Good studies will also seek to disprove the hypothesis that the method measures something other than its stated purpose, rather than merely assembling information on what it does measure. A variety of approaches should be used in testing any index, rather than relying on a single type of validation procedure. Future developments will probably see greater use of recently developed structural modelling techniques that allow theoretical (and unmeasured) variables to enter into multivariate analyses of the links between a series of measurements. An example of this approach to construct validation is given by Andrews (46).

ASSESSING RELIABILITY

Regardless of how the measurement scores should be interpreted, reliability is concerned with the degree to which they can be replicated. In traditional measurement theory the score obtained from any measurement is a combination of two components: an underlying true score and some degree of error. Many types of error occur in measurement, including the biases discussed above and random errors (47). Reliability is concerned only with random errors; bias is assessed by validity testing.

Random errors have several defining characteristics: being randomly distributed they are as likely to increase the observed score as to decrease it, the magnitude of random error is not related to the magnitude of the true score (i.e., this type of error is not greater in extreme scores), and the observed score is the arithmetic sum of the error component and the underlying true score that we are attempting to measure. The true score may be considered as the average score a person would obtain if tested repeatedly. The reliability of a measurement is then defined as the proportion of observed variation in scores that reflect actual variation in health levels (if any), while unreliability is the proportion of variation that is random error in measurement. The approach described here is that of traditional reliability theory and is the approach used in testing most health measurements. There are, however, newer approaches to reliability that may in future be applied to testing health indices (48).

Two types of inconsistency are commonly distinguished: whether different raters using the method to assess the same respondent obtain the same result (inter-rater agreement or observer variation) and, if the measurement is applied a second time to the same respondent, whether the same result is obtained (repeatability).

Inter-rater Reliability

This is generally assessed from correlations between different raters' judgments of a sample of respondents. The intraclass correlation or Kendall's index of concordance (W) are commonly used where responses of more than two raters or patients are being compared. To ensure that the persons being rated did not change their replies it may be possible to have different raters each rate a video recording of an interview. Typical values for inter-rater reliability fall in the range 0.65 to 0.95, and values above 0.85 may be considered satisfactory.

Repeatability, Stability, or "Test-retest Reliability"

The stability of the rating is especially relevant when the measurement is being used to make comparisons over time, and it is therefore necessary to eliminate or control extraneous factors influencing the measurement. Repeatability is estimated by applying the measurement twice and comparing the results, usually expressing the result as a correlation. Typical repeatability values for the measurements included in this book are relatively high, many falling between 0.85 and 0.90. Helmstadter quotes typical values for various types of psychological test, with the median for personality tests being 0.85, that for ability tests being 0.90 and for attitude tests, 0.79 (41, p85). A higher repeatability of measurement is required when assessing an individual than is necessary when comparing two groups of repondents.

While apparently simple, the test-retest procedure suffers some logical problems. It must be assumed that the characteristic being measured did not change, so the delay between measurements is kept brief. This, however, incurs the problem that recall by respondent or rater may influence the second application: the two assessments are not independent. A series of maneuvers have been used to overcome this problem, and a description of the logic underlying them will introduce a third form of reliability. Theoretically, if two versions of the test could be developed that are precisely equivalent, they could be applied in one measurement session, avoiding the problem of a real change in health and focusing only on inconsistency in the respondent's replies. To use this clever trick, however, it is first necessary to prove that the two versions of the measurement are, in fact, equivalent. This introduces the theme of internal consistency.

Internal Consistency

High correlations among the items may be used to demonstrate that two versions of a test are equivalent. A test with high inter-item correlations is homogeneous and is also likely to produce consistent responses. If used to estimate reliability by forming two subscales, the high correlations suggest that the two subscales will, indeed, be equivalent. Checking the equivalence of two halves of a measurement may be done by correlating the two sets of questions (for example, by correlating odd and even numbered questions), but a more general approach would be to estimate the correlations between all possible pairs of items. Several formulae are proposed by Kuder and Richardson for this, their formula 20 being frequently used to indicate internal consistency reliability or homogeneity. Cronbach's coefficient alpha is another frequently used indicator of internal consistency (21, pp380–385). Such formulae indicate what the correlation would be between different versions of the same measurement, and therefore estimate what the repeatability of the test is likely to be.

As with validity coefficients, there is no fixed level of correlation that indicates reliability, but internal consistency coefficients of 0.85 or above are commonly taken as acceptable. Various results help us to interpret the level of agreement implied by a particular correlation coefficient; Andrews obtained a test-retest coefficient of 0.68 where 54% of respondents gave identical answers on retest and a further 38% scored within one point of their previous answer on seven-point scales (49, p192).

Although there is a logical relationship among these various types of reliability, they are suited to somewhat different applications. A health measurement may be broad or narrow in scope, and it is not reasonable to expect a high internal consistency if the measurement covers several dimensions of health. A broad measurement may be expected to show lower repeatability as there are more ways in which the scores vary from test to retest. The relevance of internal consistency is that as health changes over time, the stability of a health measurement may be low, and under these circumstances the important issue is to indicate consistency at one time. If the health index is to be used to predict outcomes, it must be able accurately to predict itself, and so test-retest reliability is crucial. If, however, it is intended mainly to measure current status, the internal structure of the measurement is its most crucial characteristic. This is especially true when the measurement is designed to reflect a specific concept of health. In this instance, greater reliability will imply greater validity. The preceding sections have reviewed the most commonly used approaches to developing and testing a health measurement. The reviews that follow will illustrate the application of each of these techniques.

References

(1) Ware JE, Brook RH, Davies AR, Lohr KN. Choosing measures of health status for individuals in general populations. Am J Public Health 1981;71:620–625.

(2) Chapman CR. Measurement of pain: problems and issues. In: Bonica JJ, Albe-Fessard D, eds. Advances in pain research and therapy. Vol. I. New York: Raven Press, 1976;345–353.

(3) Morris JN. Uses of epidemiology. 3rd ed. London: Churchill Livingstone, 1975.

(4) Gruenberg EM. The failures of success. Milbank Mem Fund Q 1977;55:1–24.

(5) Wilkins R, Adams OB. Health expectancy in Canada, late 1970s: demographic, regional and social dimensions. Am J Public Health 1983;73:1073–1080.

(6) Moriyama IM. Problems in the measurement of health status. In: Sheldon EB, Moore W, eds. Indicators of social change: concepts and measurements. New York: Russell Sage, 1968;573–599.

(7) World Health Organization. The first ten years of the World Health Organization. Geneva: World Health Organization, 1958.

(8) Goldsmith SB. The status of health status indicators. Health Serv Rep 1972; 87:212–220.

(9) Goldsmith SB. A reevaluation of health status indicators. Health Serv Rep 1973;88:937–941.

(10) Wilson RW. Do health indicators indicate health? Am J Public Health 1981;71:461–463.

(11) Colvez A, Blanchet M. Disability trends in the United States population 1966–76: analysis of reported causes. Am J Public Health 1981;71:464–471.

(12) Chen MK, Bryant BE. The measurement of health—a critical and selective overview. Int J Epidemiol 1975;4:257–264.

(13) Elinson J. Introduction to the theme: sociomedical health indicators. Int J Health Serv 1978;6:385–391.

(14) Katz S, Akpom CA, Papsidero JA, Weiss ST. Measuring the health status of populations. In: Berg RL, ed. Health status indexes. Chicago: Hospital Research and Educational Trust, 1973:39–52.

(15) Moskowitz E, McCann CB. Classification of disability in the chronically ill and aging. J Chronic Dis 1957;5:342–346.

(16) Stevens SS. The surprising simplicity of sensory metrics. Am Psychol 1962;17:29–39. Reprinted in: Stone LA, ed. Readings in contemporary psychophysics and scaling. New York: MSS Educational Publishing, 1969.

(17) Baird JC, Noma E. Fundamentals of scaling and psychophysics. New York: Wiley, 1978.

(18) Lodge M. Magnitude scaling: quantitative measurement of opinions. Beverly Hills, California: Sage Publications, 1981. (Sage University Papers, Series on Quantitative Applications in the Social Sciences, No. 07-001).

(19) Nunnally, JC. Psychometric theory. 2nd ed. New York: McGraw-Hill, 1978.

(20) Torgerson WS. Theory and methods of scaling. New York: Wiley, 1958.

(21) Guilford JP. Psychometric methods. 2nd ed. New York: McGraw-Hill, 1954.

(22) Young FW. Scaling. Ann Rev Psychol 1984;35:55–81.

(23) McClatchie G, Schuld W, Goodwin S. A maximized-ADL index of functional status for stroke patients. Scand J Rehabil Med 1983;15:155–163.

(24) Bradburn NM, Miles C. Vague quantifiers. Public Opinion Q 1979;43:92–101.

(25) Stevens SS. Measurement, psychophysics and utility. In: Churchman CW, Ratoosh P, eds. Measurement, definitions and theories. New York: Wiley, 1959:18–63.

(26) Edwards AL. Techniques of attitude scale construction. New York: Appleton-Century-Crofts, 1975.

(27) Bradburn NM, Sudman S, Blair E, Stocking C. Question threat and response bias. Public Opinion Q 1978;42:221–234.

(28) Goldberg DP. The detection of psychiatric illness by questionnaire. London: Oxford University Press, 1972. (Maudsley Monograph No. 21).

(29) Swets JA. The relative operating characteristic in psychology. Science 1973;182:990–1000.

(30) Clark WC. Pain sensitivity and the report of pain: an introduction to sensory decision theory. In: Weisenberg M, Tursky B, eds. Pain: new perspectives in therapy and research. New York: Plenum Press, 1976:195–222.

(31) Rollman GB. Signal detection theory assessment of pain modulation: a critique. In: Bonica JJ, Able-Fessard D, eds. Advances in pain research and therapy. Vol. I. New York: Raven Press, 1976:355–362.

(32) McNeil BJ, Keeler E, Adelstein SJ. Primer on certain elements of medical decision making. New Eng J Med 1975;293:211–215.

(33) Gallin RS, Given CW. The concept and classification of disability in health interview surveys. Inquiry 1976;13:395–407.

(34) Slater SB, Vukmanovic C, Macukanovic P, Prvulovic T, Cutler JL. The definition and measurement of disability. Soc Sci Med 1974;8:305–308.

(35) World Health Organization. International classification of impairments, disabilities, and handicaps. A manual of classification relating to the consequences of disease. Geneva: World Health Organization, 1980.

(36) Duckworth D. The need for a standard terminology and classification of disablement. In: Granger CV, Gresham GE, eds. Functional assessment in rehabilitation medicine. Baltimore: Williams & Wilkins, 1984:1–13.

(37) Harris A. Handicapped and impaired in Great Britain. London: HMSO, 1971.

(38) Haber LD. Identifying the disabled: concepts and methods in the measurement of disability. Social Security Bull, December 1967:17–34.

(39) Ahlbom A, Norell S. Introduction to modern epidemiology. Chestnut Hill, Montana: Epidemiology Resources, 1984.

(40) Anastasi A. Psychological testing. New York: Macmillan, 1968.

(41) Helmstadter GC. Principles of psychological measurement. London: Methuen, 1966.

(42) American Psychological Association. Standards for educational and psychological tests. Washington, DC: American Psychological Association, 1974.

(43) Seiler LH. The 22-item scale used in field studies of mental illness: a question of method, a question of substance, and a question of theory. J Health Soc Behav 1973;14:252–264.

(44) Hanley JA, McNeil BJ. The meaning and use of the area under a receiver operating characteristic (ROC) curve. Radiology 1982;143:29–36.

(45) Comrey AL. Common methodological problems in factor analytic studies. J Consult Clin Psychol 1978;46:648–659.

(46) Andrews FM. Construct validity and error components of survey measures: a structural modeling approach. Public Opinion Q 1984;48:409–442.

(47) Wittenborn JR. Reliability, validity, and objectivity of symptom-rating scales. J Nerv Ment Dis 1972;154:79–87.

(48) Evans WJ, Cayten CG, Green PA. Determining the generalizability of rating scales in clinical settings. Med Care 1981;19:1211–1220.

(49) Andrews FM, Withey SB. Social indicators of well-being: Americans' perceptions of life quality. New York: Plenum Press, 1976.

3

Functional Disability and Handicap

Because they cover a topic of such fundamental concern in health care, there has been a proliferation of scales to measure physical disability and handicap. The available measurement methods serve a variety of purposes: some apply to particular diseases while others are broadly applicable; some assess impairments, others cover disability, handicap or the social environment; there are research instruments, screening tests and clinical rating scales; some methods are designed for severely ill inpatients, while others are for outpatients with lower levels of disability. A major problem in writing this chapter therefore lay in selecting a manageable number of instruments to describe. We have tried throughout to review the best measurement methods available, and have omitted little-used scales and those for which there is no published evidence for validity and reliability. Thus, of more than fifty activities of daily living scales described in the literature (1–8), we review only six. As it turns out, our selection is comparable to that made quite independently in another recent review article (9). The main surprise, perhaps, will be the inclusion of several older scales in our selection—many of the newer methods lack the information on reliability and validity that is available for the older instruments, and we have not included methods simply because they are new. To introduce the basis for our selection, we begin with a brief historical overview of the recent development of the field. This identifies the main categories of functional disability measurement, and the chapter will review examples of each type.

THE EVOLUTION OF FUNCTIONAL DISABILITY MEASUREMENTS

The concepts of impairment, disability and handicap were introduced in Chapter 2 and this conceptual framework has been reflected in the evolution of measurements of physical functioning. From the early impairment scales (covering physical capacities such as balance, sensory abilities or range of motion), attention shifted towards measuring disability (gross body movements and self-care) and later to handicap (fulfilment of social roles, working ability and household activities).

Formal measurements of physical impairments originated from diagnostic tests and from standardized medical summaries of a patient's condition, typically used with elderly or chronically ill patients. These were mostly rating scales applied by a clinician; they are represented in this chapter by the PULSES Profile. These measurements were often used in assessing fitness for work or in reviewing claims for accident and injury compensation; the emphasis was on rigorous, standardized ratings that could withstand legal examination. It was later recognized that although impairment may be accurately assessed, it is by no means the only factor that predicts a patient's need for care: environmental factors, the availability of social support and the patient's determination all affect how far an impairment will be translated into a disability or handicap. As the scope of rehabilitation expanded to include the return of patients to an independent existence, the assessment of physical impairment was no longer sufficient and it became important to measure disability and handicap as well. Assessment methods were enlarged to consider the activities a patient could or did perform at his level of physical capacity. Assessments of this type are generally termed "functional disability" indicators, typified by the activities of daily living (ADL) scales such as Katz's index. This was developed in 1957 to study the effects of treatment on the elderly and chronically ill. It summarizes the patient's degree of independence in bathing, dressing, using the toilet, moving around the house and eating—topics that Katz selected to represent "primary biological functions." Katz's scale is one of the few instruments to provide a theoretical justification for the topics it includes. Unfortunately, most other ADL scales are not built on any conceptual approach to disability, and there is little systematic effort to specify what topics should be covered in such scales. In part because of this, progress in the field is uncoordinated and scales proliferate apparently at the whim of their creators. Furthermore, scant attention has been paid to formal testing of the ADL methods and we know little about their comparative validity and reliability.

The ADL scales are concerned with severe levels of disability, relevant mainly to institutionalized patients and to the elderly. During the 1970s, the ADL concept was extended to consider problems more typically experienced by those living in the community: shopping, cooking and managing money, a field that has come to be termed "Instrumental Activities of Daily Living" (IADL). By broadening the scope of ADL scales, the IADL methods offer indicators of "applied" problems that extend the disability theme of ADL scales to include some elements of the handicap concept. This forms the second major category of measurements described in this chapter. Again, as with ADL scales, there is often little conceptual justification or theory to guide their content, although the IADL scales are newer and appear to have been somewhat better tested than the ADL instruments.

The development of IADL scales was stimulated in part by the movement towards community care for the elderly. Rehabilitation medicine has increasingly stressed the need to restore patients to meaningful social roles and this has fostered measurement scales that cover social adjustment as well as physical abilities. To assess a patient's ability to live in the community requires information on the level of disability, on the environment in which the patient has to live, the amount of social support that may be available, and on some of the compensating factors that determine whether or not a disability becomes a handicap. The IADL scales cover one part of this area, but other, more extensive scales have been developed to record factors that may explain different levels of handicap for a given disability such as the type of work the patient does, his housing, his personality and the social support available. Such extensions of this type to the original theme of functional disability produce measurements that are conceptually close to the indices of social functioning described in Chapter 5. We review scales that cover a combination of physical, social and emotional functioning in Chapter 8 on general health measurements. Examples include the Multidimensional Functional Assessment Questionnaire and the Sickness Impact Profile, both of which contain sections very similar in content to the scales described in this chapter.

The distinction between a person's physical capacity and his actual performance in managing his life in the face of physical limitations has been mentioned. Reflecting this contrast, there are two ways of phrasing questions on functional disability. One can ask what a person *can* do (termed "capacity" wording) or what he *does* do ("performance" wording). Both are common and both hold advantages and disadvantages. Asking a patient what he can do may provide a hypothetical answer, suggesting what the patient thinks he can do even though he does not normally attempt to do it. An index using such questions may exaggerate the healthiness of the respondent—possibly by as much as 15% to 20% (10, p70). Asking the respondent what he does or does not do overcomes this and so appears to offer a more realistic appraisal of the actual disability. A problem with performance wording, however, is that there are reasons other than ill health that restrict behavior, and performance wording should select only the health reasons why a person did not do the activity. Both physical and psychological problems may limit physical activities, and either may be exacerbated by external circumstances, such as the weather. For these reasons performance questions tend to give a lower score than capacity questions. Most recent indices favor the performance wording, although questions of both types can be asked, or an intermediate phrasing could be used, such as "Do you have difficulty with . . .?" as used in the Lambeth and Organization for Economic Cooperation and Development (OECD) questionnaires.

It would be misleading to present the general evolution of functional disability measurements in a way that suggests the field is well-established, for the actual quality of the measurements is, regrettably, far from impressive. In terms of psychometric properties—reliability, validity and conceptual clarity—the field of functional assessment has been described as being in a state of infancy (11). This is immediately clear upon comparing the indices in this chapter with others in the book: the functional disability measurements are much less rigorously developed and tested. Items are commonly selected on the basis of clinical judgment without broader reference to a body of theory. Little or no attention is paid to the psychometric properties of the scales, scoring is often rudimentary, and reliability and validity are inadequately assessed. The resulting uncertainty leaves the potential user with a wide choice of scales but an inadequate basis from which to choose among them (12).

The uncertain quality of many of the available scales did, however, provide an approach to narrowing our selection. Because our emphasis is on instruments that can be used in research studies, we stress the importance of reliability and validity results in selecting measurements. As very few disability measurements have been thoroughly tested, we reached a slightly uncomfortable compromise between describing large numbers of measurement methods that we could not really recommend because their quality remains unknown, and the opposite extreme of reviewing an exceedingly small number of scales of proven quality. Because so little is known about many methods, we have described several scales that appear to hold potential, although this is not fully established. We have classified the available measurements into those that cover physical functioning alone (ADL scales) and those that are broader in scope (IADL scales). Within each category we considered a very large number of methods and retained only those for which the questionnaire is available, for which there is some evidence on reliability or validity, and which have been used in published studies. We have sought to keep the scope of the chapter broad, and have included methods whose purpose is primarily clinical as well as those intended for survey research.

Before describing individual scales, we provide two summary tables designed to help the reader review the alternative measurements and select at a glance those that may be of particular interest. Table 3.1 summarizes the format, length and use of each scale, in addition to published evidence on its reliability and validity. Table 3.2 compares the topics covered by each measurement method.

References

(1) Berg RL, ed. Health status indexes. Chicago: Hospital Research and Educational Trust, 1973.
(2) Bruett TL, Overs RP. A critical review of 12 ADL scales. Physical Therapy 1969;49:857–862.
(3) Donaldson SW, Wagner CC, Gresham GE. A unified ADL evaluation form. Arch Phys Med Rehabil 1973;54:175–179, 185.
(4) Forer SK. Functional assessment instruments in medical rehabilitation. J Organization Rehabil Evaluators 1982;2:29–41.
(5) Linn MW, Linn BS. Problems in assessing response to treatment in the elderly by physical and social function. Psychopharmacology Bull 1981;17:74–81.
(6) Liang MH, Jette AM. Measuring functional disability in chronic arthritis: a critical review. Arth Rheum 1981;24:80–86.
(7) Brown M, Gordon WA, Diller L. Functional assessment and outcome measurement: an integrative view. In: Pan EL, Backer TE, Vasch CL, eds. Annual review of rehabilitation. Vol. 3. New York: Springer, 1983:93–120.
(8) Katz S, Hedrick SC, Henderson NS. The measurement of long-term care needs and impact. Health Med Care Serv Rev 1979;2:1, 3–21.
(9) Gresham GE, Labi MLC. Functional assessment instruments currently available for documenting outcomes in rehabilitation medicine. In: Granger CV, Gresham GE, eds. Functional assessment in rehabilitation medicine. Baltimore: Williams & Wilkins, 1984:65–85.
(10) Patrick DL, Darby SC, Green S, Horton G, Locker D, Wiggins RD. Screening for disability in the inner city. J Epidemiol Community Health 1981;35:65–70.

Table 3.1 Comparison of the Quality of Disability Indices*

ADL Scales	Scale	Number of items	Application	Administered by (time)	Studies using method	Reliability		Validity	
						Testing thoroughness	Results	Testing thoroughness	Results
PULSES Profile (Moskowitz & McCann)	ordinal	6	clinical	expert	many	++	++	+	++
Barthel Index (Mahoney & Barthel)	ordinal	10	clinical	expert	many	++	++	++	++
Index of Independence in Activities of Daily Living (Katz)	ordinal	6	clinical	expert	many	++	+	++	+
Kenny Self-Care Evaluation (Schoening)	ordinal	85	clinical	interviewer	several	+	+	+	++
Physical Self-Maintenance Scale (Lawton & Brody)	ordinal (Guttman)	6	survey, research	expert	few	++	++	+	++
Functional Status Rating System (Forer)	ordinal	30	clinical	expert (15–20 min)	few	+	++	+	0

| | | | | | | Reliability | | Validity | |
IADL scales	Scale	Number of items	Application	Administered by (time)	Studies using method	Testing thoroughness	Results	Testing thoroughness	Results
Rapid Disability Rating Scale-2 (Linn)	ordinal	18	research	expert (2 min)	several	++	+++	++	++
Functional Status Index (Jette)	ordinal	45†	clinical, survey	interviewer (60–90 min)	few	+++	++	++	+
Patient Evaluation Conference System (Harvey & Jellinek)	ordinal	79	clinical	expert	few	+	+	0	0
Functional Activities Questionnaire (Pfeffer)	ordinal	10	survey	interviewer	few	+	+	++	+++
OECD Long-Term Disability Questionnaire	ordinal	16	survey	self	many	++	+	++	+
Lambeth Disability Screening Questionnaire (Patrick)	ordinal	25	survey	self	few	+	?	++	++
Disability and Impairment Interview Schedule (Bennett & Garrad)	ordinal	17 (Section 1)	survey	interviewer	few	++	+	+	+

*For an explanation of the categories used, see Chapter 1, pages 8–9.

†Note that the FSI makes separate ratings of the difficulty, degree of dependency and pain experienced in performing each of the 45 activities.

Table 3.2 Comparison of the Content of Disability Indices (Showing Numbers of Questions on Each Topic)

ADL Scales	Self-care	Mobility	Travel	Body movement	Home management	Medical condition	Senses	Mental capacity	Work	Resources	Social interaction	Hobbies	Communication	Behavior problems	Total questions
PULSES Profile (Moskowitz & McCann)	1	1		1		1	1	1							6
Barthel Index (Mahoney & Barthel)	7	3													10
Index of Independence in Activities of Daily Living (Katz)	5	1													6
Kenny Self-Care Evaluation (Schoening)	56	19		10											85
Physical Self-Maintenance Scale (Lawton & Brody)	5	1													6
Functional Status Rating System (Forer)	9	5						7			2		7		30

IADL Scales	Self-care	Mobility	Travel	Body movement	Home management	Medical condition	Senses	Mental capacity	Work	Resources	Social interaction	Hobbies	Communication	Behavior problems	Total questions
Rapid Disability Rating Scale-2 (Linn)	6	2		1	1	2	2	2					1	1	18
Functional Status Index (Jette)	14	10	1	7	11				1			1			45*
Patient Evaluation Conference System (Harvey & Jellinek)	8	5	3	3	1	23	2	9	5	4	6	2	8		79
Functional Activities Questionnaire (Pfeffer)			1		5			3				1			10
OECD Long-Term Disability Questionnaire	3	5		3			4						1		16
Lambeth Disability Screening Questionnaire (Patrick)	4	5	1	2	1	6	3		2		1				25
Disability and Impairment Interview Schedule (Bennett & Garrad)	5	5	2		4				1						17 (Section 1)

*Note that the FSI makes separate ratings of the difficulty, degree of dependency and pain experienced in performing each of the 45 activities.

Key to topic lables.

Self-care includes: dressing, grooming, feeding, bathing, toileting, bladder and/or bowel control

Mobility includes: lower limb abilities, standing, walking, running, stair climbing, transferring

Travel includes: use of transport, driving

Body movement includes: upper limb abilities (e.g., reaching, lifting), bending, moving in bed or confined to bed, hand dexterity (e.g. cutting toenails, turning faucets), carrying, dialing a phone

Home management includes: housework, meal preparation, shopping, managing money

Medical condition includes: diagnosis, signs, symptoms, limb abnormalities, medication, pain, diet

Senses includes: sight, hearing

Mental capacity includes: cognition, anxiety, depression

Work includes: education, retirement, housework (as an occupational category)

Resources includes: social, economic, environmental resources

Hobbies includes: leisure activities, sports

Communication includes: speech, reading

43

(11) Frey WD. Functional assessment in the '80s: a conceptual enigma, a technical challenge. In: Halpern AS, Fuhrer MJ, eds. Functional assessment in rehabilitation. Baltimore: Paul H. Brookes, 1984.

(12) Keith RA. Functional assessment measures in medical rehabilitation: current status. Arch Phys Med Rehabil 1984;65:74–78.

ADL SCALES

This section provides descriptions of six ADL scales: the PULSES, Barthel, Katz and Kenny scales, a less widely known scale by Lawton and Brody, and a more recent one by Forer. It was not originally our intention to include so many older scales but in general they have been more fully tested than the newer methods. Testing, of course, does not guarantee quality, but at least we have information on their performance, information that is sorely lacking for several dozen other ADL scales that we also considered for inclusion in the book. Some of the scales that we considered but did not include are described briefly in the conclusion to this section.

The first of the ADL scales we review, the PULSES Profile, is an example of the physical impairment and disability assessment methods from which the subsequent functional disability scales were derived. As mentioned in Chapter 2, the need to assess the physical fitness of recruits in World War II led to the development of a number of assessment scales, mostly known by acronyms that indicate their content. Thus, the PULSES Profile was developed from the Canadian Army's "Physical Standards and Instructions" for the medical examination of soldiers and army recruits (1943), known as the PULHEMS Profile. In this acronym, P = physique, U = upper extremity, L = lower extremity, H = hearing and ears, E = eyes and vision, M = mental capacity and S = emotional stability, with ratings in each category ranging from normal to totally unfit. A subsequent revision was known as PLUMSHEAF. The United States Army later adapted the PULHEMS system, and merged the mental and emotional categories under the acronym PULHES. Moskowitz and McCann made further modifications to produce the PULSES Profile described here. Although the PULSES Profile is old and is included primarily for its historical significance, it continues to be used (often in conjunction with other ADL scales such as the Barthel) and is also used occasionally as a validation criterion scale. The PULSES Profile and the Barthel Index have both influenced the design of the other scales we review here.

THE PULSES PROFILE
(Eugene Moskowitz and Cairbre B. McCann, 1957)

Purpose

The PULSES Profile was designed to evaluate functional independence in the activities of daily living of a chronically ill and elderly, institutionalized population (1,2). The profile is used to predict rehabilitation potential, to evaluate patient progress, and to assist in program planning (3).

Conceptual Basis

No information is available.

Description

The PULSES Profile was derived from previous assessment methods developed for estimating fitness for military duty. It is therefore primarily an indicator of impairment, described in terms of physical abnormalities, unrelated to their actual functional impact. The components of the acronym are as follows:

P = physical condition
U = upper limb functions
L = lower limb functions
S = sensory components (speech, vision, hearing)
E = excretory functions
S = mental and emotional status

Four levels of impairment are specified in each category, scored as shown in Exhibit 3.1. The six categories receive equal weighting, resulting in a range of scores from 6, indicating unimpaired independence, to 24, indicating full dependence. Subsequently, Moskowitz recommended presenting the six scores separately, as combining them may obscure changes in one category that are balanced by opposite changes in another. Category scores are therefore presented as "L-3," indicating a person who can walk under supervision, or "E-3," indicating frequent incontinence (4).

Originally, administering the profile required "an examination of the patient by a physician with full access to all pertinent medical information and social data" (1, p343). Later, however, Granger et al. trained nurses to complete the profile retrospectively from medical records, or from interviews and observation of the patient (5, p146). Moskowitz conceived the profile "as a vehicle for consolidation of fragments of clinical information gathered in a rehabilitation setting by various staff members involved in the patient's daily care. It thereby became an expression of the consensus of opinion with regard to the functional performance of the individual" (4, p647). The original descriptions of the categories on the six scales, shown in Exhibit 3.1, were later abbreviated, and printed on a color coded chart (4). The abbreviated category labels are shown in the lower half of Exhibit 3.1.

Reliability

Granger et al. reported a test-retest reliability of 0.87 and an inter-rater reliability exceeding 0.95, almost identical to the rates they found for the Barthel Index (5, p150).

Validity

In a study of 307 severely disabled adults in ten rehabilitation centers across the United States, Granger et al. showed the PULSES Profile to be capable of

Exhibit 3.1 The PULSES Profile

P. *Physical* condition including diseases of the viscera (cardiovascular, pulmonary, gastrointestinal, urologic, and endocrine) and cerebral disorders which are not enumerated in the lettered categories below.
 1. No gross abnormalities considering the age of the individual.
 2. Minor abnormalities not requiring frequent medical or nursing supervision.
 3. Moderately severe abnormalities requiring frequent medical or nursing supervision yet still permitting ambulation.
 4. Severe abnormalities requiring constant medical or nursing supervision confining individual to bed or wheelchair.

U. *Upper* extremities including shoulder girdle, cervical and upper dorsal spine.
 1. No gross abnormalities considering the age of the individual.
 2. Minor abnormalities with fairly good range of motion and function.
 3. Moderately severe abnormalities but permitting the performance of daily needs to a limited extent.
 4. Severe abnormalities requiring constant nursing care.

L. *Lower* extremities including the pelvis, lower dorsal and lumbosacral spine.
 1. No gross abnormalities considering the age of the individual.
 2. Minor abnormalities with fairly good range of motion and function.
 3. Moderately severe abnormalities permitting limited ambulation.
 4. Severe abnormalities confining the individual to bed or wheelchair.

S. *Sensory* components relating to speech, vision, and hearing.
 1. No gross abnormalities considering the age of the individual.
 2. Minor deviations insufficient to cause any appreciable functional impairment.
 3. Moderate deviations sufficient to cause appreciable functional impairment.
 4. Severe deviations causing complete loss of hearing, vision or speech.

E. *Excretory* function, i.e., bowel and bladder control.
 1. Complete control.
 2. Occasional stress incontinence or nocturia.
 3. Periodic bowel and bladder incontinence or retention alternating with control.
 4. Total incontinence, either bowel or bladder.

S. *Mental and emotional status.*
 1. No deviations considering the age of the individual.
 2. Minor deviations in mood, temperament and personality not impairing environmental adjustment.
 3. Moderately severe variations requiring some supervision.
 4. Severe variations requiring complete supervision.

Reprinted from Moskowitz E, McCann CB. Classification of disability in the chronically ill and aging. J Chronic Dis 1957;5:343. Pergamon Press Ltd. With permission.

	P Physical Condition cardiovascular pulmonary and other visceral disorders	U Upper Extremities shoulder girdles, cervical and upper dorsal spine	L Lower Extremities pelvis, lower dorsal and lumbosacral spine	S Sensory Function vision hearing speech	E Excretory Functions bowel and bladder	S Social and Mental Status emotional and psychiatric disorders
NORMAL	1 Health maintenance	1 Complete function	1 Complete function	1 Complete function	1 Continent	1 Compatible with age
MILD	2 Occasional medical supervision	2 No assistance required	2 Fully ambulatory despite some loss of function	2 No appreciable functional impairment	2 Occasional stress incontinence or nocturia	2 No supervision required
MODERATELY SEVERE	3 Frequent medical supervision	3 Some assistance necessary	3 Limited ambulation	3 Appreciable bilateral loss or complete unilateral loss of vision or hearing. Incomplete aphasia	3 Periodic incontinence or retention	3 Some supervision necessary
SEVERE	4 Total care Bed or chair confined	4 Nursing care	4 Confined to wheelchair or bed	4 Total blindness Total deafness Global aphasia or aphonia	4 Total incontinence or retention (including catheter and colostomy)	4 Complete care in psychiatric facility

Adapted from Moskowitz E. PULSES Profile in retrospect. Arch Phys Rehabil 1985;66:648.

reflecting change between admission and discharge. Discharge scores corresponded to the referral patterns of patients discharged from rehabilitation units: those returning home were rated significantly higher than those referred to long-term institutions, who in turn scored significantly higher than those referred for acute care (3,5,6). Pearson correlation coefficients between PULSES and Barthel scores ranged from -0.74 to -0.80 ($p < 0.001$) (5, pp146–147). (The negative correlations result from the inverse scoring of the two scales).

Alternative Forms

Granger et al. made several minor modifications to the PULSES Profile, for example by including self-care under the upper limb category and mobility under the lower limb category (5, p153; 6, Table 12-3). Warren developed a modified version called PULHEEMS and used this to screen for disability in the general population (8).

Reference Standards

PULSES scores above 12 reflect serious limitations in personal care independence, and scores over 16 represent severe disability (5, p152).

Commentary

The PULSES scale is the last of the various physical measurement scales developed during the war years that still sees some use. Granger and McNamara incorporated a modified version of it in their Long-Range Evaluation System (7, 9) which also employs the Barthel and ESCROW scales. PULSES has the advantages of widespread use and available reference standards. Although it is often compared with the Barthel Index, the two are not strictly equivalent. Granger et al. have noted:

> The obvious difference between the Barthel and PULSES scales is that the Barthel subscores can measure more discrete functions (eg, eating and ambulation) which have implications for use by providers of direct care to the long-term patient; PULSES cannot do this. However, the PULSES Profile taps communication, psychosocial and support aspects, which the Barthel does not. (5, p146).

The comparative summary presented in Table 3.1 suggests that the reliability and validity of the PULSES are similar to those of most of the alternative scales, with the exception of Linn's Rapid Disability Rating Scale, which is superior. Because the scale covers physical impairments there seems little disadvantage in the fact that the scale is so old, and as a brief rating method it appears adequate.

Address

Eugene Moskowitz, MD, 212 N Columbus Avenue, Mount Vernon, New York, USA 10552

References

(1) Moskowitz E, McCann CB. Classification of disability in the chronically ill and aging. J Chronic Dis 1957;5:342–346.

(2) Moskowitz E, Fuhn ER, Peters ME, Kearley AS. Aged infirm residents in a custodial institution: two-year medical and social study. JAMA 1959;169:2009–2012.

(3) Granger CV, Greer DS. Functional status measurement and medical rehabilitation outcomes. Arch Phys Med Rehabil 1976;57:103–109.

(4) Moskowitz E. PULSES Profile in retrospect. Arch Phys Med Rehabil 1985;66:647–648.

(5) Granger CV, Albrecht GL, Hamilton BB. Outcome of comprehensive medical rehabilitation: measurement by PULSES Profile and the Barthel Index. Arch Phys Med Rehabil 1979;60:145–154.

(6) Granger CV, Sherwood CC, Greer DS. Functional status measures in a comprehensive stroke care program. Arch Phys Med Rehabil 1977;58:555–561.

(7) Granger CV. Health accounting—functional assessment of the long-term patient. In: Kottke FJ, Stillwell GK, Lehmann FJ, eds. Krusen's handbook of physical medicine and rehabilitation. 3rd ed. Philadelphia: WB Saunders, 1982:253–274.

(8) Warren MD. The use of the PULHEEMS system of medical classification in civilian practice. Br J Ind Med 1956;13:202–209.

(9) Granger CV, McNamara MA. Functional assessment utilization: the Long-Range Evaluation System (LRES). In: Granger CV, Gresham GE, eds. Functional assessment in rehabilitation medicine. Baltimore: Williams & Wilkins, 1984:99–121.

THE BARTHEL INDEX (Formerly The Maryland Disability Index) (Florence I. Mahoney and Dorothea W. Barthel; In Use Since 1955, First Published by Originators in 1965)

Purpose

The index was developed to monitor functional independence before and after treatment, and to indicate the amount of nursing care needed (1). It was intended for long-term patients in hospital with neuromuscular or musculoskeletal disorders, but has also been used to identify patients who could benefit from a rehabilitation program, to predict length of stay, estimate prognosis, anticipate discharge outcomes, and as an evaluative instrument.

Conceptual Basis

No information is available.

Description

The Barthel Index is a rating scale completed by a nurse, physiotherapist or doctor from medical records or from direct observation (2). The ten activities assessed are shown in Exhibit 3.2, with the corresponding scores. Mahoney and Barthel provided extensive definitions of the levels of independence included in the index (see Exhibit 3.3). A score of 0, 5, 10 or 15 is assigned to each level;

Exhibit 3.2 The Barthel Index

Note: A score of zero is given where patients cannot meet the defined criterion.

	With help	Independent
1. Feeding (if food needs to be cut up = help)	5	10
2. Moving from wheelchair to bed and return (includes sitting up in bed)	5–10	15
3. Personal toilet (wash face, comb hair, shave, clean teeth)	0	5
4. Getting on and off toilet (handling clothes, wipe, flush)	5	10
5. Bathing self	0	5
6. Walking on level surface (or if unable to walk, propel wheelchair)	10	15
*score only if unable to walk	0*	5*
7. Ascend and descend stairs	5	10
8. Dressing (includes tying shoes, fastening fasteners)	5	10
9. Controlling bowels	5	10
10. Controlling bladder	5	10

Reproduced from Mahoney FI, Barthel DW. Functional evaluation: the Barthel Index. Maryland State Med J 1965;14:62. With permission.

Exhibit 3.3 Instructions for Scoring the Barthel Index

Note: A score of zero is given when the patient cannot meet the defined criterion.

1. Feeding

   10 = Independent. The patient can feed himself a meal from a tray or table when someone puts the food within his reach. He must put on an assistive device if this is needed, cut up the food, use salt and pepper, spread butter, etc. He must accomplish this in a reasonable time.

   5 = Some help is necessary (when cutting up food, etc., as listed above).

2. Moving from wheelchair to bed and return

   15 = Independent in all phases of this activity. Patient can safely approach the bed in his wheelchair, lock brakes, lift footrests, move safely to bed, lie down, come to a sitting position on the side of the bed, change the position of the wheelchair, if necessary, to transfer back into it safely, and return to the wheelchair.

   10 = Either some minimal help is needed in some step of this activity or the patient needs to be reminded or supervised for safety of one or more parts of this activity.

   5 = Patient can come to a sitting position without the help of a second person but needs to be lifted out of bed, or if he transfers with a great deal of help.

3. Doing personal toilet

   5 = Patient can wash hands and face, comb hair, clean teeth, and shave. He may use any kind of razor but must put in blade or plug in razor without help as well as get it from drawer or cabinet. Female patients must put on own make-up, if used, but need not braid or style hair.

4. Getting on and off toilet

   10 = Patient is able to get on and off toilet, fasten and unfasten clothes, prevent soiling of clothes, and use toilet paper without help. He may use a wall bar or other stable object of support if needed. If it is necessary to use a bed pan instead of a toilet, he must be able to place it on a chair, empty it, and clean it.

   5 = Patient needs help because of imbalance or in handling clothes or in using toilet paper.

5. Bathing self
    5 = Patient may use a bathtub, a shower, or take a complete sponge bath. He must be able to do all the steps involved in whichever method is employed without another person being present.

6. Walking on a level surface
    15 = Patient can walk at least 50 yards without help or supervision. He may wear braces or prostheses and use crutches, canes, or a walkerette but not a rolling walker. He must be able to lock and unlock braces if used, assume the standing position and sit down, get the necessary mechanical aides into position for use, and dispose of them when he sits. (Putting on and taking off braces is scored under dressing.)
    10 = Patient needs help or supervision in any of the above but can walk at least 50 yards with a little help.

6a. Propelling a wheelchair
    5 = If a patient cannot ambulate but can propel a wheelchair independently. He must be able to go around corners, turn around, maneuver the chair to a table, bed, toilet, etc. He must be able to push a chair at least 50 yards. Do not score this item if the patient gets score for walking.

7. Ascending and descending stairs
    10 = Patient is able to go up and down a flight of stairs safely without help or supervision. He may and should use handrails, canes, or crutches when needed. He must be able to carry canes or crutches as he ascends or descends stairs.
    5 = Patient needs help with or supervision of any one of the above items.

8. Dressing and undressing
    10 = Patient is able to put on and remove and fasten all clothing, and tie shoe laces (unless it is necessary to use adaptations for this). The activity includes putting on and removing and fastening corset or braces when these are prescribed. Such special clothing as suspenders, loafer shoes, dresses that open down the front may be used when necessary.
    5 = Patient needs help in putting on and removing or fastening any clothing. He must do at least half the work himself. He must accomplish this in a reasonable time.
    Women need not be scored on use of a brassiere or girdle unless these are prescribed garments.

9. Continence of bowels
    10 = Patient is able to control his bowels and have no accidents. He can use a suppository or take an enema when necessary (as for spinal cord injury patients who have had bowel training).
    5 = Patient needs help in using a suppository or taking an enema or has occasional accidents.

10. Controlling bladder
    10 = Patient is able to control his bladder day and night. Spinal cord injury patients who wear an external device and leg bag must put them on independently, clean and empty bag, and stay dry day and night.
    5 = Patient has occasional accidents or cannot wait for the bed pan or get to the toilet in time or needs help with an external device.

Reproduced from Mahoney FI, Barthel DW. Functional evaluation: the Barthel Index. Maryland State Med J 1965;14:62–65. With permission.

overall scores range from 0 to 100. The scores are intended to reflect the amount of time and assistance a patient requires (3, p61). While the maximum score indicates independence in all ten areas, the authors emphasized that this does not necessarily mean that the person could live alone without help: cooking or cleaning assistance may be needed. In scoring, full credit is not given if even minimal supervision or assistance is required and, where applicable, the score is to be accompanied by an explanation of the patient's requirements.

Reliability

Granger et al. reported a test-retest reliability of 0.89 with severely disabled adults; the inter-rater agreement exceeded 0.95 (2, p150).

Validity

There have been many studies of the predictive validity of the Barthel Index. In two studies of stroke patients the percentages of patients who died within six months of admission fell significantly ($p < 0.001$) as the Barthel scores recorded at admission rose (4, p836; 5, p799). Among survivors, intake scores also predicted the length of stay and the patient's subsequent progress as rated by a physician. Thirty-six percent of those scoring 0 to 15 points at admission were later said to have improved, whereas 77% of those scoring 60 to 100 were so judged (5, p800; 6, p894). Most discrepancies between the change scores and the physician's impression occurred because of the omission of speech and mental functioning from the index (4, p838). Similar results were obtained by Granger et al. in four further studies of predictive validity (7-10). They concluded " . . . 60 appears to be a pivotal score where patients move from dependency to assisted independence" (7, p14).

Evidence on the correlational validity of the Barthel Index comes mainly from correlations with the PULSES Profile; the Pearson coefficients range from -0.74 to -0.90 ($p < 0.001$). (The negative sign results because the two scales are inversely scored).

Alternative Forms

Granger has outlined an extension of the Barthel Index to cover 15 topics, each scored on a four-point scale, giving a range of scores from 0 to 100 (see reference 8, Table 12-2; reference 9, Table 1). This revision is outlined in Exhibit 3.4. Fortinsky et al. reported correlations between Barthel scores and the patient's actual behavior at home for some 72 tasks. The overall correlation was 0.91, with the closest agreement for personal care tasks (9, p492). Barthel scores were also found to be significantly associated with age, psychological problems and role performance (9, p495).

Reference Standards

Granger et al. reported that a cutting point of 60 on the index represents the threshold between independence and more marked dependence, 40 or below

Exhibit 3.4 Modified Barthel Index Scoring

Independent		Dependent		
I Intact	II Limited	III Helper	IV Null	
10	5	0	0	Drink from cup/feed from dish
5	5	3	0	Dress upper body
5	5	2	0	Dress lower body
0	0	−2		Don brace or prosthesis
5	5	0	0	Grooming
4	4	0	0	Wash or bathe
10	10	5	0	Bladder continence
10	10	5	0	Bowel continence
4	4	2	0	Care of perineum/clothing at toilet
15	15	7	0	Transfer, chair
6	5	3	0	Transfer, toilet
1	1	0	0	Transfer, tub or shower
15	15	10	0	Walk on level 50 yards or more
10	10	5	0	Up and down stairs for one flight or more
15	5	0	0	Wheelchair/50 yards—only if not walking

Reproduced from Fortinsky RH, Granger CV, Seltzer GB. The use of functional assessment in understanding home care needs. Med Care 1981;19:489,Table 1. With permission.

indicates severe dependence, and 20 or below reflects total dependence in self-care and mobility (2, p152; 7, p16).

Commentary

Although old, the Barthel Index continues to be used and refined, especially by Granger and his colleagues, who have used modified versions of the Barthel and PULSES methods in their Long-Range Evaluation System (8, 10). This also incorporates the ESCROW profile, a rating scale that summarizes the social and economic resources available to a patient, his ability to make decisions, his working ability and social interaction. The ESCROW appears conceptually valuable, but the small amount of validity data that we have on it suggests that it does not succeed in its purpose; therefore we are not reviewing it separately. The validity data on the Barthel Index are more extensive than those available for many other ADL scales, and the results appear slightly superior to those of the other scales we review, with the exception of Linn's and Jette's scales.

Several criticisms have been made of the Barthel Index. First, it uses a rudimentary scoring system: changes by a given number of points do not reflect equivalent changes in disability across different activities. Second, the scale is restricted in its scope, such that deterioration and improvement can occur beyond the end points of the scale, an issue mentioned by the originators. Third, several authors have suggested that the index could be improved by adding speech and mental functions (4, 6); these are considered in several IADL scales, such as Linn's Rapid Disability Rating Scale, which may prove superior for some applications. Likewise, Granger et al. commented that limitations result from the exclusion of other factors influential to progress such as medical, mental, emotional, communication, or family problems (7). This, of course, is a limitation of all ADL scales; broader measurements that include such factors are described in Chapter 8. We anticipate that this scale will come to be used principally as a benchmark against which to judge improved scales: they should overcome the weaknesses noted above and should be capable of showing greater predictive validity than the Barthel Index, which occupies an important place in the history of the development of this field.

Address

Carl V. Granger, MD, Professor of Rehabilitation Medicine, The Buffalo General Hospital, Buffalo, New York, USA 14203

References

(1) Mahoney FI, Wood OH, Barthel DW. Rehabilitation of chronically ill patients: the influence of complications on the final goal. South Med J 1958;51:605–609.

(2) Granger CV, Albrecht GL, Hamilton BB. Outcome of comprehensive medical rehabilitation: measurement by PULSES Profile and the Barthel Index. Arch Phys Med Rehabil 1979;60:145–154.

(3) Mahoney FI, Barthel DW. Functional evaluation: the Barthel Index. Md State Med J 1965;14:61–65.

(4) Wylie CM, White BK. A measure of disability. Arch Environ Health 1964;8:834–839.

(5) Wylie CM. Gauging the response of stroke patients to rehabilitation. J Am Geriatr Soc 1967;15:797–805.

(6) Wylie CM. Measuring end results of rehabilitation of patients with stroke. Public Health Rep 1967;82:893–898.

(7) Granger CV, Dewis LS, Peters NC, Sherwood CC, Barrett JE. Stroke rehabilitation: analysis of repeated Barthel Index measures. Arch Phys Med Rehabil 1979;60:14–17.

(8) Granger CV. Health accounting—functional assessment of the long-term patient. In: Kottke FJ, Stillwell GK, Lehmann JF, eds. Krusen's handbook of physical medicine and rehabilitation. 3rd ed. Philadelphia: WB Saunders, 1982:253–274.

(9) Fortinsky RH, Granger CV, Seltzer GB. The use of functional assessment in understanding home care needs. Med Care 1981;19:489–497.

(10) Granger CV, McNamara MA. Functional assessment utilization: the Long-Range Evaluation System (LRES). In: Granger CV, Gresham GE, eds. Functional assessment in rehabilitation medicine. Baltimore: Williams & Williams, 1984:99–121.

THE INDEX OF INDEPENDENCE IN ACTIVITIES OF DAILY LIVING, OR INDEX OF ADL
(Sidney Katz, 1959, Revised 1976)

Purpose

The Index of ADL was originally developed to measure the physical functioning of elderly and chronically ill patients with strokes or fractured hips. The index has frequently been used to measure the severity of chronic illness and to evaluate the effectiveness of treatment; it has also been used to provide predictive information on the course of specific illnesses (1–3).

Conceptual Basis

In empirical studies of aging, Katz noted that the loss of functional skills occurs in a particular order, in which the most complex functions are lost first and the least complex later. The six activities covered in the index were found to lie in a hierarchical order of this Guttman type, while other items, such as mobility, walking or stair climbing did not fit into this pattern (4). Katz further suggested that, during rehabilitation, patients regain skills in order of ascending complexity, in the same order that children initially acquire the skills (1, pp917–918). He concluded that the Index of ADL appears to be based on primary biological and psychosocial function and reflects the adequacy of organized neurological and locomotor response (1, 4–6).

Description

The index is a rating form that is completed by the therapist or other observer. It assesses independence in six activities: bathing, dressing, toileting, transferring from bed to chair, continence and feeding. By observing the patient and by asking questions, the patient is rated on a three-point scale of independence for each activity. The ratings are defined by brief, descriptive phrases on the evaluation form, as presented in Exhibit 3.5. The observer records the most dependent degree of performance during a two-week period (5, p22).

The first stage in scoring involves translating the above, three-point scales into a "dependent/independent" classification. This is done using the guidelines shown in the lower half of Exhibit 3.6: the middle categories in Exhibit 3.5 are rated as independent for bathing, dressing and feeding, but as dependent for the others. The patient's overall performance is then summarized on an eight-point scale that considers the numbers of areas of dependency and their relative importance. The scoring system and definitions are given in the upper half of Exhibit 3.6. A simplified scoring system counts the number of

Exhibit 3.5 The Index of Independence in Activities of Daily Living: Evaluation Form

Name _____ Day of evaluation _____
For each area of functioning listed below, check description that applies. (The word "assistance" means supervision, direction, or personal assistance.)

Bathing—either sponge bath; tub bath, or shower

☐	☐	☐
Receives no assistance (gets in and out of tub by self if tub is usual means of bathing)	Receives assistance in bathing only one part of the body (such as back or a leg)	Receives assistance in bathing more than one part of the body (or not bathed)

Exhibit 3.5 (*continued*)

Dressing—gets clothes from closets and drawers—including underclothes, outer garments and using fasteners (including braces if worn)

☐

☐

☐

Gets clothes and gets completely dressed without assistance

Gets clothes and gets dressed without assistance except for assistance in tying shoes

Receives assistance in getting clothes or in getting dressed, or stays partly or completely undressed

Toileting—going to the "toilet room" for bowel and urine elimination; cleaning self after elimination, and arranging clothes

☐

☐

☐

Goes to "toilet room," cleans self, and arranges clothes without assistance (may use object for support such as cane, walker, or wheelchair and may manage night bedpan or commode, emptying same in morning)

Receives assistance in going to "toilet room" or in cleansing self or in arranging clothes after elimination or in use of night bedpan or commode

Doesn't go to room termed "toilet" for the elimination process

Transfer—

☐

☐

☐

Moves in and out of bed as well as in and out of chair without assistance (may be using object for support such as cane or walker)

Moves in and out of bed or chair with assistance

Doesn't get out of bed

Continence—

☐

☐

☐

Controls urination and bowel movement completely by self

Has occasional "accidents"

Supervision helps keep urine or bowel control; catheter is used, or is incontinent

Feeding—

☐

☐

☐

Feeds self without assistance

Feeds self except for getting assistance in cutting meat or buttering bread

Receives assistance in feeding or is fed partly or completely by using tubes or intravenous fluids

Reproduced from Katz S, Downs TD, Cash HR, Grotz RC. Progress in development of the Index of ADL. Gerontologist 1970;10:21. With permission.

Exhibit 3.6 The Index of Independence in Activities of Daily Living: Scoring and Definitions

---

The Index of Independence in Activities of Daily Living is based on an evaluation of the functional independence or dependence of patients in bathing, dressing, going to toilet, transferring, continence, and feeding. Specific definitions of functional independence and dependence appear below the index.

A—Independent in feeding, continence, transferring, going to toilet, dressing and bathing.

B—Independent in all but one of these functions.

C—Independent in all but bathing and one additional function.

D—Independent in all but bathing, dressing, and one additional function.

E—Independent in all but bathing, dressing, going to toilet, and one additional function.

F—Independent in all but bathing, dressing, going to toilet, transferring, and one additional function.

G—Dependent in all six functions.

Other—Dependent in at least two functions, but not classifiable as C, D, E, or F.

Independence means without supervision, direction, or active personal assistance, except as specifically noted below. This is based on actual status and not on ability. A patient who refuses to perform a function is considered as not performing the function, even though he is deemed able.

Bathing (sponge, shower or tub)
> Independent: assistance only in bathing a single part (as back or disabled extremity) or bathes self completely
> Dependent: assistance in bathing more than one part of body; assistance in getting in or out of tub or does not bathe self

Dressing
> Independent: gets clothes from closets and drawers; puts on clothes, outer garments, braces; manages fasteners; act of tying shoes is excluded
> Dependent: does not dress self or remains partly undressed

Going to toilet
> Independent: gets to toilet; gets on and off toilet; arranges clothes; cleans organs of excretion; (may manage own bedpan used at night only and may or may not be using mechanical supports)
> Dependent: uses bedpan or commode or receives assistance in getting to and using toilet

Transfer
> Independent: moves in and out of bed independently and moves in and out of chair independently (may or may not be using mechanical supports)
> Dependent: assistance in moving in or out of bed and/or chair; does not perform one or more transfers

Continence
> Independent: urination and defecation entirely self-controlled
> Dependent: partial or total incontinence in urination or defecation; partial or total control by enemas, catheters, or regulated use of urinals and/or bedpans

Feeding
> Independent: gets food from plate or its equivalent into mouth; (precutting of meat and preparation of food, as buttering bread, are excluded from evaluation)
> Dependent: assistance in act of feeding (see above): does not eat at all or parenteral feeding

---

Reproduced from Katz S, Downs TD, Cash HR, Grotz RC. Progress in development of the Index of ADL. Gerontologist 1970;10:23. With permission.

activities in which the individual is dependent, providing a scale from 0 through 6, i.e., 0 = independent in all six functions; 6 = dependent in all functions (4, p497). This method obviates the need for the miscellaneous category, "other."

Full definitions of bathing, dressing, toileting, transferring from bed to chair, continence and feeding are given by Katz et al. (5, pp22–24). The following quotation summarizes how the index is applied:

> The observer asks the subject to show him (1) the bathroom, and (2) medications in another room (or a meaningful substitute object). These requests create test situations for direct observation of transfer, locomotion, and communication and serve as checks on the reliability of information about bathing, dressing, going to toilet, and transfer. Data that is recorded on the form is then converted into an over-all ADL grade with the aid of definitions presented in [Exhibit 3.6]. (Note from the definitions in [Exhibit 3.6] that the intermediate description is classified as dependent for certain functions and independent for others.) . . .
>
> Environmental artifacts that tend to influence ADL levels are occasionally encountered. For safety reasons, some hospitals require nurses to supervise patients who shower or get into tubs. During the first few days in the hospital, patients are sometimes kept in bed until the staff can assess their behavior and the degree of dependence permissible. . . . All these special conditions can result in ADL ratings that are lower than they might be in absence of such restrictions. A test of actual functional level is possible and is indicated for certain studies. (1, pp915–916; 5, p24).

Reliability

Little formal reliability testing has been reported. Katz et al. assessed inter-rater reliability, reporting that differences between observers occurred once in 20 evaluations or less frequently (1, p915). Guttman analyses on 100 patients in Sweden yielded coefficients of scalability ranging from 0.74 to 0.88, suggesting that the index forms a successful cumulative scale (7, p128).

Validity

Remarkably little evidence for the validity of the scale is available. Katz et al. applied the Index of ADL and other indices to 270 patients at discharge from a hospital for the chronically ill. The index scores were found to correlate 0.50 with a mobility scale and 0.39 with a house confinement scale (5, Table 3). The patients were followed up for two years and Katz concluded that the Index of ADL predicted long-term outcomes as well or better than selected measures of physical or mental function (5, p29). Other studies indicating the predictive validity of the scale are summarized by Katz and Akpom (4); typical of the findings of these studies were the results reported by Brorsson and Åsberg. Thirty-two of 44 patients rated independent at admission to a hospital ward were living at home one year later, and 8 had died. By contrast, 23 of 42 patients initially rated as dependent had died, and only 8 were living in their homes (7, p130).

Commentary

The Index of ADL is unquestionably the most widely used of all functional indices. It has been used with children and with adults, with the mentally retarded and with physically disabled, with ambulatory and with institutionalized people (4,6). It has been used in studies of many conditions, including cerebral palsy, strokes, multiple sclerosis, paraplegia, quadriplegia and rheumatoid arthritis (2–4, 8–12).

Given its widespread use, it is surprising that so little evidence has been published on the reliability and validity of Katz's ADL scale. The recent study of Brorsson and Åsberg begins to fill this need, although we feel that more evidence for the validity and reliability of this method should be presented before we can fully support its use. Among the various critiques of the scale, we can direct potential users of this scale to criticisms of the scoring system made by Chen and Bryant (13, p261). We believe that the other scales should be reviewed closely before the reader selects the Index of ADL.

Address

Sidney Katz, MD, Professor and Chairman, Department of Community Health Science, Michigan State University, East Lansing, Michigan, USA 48824

References

(1) Katz S, Ford AB, Moskowitz RW, Jackson BA, Jaffe MW. Studies of illness in the aged. The Index of ADL: a standardized measure of biological and psychosocial function. JAMA 1963;185:914–919.

(2) Katz S, Ford AB, Chinn AB, Newill VA. Prognosis after strokes: II. Long-term course of 159 patients with stroke. Medicine 1966;45:236–246.

(3) Katz S, Heiple KG, Downs TD, Ford AB, Scott CP. Long-term course of 147 patients with fracture of the hip. Surg Gynecol Obstet 1967;124:1219–1230.

(4) Katz S, Akpom CA. A measure of primary sociobiological functions. Int J Health Serv 1976;6:493–507.

(5) Katz S, Downs TD, Cash HR, Grotz RC. Progress in development of the Index of ADL. Gerontologist 1970;10:20–30.

(6) Katz S, Akpom CA. Index of ADL. Med Care 1976;14:116–118.

(7) Brorsson B, Åsberg KH. Katz Index of Independence in ADL: reliability and validity in short-term care. Scand J Rehabil Med 1984;16:125–132.

(8) Steinberg FU, Frost M. Rehabilitation of geriatric patients in a general hospital: a follow-up study of 43 cases. Geriatrics 1963;18:158–164.

(9) Katz S, Vignos PJ, Moskowitz RW, Thompson HM, Sveck KH. Comprehensive outpatient care in rheumatoid arthritis: a controlled study. JAMA 1968;206:1249–1254.

(10) Grotz RT, Henderson ND, Katz S. A comparison of the functional and intellectual performance of phenylketonuric, anoxic, and Down's Syndrome individuals. Am J Ment Defic 1972;76:710–717.

(11) Katz S, Ford AB, Downs TD, Adams M, Rusby DI. Effects of continued care: a study of chronic illness in the home. Washington, DC: U.S. Government Printing Office, 1972. (DHEW Publication No. (HSM) 73-3010).

(12) Katz S, Hedrick S, Henderson NS. The measurement of long-term care needs and impact. Health Med Care Serv Rev 1979;2:1–21.
(13) Chen MK, Bryant BE. The measurement of health—a critical and selective overview. Int J Epidemiol 1975;4:257–264.

THE KENNY SELF-CARE EVALUATION
(Herbert A. Schoening and Staff of the Sister Kenny Institute, 1965, Revised 1973)

Purpose

The Kenny Self-Care Evaluation records functional performance to estimate a patient's ability to live independently at home or in a protected environment. The method was intended to be used in setting treatment goals and in evaluating progress and was designed to offer a "more precise measuring device than the traditional ADL form" (1, p690).

Conceptual Basis

The topics covered in the instrument are considered to represent the minimum requirements for an individual to live independently (2, p2).

Description

The structure of the Kenny evaluation is hierarchical. At the most general level, the 1973 version contains seven categories of self-care activities: bed activities, transfers, locomotion, dressing, personal hygiene, bowel and bladder, and feeding. Within each category there are between one and four general activities, each of which is in turn divided into component tasks. These comprise the small steps involved in the activity, for example, "legs over side of bed" is one of the steps in "rising and sitting." In all, there are 17 activities and 85 tasks (see Exhibit 3.7). The questionnaire and a user's manual are available from the Sister Kenny Institute (2).

The patient's performance on each of the tasks is observed and rated on a three-point scale: "totally independent," "requiring assistance or supervision" (regardless of the amount) or "totally dependent." Actual performance is rated: every task must be observed and self-report is not accepted. If the rater believes that the patient's performance was not representative of his true ability, there is space on the score sheet to note special circumstances (e.g., acute illness) that may have affected the score. The complete scale is shown in Exhibit 3.7.

The ratings for the tasks within an activity are then combined to provide an activity score, as follows:

Four: All tasks rated independent.
Three: One or two tasks required assistance or supervision; all others are done independently.
Two: Other configurations not covered in classes 0, 1, 3 or 4.

Exhibit 3.7 The Sister Kenny Institute Self-Care Evaluation

Number	Name

O.T.	Primary Nurse	P.T.

Date of Onset	Date of Admission	Diagnosis

Activities	Tasks	Evaluation Date:	Progress Rounds:	Progress Rounds:

BED ACTIVITIES

Activities	Tasks			
Moving in Bed	Shift position			
	Turn to left side			
	Turn to right side			
	Turn to prone			
	Turn to supine			
Rising and Sitting	Come to sitting position			
	Maintain sitting balance			
	Legs over side of bed			
	Move to edge of bed			
	Legs back onto bed			

TRANSFERS

Activities	Tasks			
Sitting Transfer	Position wheelchair			
	Brakes on/off			
	Arm rests on/off			
	Foot rests on/off			
	Position legs			
	Position sliding board			
	Maintain balance			
	Shift to bed/chair			
Standing Transfer	Position wheelchair			
	Brakes on/off			
	Move feet and pedals			
	Slide forward			
	Position feet			
	Stand			
	Pivot			
	Sit			

Exhibit 3.7 (*continued*)

Activities	Tasks	Evaluation Date:	Progress Rounds:	Progress Rounds:

TRANSFERS (Cont'd)

Toilet Transfer	Position equipment			
	Manage equipment			
	Manage undressing			
	Transfer to commode/toilet			
	Manage dressing			
	Transfer back			

Bathing Transfer	Tub/shower approach			
	Use of grab bars			
	Tub/shower entry			
	Tub/shower exit			

LOCOMOTION

Locomotion	Walking			
	Stairs			
	Wheelchair			

DRESSING

Upper Trunk and Arms	Hearing aid and eyeglasses			
	Front opening on/off			
	Pullover on/off			
	Brassiere on/off			
	Corset/brace on/off			
	Equipment/prostheses on/off			
	Sweater/shawl on/off			

Lower Trunk and Legs	Slacks/skirt on/off			
	Underclothing on/off			
	Belt on/off			
	Braces/prostheses on/off			
	Girdle/garter belt on/off			

Feet	Stockings on/off			
	Shoes/slippers on/off			
	Braces/prostheses on/off			
	Wraps/support hose on/off			

62

Activities	Tasks	Evaluation Date:	Progress Rounds:	Progress Rounds:

PERSONAL HYGIENE

Activities	Tasks	Evaluation Date:	Progress Rounds:	Progress Rounds:
Face, Hair and Arms	Wash face			
	Wash hands and arms			
	Brush teeth/dentures			
	Brush/comb hair			
	Shaving/make-up			
Trunk and Perineum	Wash back			
	Wash buttocks			
	Wash chest			
	Wash abdomen			
	Wash groin			
Lower Extremities	Wash upper legs			
	Wash lower legs			
	Wash feet			

BOWEL AND BLADDER

Activities	Tasks	Evaluation Date:	Progress Rounds:	Progress Rounds:
Bowel Program	Suppository insertion			
	Digital stimulation			
	Equipment care			
	Cleansing self			
Bladder Program	Manage equipment			
	Stimulation			
	Cleansing self			
Catheter Care	Assemble equipment			
	Fill syringe			
	Inject liquid			
	Connect/disconnect			
	Sterile technique			

FEEDING*

Activities	Tasks	Evaluation Date:	Progress Rounds:	Progress Rounds:
Feeding	Adaptive equipment			
	Finger feeding			
	Use of utensils			
	Pour from container			
	Drink (cup/glass/straw)			

*If patient cannot swallow, he is to be scored 0 in feeding

Exhibit 3.7 *(continued)*

SELF CARE SCORE

Category	Activities	Activity Scores	Category Total	Category Score	Activity Scores	Category Total	Category Score	Activity Scores	Category Total	Category Score
BED ACTIVITIES	Moving in Bed		÷ 2 =	.		÷ 2 =	.		÷ 2 =	.
	Rising and Sitting									
TRANSFERS	Sitting Transfer		÷ 4 =	.		÷ 4 =	.		÷ 4 =	.
	Standing Transfer									
	Toilet Transfer									
	Bathing Transfer									
LOCOMOTION	Walking		÷ 3 =	.		÷ 3 =	.		÷ 3 =	.
	Stairs									
	Wheelchair									
DRESSING	Upper Trunk and Arms		÷ 3 =	.		÷ 3 =	.		÷ 3 =	.
	Lower Trunk and Legs									
	Feet									
PERSONAL HYGIENE	Face, Hair and Arms		÷ 3 =	.		÷ 3 =	.		÷ 3 =	.
	Trunk and Perineum									
	Lower Extremities									
BOWEL AND BLADDER	Bowel Program		÷ 2 =	.		÷ 2 =	.		÷ 2 =	.
	Bladder Program									
	Catheter Care									
FEEDING	Feeding		=	.0		=	.0		=	.0
TOTAL SELF CARE SCORE										

Reproduced from Iversen IA, Silberberg NE, Stever RC, Schoening HA. The revised Kenny Self-Care Evaluation: a numerical measure of independence in activities of daily living. Minneapolis, Minnesota: Sister Kenny Institute, 1973. With permission.

One: One or two tasks required assistance or supervision, or one was carried out independently, but in all others the patient was dependent.
Zero: All tasks were rated dependent.

Category scores are calculated as the average of the activity scores within that category (see scoring sheet provided at the end of the exhibit). The category scores may be summed to provide a total score in which the seven categories receive equal weights. Equal weights were justified on the basis of empirical observations suggesting that roughly equal nursing time was required for helping the dependent patient with each group of activities (1, pp690–693). No guidelines are given on how to interpret the scores.

Reliability

The inter-rater reliability among 43 raters for the Kenny total score was 0.67 or 0.74, according to whether it was applied before or after another rating scale. The reliability of the locomotion score (0.46 or 0.42) was markedly lower than that of the other scores, which ranged from 0.71 to 0.94 (3, Table 2). Iversen et al. commented that the locomotion category is the most difficult to score (2, p14). Gordon et al. achieved higher inter-rater reliabilities: error was only 2.5% (4, p400).

Validity

Gresham et al. compared Kenny and Barthel Index ratings of stroke patients, giving a kappa coefficient of 0.42 and a Spearman correlation of 0.73 ($p <$ 0.001) (5, Table 3). They found that the Kenny form tends to rate slightly more patients as independent than other indices. Complete independence was designated in 35.1% of 148 stroke patients by the Barthel Index, in 39.2% by the Katz Index of ADL, and in 41.9% using the Kenny instrument (differences were not statistically significant) (5, p355).

Commentary

The Kenny instrument differs from other ADL scales in that it covers a somewhat narrower scope (omitting communication and travel) but deals with each topic in considerable detail. It also requires direct observation of the patient. The available evidence suggests somewhat greater inter-rater agreement for the Kenny than is obtained using simpler ratings. As the Kenny

> breaks activities down into their component parts, raters were able to achieve higher levels of agreement because the narrower scope of the task evaluations reduced the number of behavioral components that could be subjectively weighted. (3, pp164–165).

However, the results of comparing the Kenny with simpler scales suggests that the additional detail does not provide superior discriminative ability (3, p164). The correlation of 0.73 with the Barthel Index is high, and if this were corrected for attenuation due to the imperfect reliability of the two scales, it would imply that the simpler Barthel Index provides results that are virtually identical. The quality of the Kenny scale is also comparable to that of the Katz index; there is little evidence that supports the superiority of the Kenny for research purposes. The detailed ratings it provides may, however, have clinical utility.

Address

Sister Kenny Institute, Chicago Avenue at 27th Street, Minneapolis, Minnesota, USA 55407

References

(1) Schoening HA, Anderegg L, Bergstrom D, Fonda M, Steinke N, Ulrich P. Numerical scoring of self-care status of patients. Arch Phys Med Rehabil 1965;46:689–697.
(2) Iversen IA, Silberberg NE, Stever RC, Schoening HA. The revised Kenny Self-Care Evaluation: a numerical measure of independence in activities of daily living. Minneapolis, Minnesota: Sister Kenny Institute, 1973.
(3) Kerner JF, Alexander J. Activities of daily living: reliability and validity of gross vs specific ratings. Arch Phys Med Rehabil 1981;62:161–166.
(4) Gordon EE, Drenth V, Jarvis L, Johnson J, Wright V. Neurophysiologic syndromes in stroke as predictors of outcome. Arch Phys Med Rehabil 1978;59:399–409.
(5) Gresham GE, Phillips TF, Labi MLC. ADL status in stroke: relative merits of three standard indexes. Arch Phys Med Rehabil 1980;61:355–358.

THE PHYSICAL SELF-MAINTENANCE SCALE
(M. Powell Lawton and Elaine M. Brody, 1969)

Purpose

Lawton and Brody developed the Physical Self-Maintenance Scale for use in planning and evaluating treatment for people over 60 years of age living in the community or in institutions.

Conceptual Basis

This scale is based on the theory that human behavior can be ordered in a hierarchy of complexity, from physical self-maintenance, through instrumental activities of daily living to motivation and social interaction (1), an approach similar to that used in Katz's Index of ADL.

Description

The Physical Self-Maintenance Scale (PSMS) is a modification of a scale developed at the Langley-Porter Neuropsychiatric Institute by Lowenthal et al., which is discussed, but not presented, in Lowenthal's book (2). The PSMS ratings may be made by a variety of staff members, and concentrate on observable behaviors. Five-point response scales ranging from total independence to total dependence are used for all six items, which fall on a Guttman scale. Two scoring methods may be used: a count of the numbers of items on which any degree of disability is identified, or a severity scale summing the response codes for each item, resulting in an overall score ranging from 6 to 30. The scale, showing the response codes, is presented in Exhibit 3.8.

Exhibit 3.8 The Physical Self-Maintenance Scale

A. Toilet
    1. Cares for self at toilet completely, no incontinence.
    2. Needs to be reminded, or needs help in cleaning self, or has rare (weekly at most) accidents.
    3. Soiling or wetting while asleep more than once a week.
    4. Soiling or wetting while awake more than once a week.
    5. No control of bowels or bladder.

B. Feeding
    1. Eats without assistance.
    2. Eats with minor assistance at meal times and/or with special preparation of food, or help in cleaning up after meals.
    3. Feeds self with moderate assistance and is untidy.
    4. Requires extensive assistance for all meals.
    5. Does not feed self at all and resists efforts of others to feed him.

C. Dressing
    1. Dresses, undresses and selects clothes from own wardrobe.
    2. Dresses and undresses self, with minor assistance.
    3. Needs moderate assistance in dressing or selection of clothes.
    4. Needs major assistance in dressing, but cooperates with efforts of others to help.
    5. Completely unable to dress self and resists efforts of others to help.

D. Grooming (neatness, hair, nails, hands, face, clothing)
    1. Always neatly dressed, well-groomed, without assistance.
    2. Grooms self adequately with occasional minor assistance, e.g., shaving.
    3. Needs moderate and regular assistance or supervision in grooming.
    4. Needs total grooming care, but can remain well-groomed after help from others.
    5. Actively negates all efforts of others to maintain grooming.

E. Physical Ambulation
    1. Goes about grounds or city.
    2. Ambulates within residence or about one block distant.
    3. Ambulates with assistance of (check one) a ( ) another person, b ( ) railing, c ( ) cane, d ( ) walker, e ( ) wheelchair.
        1 ____ Gets in and out without help.
        2 ____ Needs help in getting in and out.
    4. Sits unsupported in chair or wheelchair, but cannot propel self without help.
    5. Bedridden more than half the time.

F. Bathing
    1. Bathes self (tub, shower, sponge bath) without help.
    2. Bathes self with help in getting in and out of tub.
    3. Washes face and hands only, but cannot bathe rest of body.
    4. Does not wash self but is cooperative with those who bathe him.
    5. Does not try to wash self and resists efforts to keep him clean.

Reproduced from Lawton MP, Brody EM. Assessment of older people: Self-Maintaining and Instrumental Activities of Daily Living. Gerontologist 1969;9:180, Table 1. With permission.

Reliability

A Pearson correlation of 0.87 was obtained between pairs of nurses who rated 36 patients; the agreement between two research assistants who independently rated 14 patients was 0.91 (1, p182). The six items fall on a Guttman scale when cutting points are set between independent (code 1 in each item) and all levels of dependency. The rank order of the items was: feeding (77% independent), toilet (66%), dressing (56%), bathing (43%), grooming (42%) and ambulation (27% independent). A reproducibility coefficient of 0.96 was reported (N = 265) (1, Table 1).

Validity

The PSMS was tested on elderly persons, some in an institution and others living at home. It correlated 0.62 with a physician's rating of functional health (N = 130), and 0.61 with an IADL scale (N = 77) (1, Table 6). As would be expected, it correlated less highly (r = 0.38) with a mental status test covering orientation and memory, and it also correlated 0.38 with a behavioral rating of social adjustment (1, Table 6).

Commentary

A scale similar to this is incorporated in the Multilevel Assessment Instrument developed by Lawton and described in Chapter 8. The hierarchical model of disability used in the PSMS is similar to, but extends the scope of, Katz's approach in his Index of ADL. The PSMS has not been widely reported in the literature, but appears to be a reliable and valid ADL scale for clinical and survey research applications.

Address

M. Powell Lawton, PhD, Philadelphia Geriatric Center, 5301 Old York Road, Philadelphia, Pennsylvania, USA 19141

References

(1) Lawton MP, Brody EM. Assessment of older people: Self-Maintaining and Instrumental Activities of Daily Living. Gerontologist 1969;9:179–186.
(2) Lowenthal MF. Lives in distress: the paths of the elderly to the psychiatric ward. New York: Basic Books, 1964.

THE FUNCTIONAL STATUS RATING SYSTEM
(Stephen K. Forer, 1981)

Purpose

The Functional Status Rating System (FSRS) estimates the assistance required by rehabilitation patients in their daily lives. It covers independence in ADL, ability to communicate and social adjustment.

Conceptual Basis

No information is available.

Description

This rating scale was based on a method developed by the Hospitalization Utilization Project of Pennsylvania (HUP) initiated in 1974 to provide national statistics on hospital utilization and treatment outcomes (1). A preliminary version of the FSRS covered five ADL topics (2); the revised rating form described here is broader in scope: 30 items cover five topics. The items are summarized in Exhibit 3.9; the scales on which each item is rated are shown at the foot of the exhibit. An instruction manual is available that gives more detailed definitions of each item (3). Ratings are made by the treatment team member with primary responsibility for that aspect of care. Item scores are averaged to form scores for each of the five sections. The scale can be completed in 15 to 20 minutes.

Reliability

Information is available for the preliminary version only. Inter-rater agreement was high, but varied according to the professional background of the rater and the method of administration. Correlations ranged from 0.81 to 0.92 (2, p362).

Validity

Some predictive validity results are presented by Forer and Miller (2). Admission scores on bladder management and cognition were found to predict the eventual placement of the patient in home or institutional care. The instru-

Exhibit 3.9 The Functional Status Rating System

Functional Status in Self-care
A. *Eating/feeding:* Management of all aspects of setting up and eating food (including cutting of meat) with or without adaptive equipment.
B. *Personal hygiene:* Includes set up, oral care, washing face and hands with a wash cloth, hair grooming, shaving, and makeup.
C. *Toileting:* Includes management of clothing and cleanliness.
D. *Bathing:* Includes entire body bathing (tub, shower, or bed bath).
E. *Bowel management:* Able to insert suppository and/or perform manual evacuation, aware of need to defecate, has sphincter muscle control.
F. *Bladder management:* Able to manage equipment necessary for bladder evacuation (may include intermittent catheterization).
G. *Skin management:* Performance of skin care program, regular inspection, prevention of pressure sores, rashes, or irritations.
H. *Bed activities:* Includes turning, coming to a sitting position, scooting, and maintenance of balance.
I. *Dressing:* Includes performance of total body dressing except tying shoes, with or without adaptive equipment (also includes application of orthosis & prosthesis).

Exhibit 3.9 (*continued*)

Functional Status in Mobility

A. *Transfers:* Includes the management of all aspects of transfers to and from bed, mat, toilet, tub/shower, wheelchair, with or without adaptive equipment.
B. *Wheelchair skills:* Includes management of brakes, leg rests, maneuvering and propelling through and over doorway thresholds.
C. *Ambulation:* Includes coming to a standing position and walking short to moderate distances on level surfaces with or without equipment.
D. *Stairs and environmental surfaces:* Includes climbing stairs, curbs, ramps or environmental terrain.
E. *Community mobility:* Ability to manage transportation.

Functional Status in Communication

A. *Understanding spoken language*
B. *Reading comprehension*
C. *Language expression (non-speech/alternative methods):* Includes pointing, gestures, manual communication boards, electronic systems.
D. *Language expression (verbal):* Includes grammar, syntax, & appropriateness of language.
E. *Speech intelligibility*
F. *Written communication (motor)*
G. *Written language expression:* Includes spelling, vocabulary, punctuation, syntax, grammar, and completeness of written response.

Functional Status in Psychosocial Adjustment

A. *Emotional adjustment:* Includes frequency and severity of depression, anxiety, frustration, lability, unresponsiveness, agitation, interference with progress in therapies, motivation, ability to cope with and take responsibility for emotional behavior.
B. *Family/significant others/environment:* Includes frequency of chronic problems or conflicts in patient's relationships, interference with progress in therapies, ability and willingness to provide for patient's specific needs after discharge, and to promote patient's recovery and independence.
C. *Adjustment to limitations:* Includes denial/awareness, acceptance of limitations, willingness to learn new ways of functioning, compensating, taking appropriate safety precautions, and realistic expectations for long-term recovery.
D. *Social adjustment:* Includes frequency & initiation of social contacts, responsiveness in one to one & group situations, appropriateness of behavior in relationships, and spontaneity of interactions.

Functional Status in Cognitive Function

A. *Attention span:* Includes distractability, level of alertness and responsiveness, ability to concentrate on a task, ability to follow directions, immediate recall as the structure, difficulty and length of the task varies.
B. *Orientation*
C. *Judgment reasoning*
D. *Memory:* Includes short and long-term.
E. *Problem-solving*

Summary of Rating Scales

Self-care and mobility items	Communication, psychosocial and cognitive function items
1.0 = Unable—totally dependent	1.0 = Extremely severe
1.5 = Maximum assistance of 1 or 2 people	1.5 = Severe
2.0 = Moderate assistance	2.0 = Moderately severe
2.5 = Minimal assistance	2.5 = Moderate impairment
3.0 = Standby assistance	3.0 = Mild impairment
3.5 = Supervised	3.5 = Minimal impairment
4.0 = Independent	4.0 = No impairment

Adapted from the Rating Form obtained from Steven K. Forer.

ment was shown capable of reflecting improvement between admission and discharge for a number of diagnostic groups (2, Table 2).

Commentary

Despite the lack of validity information we have included this scale because it is one of the more recent ADL scales to be published and because of its broad scope and detailed ratings. As a clinical instrument the scale appears relevant and valuable, but the paucity of formal reliability and validity testing of the revised version underscores the need for caution in using it.

Address

Stephen K. Forer, Rehabilitation Services Manager, Administration Office, Santa Clara Valley Medical Center, 751 South Bascom Avenue, San Jose, California, USA 95128

References

(1) Breckenridge K. Medical rehabilitation program evaluation. Arch Phys Med Rehabil 1978;59:419–423.
(2) Forer SK, Miller LS. Rehabilitation outcome: comparative analysis of different patient types. Arch Phys Med Rehabil 1980;61:359–365.
(3) Forer SK. Revised functional status rating instrument. Glendale, California: Rehabilitation Institute, Glendale Adventist Medical Center, December 1981.

CONCLUSION: ADL SCALES

It is unfortunate that the development of ADL scales has been so uncoordinated. More recent scales have not been planned explicitly on a careful review of the strengths and weaknesses of previous instruments, and the definition of disability itself seems usually to be taken for granted rather than clearly stated. There is no evidence for an accumulation of a body of scientific knowledge concerning the concept of disability, its relationship to impairment and handicap, or of the sequence in which changes in disability occur as a patient's condition deteriorates or improves. We know relatively little about the overlap among the various measurement methods, and the few comparative studies that exist mainly review the older scales. For example, Donaldson et al. designed a unified ADL evaluation form that incorporates the Barthel, Katz and Kenny ratings (1). This was applied to 100 patients at admission and one month later. For 68 of the 100 patients the change (or lack of it) between scores was reflected in all three scales. Of the 32 cases in which a discrepancy occurred, 19 showed no change on the Katz, but change on the other two scales; in 5 cases the Kenny score had changed and the others had not. These and other results led Donaldson to conclude that the Katz scale is the least sensitive of the three methods, followed by the Barthel, with the Kenny being most sensitive to change. The Kenny's omission of continence explains some of the discrepancies between its results and those of the other scales. Gresham et al. also found that these three indices "are documenting the same basic group of functional skills and classifying the overall degree of independence in ADL in a very similar manner"(2, p357). They noted that the Barthel Index had several practical advantages: widespread use, clarity of scoring system, and completeness. While these three are among the most widely used scales, they are also old and the available validity results are not impressive, although the majority of newer scales contain even less evidence for reliability and validity, and few studies have compared their results.

In preparing this chapter we examined a large number of other ADL scales, most of which we excluded on the grounds of inadequate evidence for validity and reliability. Some of the scales are, however, worthy of mention because of characteristics that may commend them for particular applications. The ADL scale of Pool and Brown, for example, offers considerable coverage in the area of locomotion: 13 of the 23 questions are devoted to walking, managing wheelchairs and transport. No validity results are available, but an inter-rater concordance of 0.87 was reported (3). A scale that Sainsbury outlined (but did not present in detail) is imaginative in the way that each disability item is explicitly linked with the types of impairment it reflects. For example, doing the shopping and carrying groceries reflect coordination, sustained effort, mobility and reach (4). Several scales combine questions on ADL with psychosocial factors, but lack reliability and validity data (5–7). Susset describes, but does not present, the questions on a scale of this type. The ADL form described by Rinzler et al. pays close attention to objectivity by standardizing the activities: performance is timed and exact distances are specified (8).

Several of the scales described in Chapter 8 include ADL-type questions, usually in the context of a broader-ranging instrument. This makes it questionable whether the ADL sections of the scales can be applied alone. However, the quality of validity results is superior for most of the scales in Chapter 8, and we recommend that readers looking for an ADL scale consider those also.

Since this chapter was written, some early descriptions have become available of the Functional Independence Measure, a 19-item rating scale that covers self-care, mobility, communication, cognition and social adjustment. The instrument was proposed by a task force working on the development of a uniform data system for rehabilitation, whose project office is in the Department of Rehabilitation Medicine at Buffalo General Hospital, 100 High Street, Buffalo, New York, USA 14203. The scale is similar in design to Forer's Functional Status Rating System; no numerical indications of validity or reliability are available yet.

References

(1) Donaldson SW, Wagner CC, Gresham GE. A unified ADL evaluation form. Arch Phys Med Rehabil 1973;54:175–179.
(2) Gresham GE, Phillips TF, Labi MLC. ADL status in stroke: relative merits of three standard indexes. Arch Phys Med Rehabil 1980;61:355–358.
(3) Pool DA, Brown RA. A functional rating scale for research in physical therapy. Tex Rep Biol Med 1968;26:133–136.

(4) Sainsbury S. Measuring disability. London: G. Bell, 1973.
(5) Gauger AB, Brownell WM, Russell WW, Retter RW. Evaluation of levels of subsistence. Arch Phys Med Rehabil 1964;45:286–292.
(6) Susset V, Vobecky J, Black R. Disability outcome and self-assessment of disabled persons: an analysis of 506 cases. Arch Phys Med Rehabil 1979;60:50–56.
(7) Scranton J, Fogel ML, Erdman WJ. Evaluation of functional levels of patients during and following rehabilitation. Arch Phys Med Rehabil 1970;51:1–21.
(8) Rinzler SH, Brown H, Benton JG. A method for the objective evaluation of physical and drug therapy in the rehabilitation of the hemiplegic patient. Am Heart J 1951;42:710–718.

IADL SCALES

Instrumental Activities of Daily Living scales extend the ADL theme to cover tasks that require a finer level of motor coordination than is necessary for the relatively gross activities covered in ADL scales. IADL scales are commonly used with less severely handicapped populations, often as survey instruments for use in the general population, and cover activities needed for continued community residence. They were intended to improve on the sensitivity of ADL scales that were found not to identify low levels of disability, nor minor changes in level of disability. It should be noted that several scales include both ADL and IADL questions; our classification is therefore somewhat arbitrary and was made according to what appears to be the primary orientation of the scale.

We describe seven IADL scales, three that are used in clinical settings, one research scale, and three population survey instruments. The survey instruments include the questionnaire developed by the international Organization for Economic Cooperation and Development and two disability screening scales developed in England: the Lambeth scale and Bennett and Garrad's interview schedule. The research scale we review, Linn's Rapid Disability Rating Scale, is seeing growing use in published studies. The clinical scales include the Functional Status Index of Jette, a brief rating scale by Pfeffer, and the fuller Patient Evaluation Conference System developed by Harvey and Jellinek. In addition to these scales the reader should consult Chapter 8, which presents several scales such as the Multidimensional Functional Activities Questionnaire that include sections with IADL themes.

A RAPID DISABILITY RATING SCALE
(Margaret W. Linn, 1967, Revised 1982)

Purpose

The Rapid Disability Rating Scale (RDRS) was developed as a research tool for summarizing the functional capacity and mental status of elderly chronic patients. It may be used with hospitalized patients and with people living in the community.

Conceptual Basis

No information is available.

Description

The 1967 version of the RDRS contained 16 items covering physical and mental functioning and independence in self-care. A revised scale of 18 items was published by Linn and Linn as the RDRS-2 in 1982 (1). Changes included the addition of three items covering mobility, toileting and adaptive tasks (i.e., managing money, telephoning, shopping); the question on safety supervision was dropped (1, p379). Four-point response scales replaced the earlier three-point scales. The RDRS-2 has eight questions on activities of daily living, three on sensory abilities, three on mental capacities and one question on each of dietary changes, continence, medications, and confinement to bed (see Exhibit 3.10). The following review refers mainly to the revised version.

The rating scale is completed by a nurse or a person familiar with the patient. Because the scale describes performance, the rater must observe the patient carrying out the various tasks rather than rely on self-report. Once the rater has made the observations, it takes about two minutes to complete the scale.

Response categories are phrased in terms of the amount of assistance the patient requires so that the instrument indicates handicap rather than impairment. Each item is weighted equally in calculating an overall score. The scores range from 18 to 72, with higher values indicating greater disability; items may be combined to provide three subscores indicating degree of assistance with activities of daily living, physical disabilities and psychosocial problems (1, p380).

Reliability

Inter-rater reliability of the preliminary version was assessed by comparing ratings of 20 patients made independently by three raters; a coefficient of 0.91 was obtained using Kendall's W index of concordance (2, p213). Test-retest reliability was investigated by repeating ratings of 238 patients before and after admission to nursing homes. With a mean delay of three and a half days, the correlation between ratings was 0.83, and the mean scores of the two sets of ratings were within one point of each other (2, p213). Linn and Linn reported item reliability results for the revised version: two nurses independently rated 100 patients and item correlations ranged from 0.62 to 0.98; the three lowest correlations were for the mental status items (1, Table 2). Test-retest reliability on 50 patients after an interval of three days produced correlations between 0.58 and 0.96 (1, pp380–381).

Validity

A factor analysis of ratings of 120 hospitalized patients provided a three-factor solution (1, p381). Linn and Linn interpreted the factors as reflecting activities

Exhibit 3.10 The Rapid Disability Rating Scale-2

Directions: Rate what the person *does* to reflect current behavior. Circle one of the four choices for each item. Consider rating with any aids or prostheses normally used. None = completely independent or normal behavior. Total = that person cannot, will not or may not (because of medical restriction) perform a behavior or has the most severe form of disability or problem.

Assistance with activities of daily living

Eating	None	A little	A lot	Spoon-feed; intravenous tube
Walking (with cane or walker if used)	None	A little	A lot	Does not walk
Mobility (going outside and getting about with wheelchair, etc., if used)	None	A little	A lot	Is housebound
Bathing (include getting supplies, supervising)	None	A little	A lot	Must be bathed
Dressing (include help in selecting clothes)	None	A little	A lot	Must be dressed
Toileting (include help with clothes, cleaning, or help with ostomy, catheter)	None	A little	A lot	Uses bedpan or unable to care for ostomy/catheter
Grooming (shaving for men, hairdressing for women, nails, teeth)	None	A little	A lot	Must be groomed
Adaptive tasks (managing money/possessions; telephoning; buying newspaper, toilet articles, snacks)	None	A little	A lot	Cannot manage

Degree of disability

Communication (expressing self)	None	A little	A lot	Does not communicate
Hearing (with aid if used)	None	A little	A lot	Does not seem to hear
Sight (with glasses, if used)	None	A little	A lot	Does not see
Diet (deviation from normal)	None	A little	A lot	Fed by intravenous tube
In bed during day (ordered or self-initiated)	None	A little (<3 hrs)	A lot	Most/all of time
Incontinence (urine/feces, with catheter or prosthesis, if used)	None	Sometimes	Frequently (weekly +)	Does not control
Medication	None	Sometimes	Daily, taken orally	Daily; injection; (+ oral if used)

Exhibit 3.10 *(continued)*

Degree of special problems				
Mental confusion	None	A little	A lot	Extreme
Uncooperativeness	None	A little	A lot	Extreme
(combats efforts				
to help with care)				
Depression	None	A little	A lot	Extreme

Reprinted with permission from the American Geriatrics Society, The Rapid Disability Rating Scale-2, by Linn MW and Linn BS (Journal of the American Geriatrics Society, Vol 30, p 380, 1982).

of daily living, disability and psychological problems. The latter were labeled "special problems" by the authors, as shown in Exhibit 3.10.

Ratings of 845 men (mean age, 68 years) were used to predict subsequent mortality using multiple regression and discriminant function analyses. Twenty percent of the variance in mortality was explained, correctly classifying 72% of patients who would die (1, p382).

Correlations of 0.27 were obtained between the RDRS-2 and a physician's 13-item rating scale of impairment of 172 elderly patients living in the community; a correlation of 0.43 was obtained with a six-point self-report scale of health (1, p382).

Reference Standards

No formal reference standards are available, but Linn and Linn noted that for the RDRS-2:

> Elderly persons living in the community with minimal disabilities have scores averaging 21 to 22. For hospitalized elderly patients the average is about 32, and for those transferred to nursing homes the average is about 36 (1, p380).

Commentary

This is a broad-ranging scale that rates the amount of assistance required in 18 activities, broader in scope than the PULSES, Barthel or most ADL scales. It has been used in several evaluative studies (3-5) and a French version was used by Jenicek et al. (6). Its research orientation is reflected in the attention paid to reliability and validity, which are superior to those of the clinical scales. Nonetheless, the validity tests could be improved. For example, correlations with physicians' ratings commonly produce low coefficients because the physician is not aware of details of the patient's functioning. The use of predictive validation is imaginative, but as this is rarely attempted with such indices it is hard to judge whether a 20% explanation variance is high or low. It would be advantageous if studies of predictive validity reported findings in a comparable manner: Granger expressed the predictive validity of the Barthel Index in terms of percentages of patients with low scores who died.

Criticisms have been made of the scoring system. For example, the same weight is assigned to different degrees of disability: "permanent confinement to bed" and "following a special diet" both rate three points (6, p345). This weakness would reduce the validity of the scale in giving absolute indications of disability, although it may be less serious if the scale is used to monitor change over time.

Despite criticisms, this is the most reliable scale reviewed in this chapter, and the validity results are second only to those of Pfeffer's Functional Activities Questionnaire.

Address

Margaret W. Linn, PhD, Director, Social Science Research, Veterans Administration Medical Center, 1201 Northwest 16th Street, Miami, Florida, USA 33125

References

(1) Linn MW, Linn BS. The Rapid Disability Rating Scale-2. J Am Geriatr Soc 1982;30:378–382.
(2) Linn MW. A Rapid Disability Rating Scale. J Am Geriatr Soc 1967;15:211–214.
(3) Ogren EH, Linn MW. Male nursing home patients: relocation and mortality. J Am Geriatr Soc 1971;19:229–239.
(4) Linn MW, Gurel L, Linn BS. Patient outcome as a measure of quality of nursing home care. Am J Public Health 1977;67:337–344.
(5) Linn MW, Linn BS, Harris R. Effects of counseling for late stage cancer patients. Cancer 1982;49:1048–1055.
(6) Jenicek M, Cléroux R, Lamoureux M. Principal component analysis of four health indicators and construction of a global health index in the aged. Am J Epidemiol 1979;110:343–349.

THE FUNCTIONAL STATUS INDEX
(Pilot Geriatric Arthritis Program, Alan M. Jette, 1978, Revised 1980)

Purpose

The Functional Status Index (FSI) assesses the functional status of adult arthritics living in the community (1). Intended both as a clinical and as an evaluative tool, the scale measures the degree of dependence, pain and difficulty experienced in performing daily activities (2).

Conceptual Basis

The FSI was developed to evaluate a Pilot Geriatric Arthritis Program (PGAP) which sought to improve the quality of life of elderly arthritics (3). The goals of the program were to prevent disability, restore activity, reduce pain, and encourage social and emotional adjustment (3).

Jette argued that the outcomes of care should not be viewed solely in terms of independence, as is the case in most ADL scales. Sometimes providing assistance to a patient, which increases his dependence, may alleviate pain and reduce difficulty. He criticized "the exclusive emphasis on level of dependence in previous work as well as the assumption that assistance in ADL constitutes a loss of health" (4, p576). Accordingly, the FSI measures pain and difficulty in performing tasks as well as the patient's level of dependence.

Description

Based on the Barthel, PULSES and Katz instruments, the staff of the Pilot Geriatric Arthritis Program developed the FSI "to provide a comprehensive assessment of the major ADL of noninstitutionalized adults" (2, 3).

> The PGAP staff also criticized previous instruments for their use of broad categories of activity (e.g. dressing) which incorporated complex series of activities involving many different joints and muscle groups. To make the instrument more sensitive to modest changes in functional ability, they expanded the instrument to include 44 [later 45] activities and increased the specificity of the activities. (4, p576).

The full-length version of the FSI included 45 questions on activities of daily living (2, Table 1); these were asked three times, to give separate ratings of the level of dependence, difficulty and pain involved in carrying out each activity. The resulting 135 questions (45 items × three dimensions) took between 60 and 90 minutes to administer (5).

The shortened version, shown in Exhibit 3.11, contains 18 items grouped under five headings: mobility, hand activities, personal care, home chores and interpersonal activities. These questions are asked three times, to assess the respondent's level of dependency, then his pain and level of difficulty. The

Exhibit 3.11 The Functional Status Index: Tasks

Gross mobility	Personal Care
walking inside	washing all parts of the body
stair climbing	putting on pants
chair transfers	putting on a shirt
	buttoning a shirt
Hand activities	Home chores
opening containers	doing laundry
writing	reaching into low cupboards
dialing a phone	doing yardwork
	vacuuming a rug

Interpersonal activities
   driving a car
   visiting family or friends
   attending meetings
   performing your job

Reproduced from Jette AM. Functional Status Index: reliability of a chronic disease evaluation instrument. Arch Phys Med Rehabil 1980;61:398,Table 4. With permission.

order in which the dimensions are presented is systematically varied; the shortened version takes 20 to 30 minutes to administer (5). Exhibit 3.11 shows the topics covered by the FSI; the question stem is the same for each topic. In assessing dependency (or level of assistance used) the respondent is asked: "How much help did you use, on the average, during the past week to. . . . " In assessing pain, the question asks the respondent to use a ladder scale to rate "the amount of pain you experienced when doing each activity on the average, last week." For difficulty, the respondent is asked to "Make a check on the rung of the ladder which best represents the degree of ease or difficulty you experienced when performing each activity, on the average during the past 7 days."

The revised FSI is administered by an interviewer, with the respondent describing his level of performance over the previous seven days. Responses are based on self-report, not observation. The 45-item version uses fixed-choice responses employing a five-point scale for the dependency dimension and four-point scales for the pain and difficulty dimensions (2, 3). For the 18-item version, four-point scales (used no help, used equipment, used human assistance, used equipment and human assistance) are still used for the dependency dimension, but the other two dimensions use either a 0 to 7 or a 0 to 13 ladder scale. Jette recommends the 0 to 7 scale (personal communication, 1983).

Reliability

Jette and Deniston studied inter-rater reliability in assessing 19 patients using the 45-item version (1). They found that as the degree of pain and difficulty increased, agreement between raters decreased (1, Table 3). The agreement among nine raters yielded intra-class correlations averaging 0.78 for the dependence dimension, 0.61 for difficulty and 0.75 for pain (1, Table 4). Liang and Jette reported equivalent figures of 0.72, 0.75 and 0.78 (6).

Liang and Jette reported test-retest reliability of 0.75 in the dependence dimension, 0.77 in the difficulty dimension and 0.69 in the pain dimension (6, p83).

Jette compared the internal consistency reliability for the five dimensions of the 18-item FSI. He also studied three different response modes: defined response options (of the type listed above), a ladder scale and a Q-sort technique (5). For 149 patients, the internal consistency of the mobility and personal care sections ranged from 0.70 to over 0.90 (5, Tables 5-7). Similar reliability results were achieved with each of the three response modes, except that the fixed answer categories proved less reliable in assessing pain levels than the other scaling techniques (5).

Validity

Deniston and Jette compared responses to the 45-item FSI with ratings made by hospital staff and with self-ratings made by 95 elderly arthritics. Correlations between the patients' judgments of their "number of good days in the past week" and the FSI scores were 0.14 for the dependence dimension, 0.41 for difficulty and 0.46 for pain (3, Table 2). Correlations of the FSI scores and a self-rating of ability to deal with disease-related problems averaged 0.24; correlations with a self-rating of joint condition averaged 0.39 (3, Table 1). In these results, the pain and difficulty dimensions again showed the stronger associations. Correlations with ratings made by the staff were lower; staff ratings of joint status and the FSI correlated 0.11 for dependence and difficulty and 0.22 for pain (3, Table 4). These correlations ranged widely according to the identity of the staff person who rated the patient. The authors discussed reasons for the low associations and suggested that the questions posed to the raters may not have been specific enough (3). Shope et al. reported correlations between FSI scores and clinical assessments of 80 patients with rheumatoid arthritis. Correlations with the American Rheumatism Association functional classification ranged from 0.40 to 0.43 ($p < 0.05$) (7).

Jette reported a factor analysis of the 18-item version, identifying the five factors shown in Exhibit 3.11 (5). In a different study analyzing 36 items, Jette again obtained five factors, but named them differently: physical mobility, kitchen chores, home chores, transfers and personal care. These factors accounted for 58.5% of the variance (2, Table 2). A factor analysis of the pain items produced six factors accounting for 60.5% of the variance, while an analysis of the difficulty questions produced eight factors accounting for 61.4% of the variance (2, p89). Jette concluded that five functional categories are common to the three dimensions: mobility, transfer, home chores, kitchen chores and personal care (2). These amplify the three categories (mobility, personal care and work) that were originally proposed.

Commentary

This instrument is similar to the Kenny scale in its intent to provide a more detailed rating of disability than the other scales. The scale is based on a conceptual analysis of disability, a strength compared with other IADL scales. The division of the FSI into three dimensions has received some empirical support: the fact that difficulty and pain showed higher correlations with independent ratings suggests that these dimensions are considered important by both staff and patients. Deniston and Jette noted that the distinction between dependence and the other two dimensions is meaningful, but that the distinction between functional pain and difficulty is still equivocal (3). Jette does not report the correlation between the pain and difficulty dimensions; it is to be hoped that future studies will examine the necessity of keeping the latter two dimensions separate.

In terms of the practical utility of the method, the administration time (60 to 90 minutes) is likely to be a drawback. The ability of the FSI to detect clinically important changes has not yet been assessed (6), nor has its application to conditions other than arthritis been studied. The results of the validity testing raise cause for concern: the correlation with the criteria are lower than for other scales that we review. It is desirable that more evidence on validity be accumulated before this scale can be fully recommended.

Address

Alan M. Jette, PT, PhD, Department of Social Medicine and Health Policy, Division on Aging, Harvard Medical School, 643 Huntington Avenue, Boston, Massachusetts, USA 02115

References

(1) Jette AM, Deniston OL. Inter-observer reliability of a functional status assessment instrument. J Chronic Dis 1978;31:573–580.
(2) Jette AM. Functional capacity evaluation: an empirical approach. Arch Phys Med Rehabil 1980;61:85–89.
(3) Deniston OL, Jette A. A functional status assessment instrument: validation in an elderly population. Health Serv Res 1980;15:21–34.
(4) Jette AM. Health status indicators: their utility in chronic-disease evaluation research. J Chronic Dis 1980;33:567–579.
(5) Jette AM. Functional Status Index: reliability of a chronic disease evaluation instrument. Arch Phys Med Rehabil 1980;61:395–401.
(6) Liang MH, Jette AM. Measuring functional ability in chronic arthritis: a critical review. Arthritis Rheum 1981;24:80–86.
(7) Shope JT, Banwell BA, Jette AM, Kulik C-L, Edwards NL. Functional status outcome following treatment of rheumatoid arthritis. (Manuscript, 1983).

THE PATIENT EVALUATION CONFERENCE SYSTEM
(Richard F. Harvey and Hollis M. Jellinek, 1981)

Purpose

The Patient Evaluation Conference System (PECS) rates the functional and psychosocial status of rehabilitation patients. It is intended for use in defining treatment goals and in evaluating progress toward them.

Conceptual Basis

Although no formal conceptual basis was given to justify the content of the instrument, Harvey and Jellinek did describe several principles that guided the design of the PECS. These included its need to be able to reflect minor changes in functional level, its multidisciplinary scope (it had to cover medical, psychological, social and vocational topics) and its simplicity of application, scoring and interpretation (1).

Description

The PECS is a broad-ranging instrument containing 79 functional assessment items grouped into 15 sections and an additional 3 sections pertaining to the results of a case conference. Each section is completed by the staff member who has primary responsibility for that aspect of care. The ratings made by each therapist are collated onto a master form that summarizes the rehabilitation

Exhibit 3.12 The Patient Evaluation Conference System

DEPARTMENT OF REHABILITATION MEDICINE
PATIENT EVALUATION CONFERENCE SYSTEM (PECS)©

Date _____

Ramac # _____ History # _____

Name _____ Location _____

Service _____ Status _____ Birthdate _____

Street _____

City _____ State _____ Zip _____

Scores range from 0 to 7, with 0 being the lowest score, or not assessed, and 7 being the highest score, such as normal or independent. Scores of 1 to 4 indicate dependent function. Scores of 5 or more indicate independent function.

Keys to scores are available in each participating discipline.

Instructions: Circle (O) the goal score   example
            X the current status score   0 1 2 ✗ 4 ⑤ 6 7
                                      Dependent | Independent

Date _____ Primary Dx _____ Secondary Dx _____

I. Rehabilitation Medicine (MED)

1. Motor loss (including muscle weakness and limb deficiency)   0 1 2 3 4 5 6 7
2. Spasticity/involuntary movement (including dystonia and ataxia)   0 1 2 3 4 5 6 7
3. Joint limitations   0 1 2 3 4 5 6 7
4. Autonomic disturbance   0 1 2 3 4 5 6 7
5. Sensory deficiency   0 1 2 3 4 5 6 7
6. Perceptual and cognitive deficit   0 1 2 3 4 5 6 7
7. Associated medical problems   0 1 2 3 4 5 6 7

II. Rehabilitation Nursing (NSG)

1. Performance of bowel program   0 1 2 3 4 5 6 7
2. Performance of urinary program   0 1 2 3 4 5 6 7
3. Performance of skin program   0 1 2 3 4 5 6 7
4. Assumes responsibility for self-care   0 1 2 3 4 5 6 7
5. Performs assigned interdisciplinary activities   0 1 2 3 4 5 6 7

III. Physical Mobility (PHY)

1. Performance of transfers   0 1 2 3 4 5 6 7
2. Performance of ambulation   0 1 2 3 4 5 6 7
3. Performance of wheelchair mobility (primary mode)   0 1 2 3 4 5 6 7
4. Ability to handle environmental barriers (e.g., stairs, rugs, elevators)   0 1 2 3 4 5 6 7
5. Performance of car transfer   0 1 2 3 4 5 6 7
6. Driving mobility   0 1 2 3 4 5 6 7
7. Assumes responsibility for mobility   0 1 2 3 4 5 6 7

IV. Activities of Daily Living (ADL)

1. Performance in feeding   0 1 2 3 4 5 6 7
2. Performance in hygiene/grooming   0 1 2 3 4 5 6 7
3. Performance in dressing   0 1 2 3 4 5 6 7
4. Performance in home management   0 1 2 3 4 5 6 7
5. Performance of mobility in home environment (including utilization of environmental adaptations for communication)   0 1 2 3 4 5 6 7

V. Communication (COM)

1. Ability to comprehend spoken language   0 1 2 3 4 5 6 7
2. Ability to produce language   0 1 2 3 4 5 6 7
3. Ability to read   0 1 2 3 4 5 6 7
4. Ability to produce written language   0 1 2 3 4 5 6 7
5. Ability to hear   0 1 2 3 4 5 6 7
6. Ability to comprehend and use gesture   0 1 2 3 4 5 6 7
7. Ability to produce speech   0 1 2 3 4 5 6 7

VI. Medications (DRG)

1. Knowledge of medications   0 1 2 3 4 5 6 7
2. Skill with medications   0 1 2 3 4 5 6 7
3. Utilization of medications   0 1 2 3 4 5 6 7

VII. Nutrition (NUT)

1. Nutritional status - body weight   0 1 2 3 4 5 6 7
2. Nutritional status - lab values   0 1 2 3 4 5 6 7
3. Knowledge of nutrition and/or modified diet   0 1 2 3 4 5 6 7
4. Skill with nutrition and diet (adherence to nutritional plan)   0 1 2 3 4 5 6 7
5. Utilization of nutrition and diet (nutritional health)   0 1 2 3 4 5 6 7

VIII. Assistive Devices (DEV)

1. Knowledge of assistive device(s)   0 1 2 3 4 5 6 7
2. Skill with assuming operating position of assistive device(s)   0 1 2 3 4 5 6 7
3. Utilization of assistive device(s)   0 1 2 3 4 5 6 7

IX. Psychology (PSY)

1. Distress/comfort   0 1 2 3 4 5 6 7
2. Helplessness/self-efficacy   0 1 2 3 4 5 6 7
3. Self-directed learning skills   0 1 2 3 4 5 6 7
4. Skill in self-management of behavior and emotions   0 1 2 3 4 5 6 7
5. Skill in interpersonal relations   0 1 2 3 4 5 6 7

X. Neuropsychology (NP)

1. Impairment of short-term memory   0 1 2 3 4 5 6 7
2. Impairment in long-term memory   0 1 2 3 4 5 6 7
3. Impairment in attention-concentration skills   0 1 2 3 4 5 6 7
4. Impairment in verbal linguistic processing   0 1 2 3 4 5 6 7
5. Impairment in visual spatial processing   0 1 2 3 4 5 6 7
6. Impairment in basic intellectual skills   0 1 2 3 4 5 6 7

XI. Social Issues (SOC)

1. Ability to problem solve and utilize resources   0 1 2 3 4 5 6 7
2. Family: communication/resource   0 1 2 3 4 5 6 7
3. Family understanding of disability   0 1 2 3 4 5 6 7
4. Economic resources   0 1 2 3 4 5 6 7
5. Ability to live independently   0 1 2 3 4 5 6 7
6. Living arrangements   0 1 2 3 4 5 6 7

goals. This is used in case conferences to record the patient's progress. The PECS form shown in Exhibit 3.12 was obtained from Dr. Harvey and is a slightly expanded version of that shown in reference 5 (Figure 2). Copies of the scale and instructions may be purchased from Dr. Harvey.

Eight-point responses are used for most items, with 0 representing unmeasured or unmeasurable function and 7 representing full independence. Scores are comparable across different scales: a cutting point of 5 distinguishes

XII. Vocational-Educational Activity (V/E)   Summary:

1. Active participation in realistic voc/ed planning   0 1 2 3 4 5 6 7
2. Realistic perception of work-related activity   0 1 2 3 4 5 6 7
3. Ability to tolerate planned number of hours of voc/ed activity/day   0 1 2 3 4 5 6 7
4. Vocational/educational placement   0 1 2 3 4 5 6 7
5. Physical capacity for work   0 1 2 3 4 5 6 7

XIII. Recreation (REC)

1. Participation in group activities   0 1 2 3 4 5 6 7
2. Participation in community activities   0 1 2 3 4 5 6 7
3. Interaction with others   0 1 2 3 4 5 6 7
4. Participation and satisfaction with individual leisure activities   0 1 2 3 4 5 6 7
5. Active participation in sports   0 1 2 3 4 5 6 7

XIV. Pain (consensus) (PAI)

1. Pain behavior   0 1 2 3 4 5 6 7
2. Physical inactivity   0 1 2 3 4 5 6 7
3. Social withdrawal   0 1 2 3 4 5 6 7
4. Pacing   0 1 2 3 4 5 6 7
5. Sitting   0 1 2 3 4 5 6 7
6. Standing tolerance   0 1 2 3 4 5 6 7
7. Walking endurance   0 1 2 3 4 5 6 7

XV. Pulmonary Rehabilitation (PUL)

1. Knowledge of pulmonary rehabilitation program   0 1 2 3 4 5 6 7
2. Skill with pulmonary rehabilitation program   0 1 2 3 4 5 6 7
3. Utilization of pulmonary rehabilitation program   0 1 2 3 4 5 6 7

XVI. Patient Participation at Conference   1   2

1. Attended   N   Y
2. Participated in goal setting   N   Y
3. Family (significant other) attended   N   Y

XVII. Preparation Completed for Pass and/or Discharge   1   2

1. Recreational Therapy pass   N   Y
2. P.R.N. pass   N   Y
3. T.L.O.A. pass   N   Y
4. Is this the discharge conference?   N   Y
5. Equipment ordered   N   Y
6. Type of assistive device   0 1 2 3 4 5 6 7
7. Phase of device development   0 1 2 3 4 5 6 7
8. Therapy schedule set according to priority   N   Y
9. Rehab. Med. Clinic standard follow-up (1, 3, 6, 12 mo.)   N   Y

XVIII. Specialty Program (Specify):

1. _____   0 1 2 3 4 5 6 7
2. _____   0 1 2 3 4 5 6 7
3. _____   0 1 2 3 4 5 6 7
4. _____   0 1 2 3 4 5 6 7
5. _____   0 1 2 3 4 5 6 7
6. _____   0 1 2 3 4 5 6 7
7. _____   0 1 2 3 4 5 6 7

Signature of M.D.

Date

Reproduced from the Patient Evaluation Conference System rating form provided by Dr. Richard F. Harvey. With permission.

between a need for human assistance and managing independently (with or without aids). A few items use four-point scales.

Reliability

Inter-rater reliability for different sections of the PECS ranged from 0.68 to 0.80 for 125 patients (1, p 459).

Validity

An abbreviated, self-administered version of the PECS was compared with the Brief Symptom Inventory, which measures emotional distress, for 22 brain-injured patients. Significant correlations in the range 0.38 to 0.47 were obtained with the self-care, mobility, living arrangements and communication scales on the PECS (2, Table 2). Two PECS scales, bladder and skin care, were assessed at time of discharge on 28 patients. The results correlated with several depression scores recorded at admission to the rehabilitation program, with coefficients between 0.37 and 0.39 (3, p361).

A study of 30 head trauma patients compared change in PECS scores between admission and discharge with the results of computerized tomography (CT) scans (4). Three patients found by CT scan to have no lesions achieved complete recovery in four out of five PECS scales; all ten patients with one-hemisphere lesions achieved independence in at least two areas, while for 17 patients with bilateral lesions, there were no areas in which all patients recovered completely (4, Table 2).

Commentary

Harvey and associates are in the process of expanding the PECS to include documentation for outpatient evaluation, with reports to referring physicians. Its use of a goal-attainment approach is distinctive, and a graphical presentation of data has been developed (5). Most of the validation studies used very small samples, however, and in some cases (3) it is not clear what the rationale for the study was. Although additional evidence on the quality of this scale is required before we can recommend it, Harvey and associates are actively involved in refining and testing the method, and it appears to hold considerable potential as a clinical measurement system for rehabilitation settings.

Address

Richard F. Harvey, MD, Vice President and Chief of Medical Staff, Marianjoy Hospital, Roosevelt Road, PO Box 795, Wheaton, Illinois, USA 60189

References

(1) Harvey RF, Jellinek HM. Functional performance assessment: a program approach. Arch Phys Med Rehabil 1981;62:456–461.
(2) Jellinek HM, Torkelson RM, Harvey RF. Functional abilities and distress levels in brain injured patients at long-term follow-up. Arch Phys Med Rehabil 1982;63:160–162.
(3) Malec J, Neimeyer R. Psychologic prediction of duration of inpatient spinal cord injury rehabilitation and performance of self-care. Arch Phys Med Rehabil 1983;64:359–363.
(4) Rao N, Jellinek HM, Harvey RF, Flynn MM. Computerized tomography head scans as predictors of rehabilitation outcome. Arch Phys Med Rehabil 1984;65:18–20.

(5) Harvey RF, Jellinek HM. Patient profiles: utilization in functional performance assessment. Arch Phys Med Rehabil 1983;64:268–271.

THE FUNCTIONAL ACTIVITIES QUESTIONNAIRE
(Robert I. Pfeffer, 1982, Revised 1984)

Purpose

This is a screening tool for assessing independence in daily activities designed for community studies of normal aging and mild senile dementia (1).

Conceptual Basis

The scale was intended to cover universal skills among older adults. Pfeffer followed the intuitively appealing concept of a hierarchy of skills proposed by Lawton and Brody and concentrated on higher level skills such as managing one's financial affairs and reading, which they had termed "social functions" (1).

Description

The Functional Activities Questionnaire (FAQ) is not self-administered, but is completed by a lay informant such as the spouse, a relative, or a close friend. The original version described in the literature shown in Exhibit 3.13, has ten items concerned with performing daily tasks necessary for independent living. In 1984, the questionnaire was slightly expanded by adding four ADL items and an item on initiative; the first ten items are the same in both versions. The expanded version will be published when validation is complete and it is not further described here. For each activity, four levels ranging from dependence (scored 3) to independence (scored 0) are specified. For activities not normally undertaken by the person, the informant must specify whether the person would be unable to undertake the task if required (scored 1) or could do so if required (0). The total score is the sum of individual item scores; higher scores reflect greater dependency.

Reliability

The item-total correlations for all items exceeded 0.80 (1, Table 4).

Validity

In a study of 158 elderly people living in the community, ratings on the FAQ correlated 0.72 with Lawton and Brody's IADL scale (1, Table 3). Correlations with mental functioning tests were mostly in excess of 0.70; the lowest correlation (0.41) was with Raven's matrices. The highest correlation (0.83) was with a neurologist's global rating on a Scale of Functional Capacity designed

Exhibit 3.13 The Functional Activities Questionnaire

Activities questionnaire to be completed by spouse, child, close friend or relative of the participant.

Instructions: The following pages list ten common activities. *For each activity,* please read all choices, then choose the *one* statement which best describes the *current* ability of the participant. Answers should apply to *that person's* abilities, not your own. Please check off a choice for *each* activity; do not skip any.

1. Writing checks, paying bills, balancing checkbook, keeping financial records
    ____ A. Someone has recently taken over this activity completely or almost completely.
    ____ B. Requires frequent advice or assistance from others (e.g. relatives, friends, business associates, banker), which was *not previously necessary.*
    ____ C. Does without any advice or assistance, but more difficult than used to be or less good job.
    ____ D. Does without any difficulty or advice.
    ____ E. Never did and would find quite difficult to start now.
    ____ F. Didn't do regularly but can do normally now with a little practice if they have to.

2. Making out insurance or Social Security forms, handling business affairs or papers, assembling tax records
    ____ A. Someone has recently taken over this activity completely or almost completely, and that someone did not used to do any or as much.
    ____ B. Requires more frequent advice or more assistance from others than in the past.
    ____ C. Does without any more advice or assistance than used to, but finds more difficult or does less good job than in the past.
    ____ D. Does without any difficulty or advice.
    ____ E. Never did and would find quite difficult to start now, even with practice.
    ____ F. Didn't do routinely, but can do normally now should they have to.

3. Shopping alone for clothes, household necessities and groceries
    ____ A. Someone has recently taken over this activity completely or almost completely.
    ____ B. Requires frequent advice or assistance from others.
    ____ C. Does without advice or assistance, but finds more difficult than used to or does less good job.
    ____ D. Does without any difficulty or advice.
    ____ E. Never did and would find quite difficult to start now.
    ____ F. Didn't do routinely but can do normally now should they have to.

4. Playing a game of skill such as bridge, other card games or chess or working on a hobby such as painting, photography, woodwork, stamp collecting
    ____ A. Hardly ever does now or has great difficulty.
    ____ B. Requires advice, or others have to make allowances.
    ____ C. Does without advice, or assistance, but more difficult or less skillful than used to be.
    ____ D. Does without any difficulty or advice.
    ____ E. Never did and would find quite difficult to start now.
    ____ F. Didn't do regularly, but can do normally now should they have to.

5. Heat the water, make a cup of coffee or tea, and turn off the stove
    ____ A. Someone else has recently taken over this activity completely, or almost completely.
    ____ B. Requires advice or has frequent problems (for example, burns pots, forgets to turn off stove).
    ____ C. Does without advice or assistance but occasional problems.
    ____ D. Does without any difficulty or advice.
    ____ E. Never did and would find quite difficult to start now.
    ____ F. Didn't usually, but can do normally now, should they have to.

6. Prepare a balanced meal (e.g., meat, chicken or fish, vegetables, dessert)
  ____ A. Someone else has recently taken over this activity completely or almost completely.
  ____ B. Requires frequent advice or has frequent problems (for example, burns pots, forgets how to make a given dish).
  ____ C. Does without much advice or assistance, but more difficult (for example, switched to TV dinners most of the time because of difficulty).
  ____ D. Does without any difficulty or advice.
  ____ E. Never did and would find quite difficult to do now even after a little practice.
  ____ F. Didn't do regularly, but can do normally now should they have to.

7. Keep track of current events, either in the neighborhood or nationally
  ____ A. Pays no attention to, or doesn't remember outside happenings.
  ____ B. Some idea about *major* events (for example, comments on presidential election, major events in the news or major sporting events).
  ____ C. Somewhat less attention to, or knowledge of, current events than formerly.
  ____ D. As aware of current events as ever was.
  ____ E. Never paid much attention to current events, and would find quite difficult to start now.
  ____ F. Never paid much attention, but can do as well as anyone now when they try.

8. Pay attention to, understand, and discuss the plot or theme of a one hour television program; get something out of a book or magazine
  ____ A. Doesn't remember, or seems confused by, what they have watched or read.
  ____ B. Aware of the *general idea,* characters, or nature while they watch or read, but may *not recall* later; may *not grasp theme* or have opinion about what they saw.
  ____ C. Less attention, or less memory than before, less likely to catch humor, points which are made quickly, or subtle points.
  ____ D. Grasps as quickly as ever.
  ____ E. Never paid much attention to or commented on T.V., never read much and would probably find very difficult to start now.
  ____ F. Never read or watch T.V. much, but read or watch as much as ever and get as much out of it as ever.

9. Remember appointments, plans, household tasks, car repairs, family occasions (such as birthdays or anniversaries), holidays, medications
  ____ A. Someone else has recently taken this over.
  ____ B. Has to be reminded some of the time (more than in the past or more than most people).
  ____ C. Manages without reminders but has to rely heavily on notes, calendars, schemes.
  ____ D. Remembers appointments, plans, occasions, etc. as well as they ever did.
  ____ E. Never had to keep track of appointments, medications or family occasions, and would probably find very difficult to start now.
  ____ F. Didn't have to keep track of these things in the past, but can do as well as anyone when they try.

10. Travel out of neighborhood; driving, walking, arranging to take or change buses and trains, planes
  ____ A. Someone else has taken this over completely or almost completely.
  ____ B. Can get around in own neighborhood but gets lost out of neighborhood.
  ____ C. Has more problems getting around than used to (for example, occasionally lost, loss of confidence, can't find car, etc.) but usually O.K.
  ____ D. Gets around as well as ever.
  ____ E. Rarely did much driving or had to get around alone and would find quite difficult to learn bus routes or make similar arrangements now.
  ____ F. Didn't have to get around alone much in past, but can do as well as ever when has to.

Reproduced from the Functional Activities Questionnaire provided by Dr. Robert I. Pfeffer. With permission.

by Pfeffer (1, Table 3). The validity coefficients obtained for the FAQ were consistently higher than those obtained for the IADL. The FAQ and the IADL were used in multiple regression analyses as predictors of mental status and functional assessments and the FAQ consistently performed better.

Comparing the FAQ to diagnoses made by attending neurologists, the sensitivity was 85% at a specificity of 81% (1). The FAQ was found to correlate 0.76 with a Mental Function Index developed by Pfeffer (2). Scores on the FAQ in a longitudinal study reflected both clinical judgments of change and cognitive measures in 54 elderly patients (2, Table 8). The FAQ also showed significant contrasts between normal, depressed and demented cases in a study of 195 respondents (3, Table 6).

Commentary

The Functional Activities Questionnaire is new, and the available validity results are promising. For the elderly population used in the validation study, the method seems clearly superior to Lawton and Brody's IADL, on which it builds. At the time of writing, validation studies of the expanded version of the scale are in progress. The method differs somewhat from other IADL scales in that the scale levels are defined primarily in terms of social function rather than physical capacities. This brings the scale close to some described in Chapter 5 on social health measurements.

Address

Robert I. Pfeffer, MD, Department of Neurology, California College of Medicine, University of California Irvine Medical Center, 101 City Drive South, Orange, California, USA 92668

References

(1) Pfeffer RI, Kurosaki TT, Harrah CH, Chance JM, Filos S. Measurement of functional activities in older adults in the community. J Gerontol 1982;37:323–329.
(2) Pfeffer RI, Kurosaki TT, Chance JM, Filos S, Bates D. Use of the Mental Function Index in older adults: reliability, validity, and measurement of change over time. Am J Epidemiol 1984;120:922–935.
(3) Pfeffer RI, Kurosaki TT, Harrah CH, Chance JM, Bates D, Detels R, Filos S, Butzke C. A survey diagnostic tool for senile dementia. Am J Epidemiol 1981;114:515–527.

THE OECD LONG-TERM DISABILITY QUESTIONNAIRE
(Organization for Economic Cooperation and Development [OECD], 1981)

Purpose

The OECD questionnaire is a survey instrument designed to summarize the impact of ill health on essential daily activities. It was intended to provide international comparisons of disability and to monitor changes in disability at a national level over time (1).

Conceptual Basis

In 1976, the OECD sponsored an international effort to develop various social and health indicators.* The health survey questionnaire was to measure disability in terms of limitations in activities essential to daily living: mobility, self-care and communication. The disruption of normal social acitivity was seen as the central theme (1).

Two aspects of disability were considered: short-term alterations in functional levels and such long-term restrictions as might arise from congenital anomalies. A person's current functional performance would reflect the presence of any long-term disability, overlaid by short-term fluctuations. Indicators of short-term disability already exist in the form of restricted activity or disability days. The OECD group considered these adequate and therefore devoted the questionnaire to measuring long-term disability among adults (2).

Description

Sixteen questions were written, ten of which can be used as an abbreviated instrument and represent a core set of items for international comparisons. They are shown in Exhibit 3.14. No time specification is attached to these ques-

*Participating countries included Canada, Finland, France, West Germany, The Netherlands, Switzerland, the United Kingdom and the United States.

Exhibit 3.14 The OECD Long-Term Disability Questionnaire

Note: The ten questions with an asterisk are included in the abbreviated version.

---

* 1. Is your eyesight good enough to read ordinary newspaper print? (with glasses if usually worn).
  2. Is your eyesight good enough to see the face of someone from 4 metres? (with glasses if usually worn).
  3. Can you hear what is said in a normal conversation with 3 or 4 other persons? (with hearing aid if you usually wear one).
* 4. Can you hear what is said in a normal conversation with one other person? (with hearing aid if you usually wear one).
* 5. Can you speak without difficulty?
* 6. Can you carry an object of 5 kilos for 10 metres?
  7. Could you run 100 metres?
* 8. Can you walk 400 metres without resting?
* 9. Can you walk up and down one flight of stairs without resting?
*10. Can you move between rooms?
*11. Can you get in and out of bed?
*12. Can you dress and undress?
 13. Can you cut your toenails?
 14. Can you (when standing), bend down and pick up a shoe from the floor?
*15. Can you cut your own food? (such as meat, fruit, etc.).
 16. Can you both bite and chew on hard foods? (for example, a firm apple or celery).

Reproduced from McWhinnie JR. Disability assessment in population surveys: results of the OECD common development effort. Rev Epidémiol Santé Publique 1981;29:417, Masson SA, Paris. With permission.

tions to signify long-term disability. Rather, the respondent is asked what she or he can usually do on a normal day, excluding any temporary difficulties. Four response categories were proposed: (1) yes, without difficulty; (2) yes, with minor difficulty; (3) yes, with major difficulty; (4) no, not able to. These were not strictly adhered to in the field trials and sometimes categories 2 and 3 were merged into "yes, with difficulty." A detailed presentation of the rationale for question selection and administration is given in the OECD report (2).

Reliability

Wilson and McNeil used 11 of the questions, slightly modified, in interviews with 223 respondents that were repeated after a two-week delay (3). It was not always possible to reinterview the original respondent, and in about half of the cases a proxy report was used. The agreement between first and second interviews was low, ranging from about 30% to 70% for the 11 items. Considering the scale as a whole, less than two thirds of those who reported disabilities on either interview reported them on both interviews. Analyses showed that the inconsistencies were not due to using proxy respondents (3).

A Dutch survey compared the responses to a self-administered version of the questionnaire (N = 940) with an interveiw version (N = 500). Although the two groups were very similar in age and sex, there was a systematic bias towards more disability being reported in the self-administered version: on average, 3.1% more people declared some level of disability in the written version (4, p466).

Validity

Twelve of the OECD questions were included in a Finnish national survey (N = 2,000). With the exception of people over 65 years of age, the great majority expressed no difficulty with any of the activities covered (5, Table 1). Similar findings were obtained in the United States and in the Netherlands (3, 4). In a Swiss study the questions were applied to 1,600 respondents aged 65 and over, and Raymond et al. reported sensitivity results for respondents suffering various types of medical complaint (6). Using the division between those reporting one or more limitations and those reporting none as a cutting point, sensitivity figures ranged from 61% to 85%; the specificity rate was 75.9% (6, p455). Sensitivity findings were highest for those with eyesight, hearing and speech problems.

In Canada, the OECD items were tested in interviews with 104 rehabilitation outpatients. Correlations between the questions concerned with physical movements and a physicians's rating of mobility ranged between 0.21 and 0.61 (7, Table II). Item-total correlations ranged from 0.54 down to 0.14.

Commentary

The OECD questionnaire represents one of the rare attempts to develop an internationally applicable set of disability items. As well as the studies cited here, the method has been used in France (8), Japan and West Germany. The questions continue to be used in Canadian surveys (9). Many of the items are similar to those included in questionnaires used by the Rand Corporation and the American Social Security Administration disability surveys.

Although the idea of an internationally standardized scale is commendable, it was not fully achieved. The studies cited all exhibit slight variations in the questions or answer categories; these are only partly attributable to inconsistencies in translation. In its design, the scale contains certain illogicalities: although it is intended to measure the behavioral consequences of disability, the questions use a capacity rather than a performance wording. The method is designed as a survey instrument, but the questions cover relatively severe levels of disability so that few people in the general adult population answer affirmatively; the questions seem most relevant to people over 65. The low test-retest reliability reported in the American study raises cause for concern; the authors suggested that the distinction between short- and long-term disability may not have been adequately explained to the respondents, who may have reported minor and transient difficulties, rather than long-term problems (3). We have the impression that the distinction between acute and chronic disability is very hard to draw, especially where a respondent has problems of both types that may interact. Perhaps the method would be more successful if this distinction were dropped. The imprecision of the instructions to the respondents also represents a weakness in this questionnaire.

The reliability and validity results are poor, probably less good than those of the Lambeth Screening Questionnaire. The OECD instrument is also narrower in scope than the Lambeth questionnaire, which covers employment and social activities as well as the ADL and IADL themes included in the OECD instrument.

Address

J.R. McWhinnie, Employment and Immigration Department, 140 Promenade du Portage, Hull, Quebec, Canada K1A OJ9

References

(1) McWhinnie JR. Disability assessment in population surveys: results of the OECD common development effort. Rev Epidémiol Santé Publique 1981;29:413–419.

(2) McWhinnie JR. Disability indicators for measuring well-being. Paris: OECD Social Indicators Programme, 1981.

(3) Wilson RW, McNeil JM. Preliminary analysis of OECD disability on the pretest of the post census disability survey. Rev Epidémiol Santé Publique 1981;29:469–475.

(4) Van Sonsbeek JLA. Applications aux Pays-Bas des questions de l'OCDE relatives à l'incapacité. Rev Epidémiol Santé Publique 1981;29:461–468.

(5) Klaukka T. Application of the OECD disability questions in Finland. Rev Epidémiol Santé Publique 1981;29:431–439.

(6) Raymond L, Christe E, Clemence A. Vers l'établissement d'un score global d'inca-

      pacité fonctionnelle sur la base des questions de l'OCDE, d'après une enquête en
      Suisse. Rev Epidémiol Santé Publique 1981;29:451–459.

(7) McDowell I. Screening for disability. An examination of the OECD survey ques-
      tions in a Canadian study. Rev Epidémiol Santé Publique 1981;29:421–429.

(8) Mizrahi A, Mizrahi A. Evaluation de l'état de santé de personnes âgées en France,
      à l'aide de plusieurs indicateurs, dont les questions de l'OCDE. Rev Epidémiol
      Santé Publique 1981;29:441–450.

(9) McDowell I, Praught E. Report of the Canadian health and disability survey, 1983–
      1984. Ottawa, Canada: Minister of Supply and Services, 1986. (Catalogue No.
      82–555E).

THE LAMBETH DISABILITY SCREENING QUESTIONNAIRE
(Donald L. Patrick and Others, 1981)

Purpose

This is a postal questionnaire designed to screen for physical disability in
adults living in the community. It provides estimates of the prevalence of disability intended for use in planning health and social services.

Conceptual Basis

Based on the impairment, disability and handicap triad, the disability questions concern mobility and self-care; they are phrased in terms of difficulty in
performing various activities rather than in terms of reduced capacity. The
questions on handicap cover housework, employment and social activities.

Description

Used in the first stage of the Lambeth Health Survey, the questionnaire was
designed to identify disabled people and to provide an estimate of the prevalence of disability in the general population. In a second stage of the survey,
the disabled persons identified by this screening instrument and nondisabled
controls were interviewed using a British version of the Sickness Impact Profile
called the Functional Limitations Profile (FLP). The data collected by the FLP
were used in validating the screening instrument described here.

    The instrument has been modified several times and published articles
report three different versions that will be referred to here as versions 1, 2 and
3. The first was used by Peach et al. and contains 31 questions (1). Twenty-five
of these were retained for the second version of the questionnaire, which was
used in the screening stage of the Lambeth Health Survey (see Exhibit 3.15).
During the subsequent stage of the survey (1980–1981) a third version of the
screening questionnaire was applied; this contains 22 items, 13 of which were
taken, unchanged, from the previous instrument, 2 were new, 2 were items
reintroduced from the first version, and 5 were reworded from the second version (3). The third version is shown in Exhibit 3.16. Although the questions
have been refined, the three versions all record difficulties with body move-

Exhibit 3.15 The Lambeth Disability Screening Questionnaire (Version 2)

The following questions apply to EVERYONE AGED 16 OR OVER living in this household. Please answer every question as well as you can, as shown in the examples below.

EXAMPLE 1 *(for when someone has difficulty)*

WHO has difficulty with any of the following?	The first names and ages of everyone having this difficulty are	No-one
Getting around the house without help	*John (65)* *Mary (56)*	

EXAMPLE 2 *(for when no-one has difficulty)*

WHO has difficulty with any of the following?	The first names and ages of everyone having this difficulty are	No-one
Getting around the house without help		✓

START HERE ➡

1. WHO has difficulty with any of the following?	The first names and ages of everyone having this difficulty are	No-one
a. Walking without help		
b. Getting outside the house without help		
c. Crossing the road without help		
d. Travelling on a bus or train without help		

2. WHO has difficulty with any of the following?	The first names and ages of everyone having this difficulty are	No-one
a. Getting in and out of bed or chair without help		
b. Dressing or undressing without help		
c. Kneeling or bending over without help		
d. Going up or down stairs without help		
e. Having a bath or all over wash without help		
f. Holding or gripping (for example a comb or a pen) without help		
g. Getting to and using the toilet without help		

Please continue on the back of this page

93

Exhibit 3.15 *(continued)*

3. WHO has any of the following problems?	The first names and ages of everyone having this difficulty are	No-one
a. Difficulty with spells of giddiness or fits		
b. Frequent falls		
c. Weakness or paralysis of arms or legs		
d. A stroke		
e. Difficulty seeing newspaper print even with glasses		
f. Difficulty recognizing people across the road even with glasses		
g. Hearing difficulties		
h. Loss of whole or *significant part* of an arm, hand, leg or foot		
i. Controlling bowels or bladder		

4. WHO is limited in doing any of the following BECAUSE OF ILLNESS OR DISABILITY?	The first names and ages of everyone having this difficulty are	No-one
a. Working at all		
b. Doing the job of their choice		
c. Doing housework		
d. Visiting family or friends		

Please continue on next page

ment, ambulation and mobility, self-care, social activity and sensory problems. The items were drawn from the questionnaires of Bennett and Garrad, of Haber and of Harris (4, 5). A section on impairments records the nature of the illnesses causing disability. There is also a section collecting household information. The questions shown in Exhibit 3.16 are scored 3 for "no difficulty," 2 for "difficulty that has lasted 2 weeks or less," and 1 for "difficulty that has lasted more than 2 weeks."

The second version (shown in Exhibit 3.15) is a self-report instrument that

5. *If you have written ANY names in Questions 1-4,* please tell us what their major illness or disability is?

First names and ages of anyone mentioned in Questions 1-4	Please describe their major illness or disability below

6. Does *anyone else* in your household have an illness or disability which affects their activities in any way?

First names and ages of anyone with illness or disability	What is the major illness or disability?	Please describe activity (e.g. playing sports, sewing, going to the pub)

Please continue on the back of this page

records information on all members of a household. Rather than collecting data from each individual, one respondent records information on all the adults living in his household. The respondent is asked to indicate the first name and age of each person who has any of the problems listed. The scoring system is as follows:

Respondents were classified as "disabled" if they reported difficulty with one or more of (a) the ambulation, mobility, body care, or movement items, except constipation or stress incontinence alone; (b) the sensory-motor items except giddiness when no associated illness condition was reported; and/or (c) the social activity items, except limitation in working at all or doing the job of choice where the respondent was over retirement age. (6, p66).

The third version is interviewer-administered and collects data on the respondent only. It uses a yes/no response format and scoring weights are available (3).

Exhibit 3.15 *(continued)*

ALL INFORMATION CONFIDENTIAL

Please complete below EVEN IF NO-ONE IS ILL OR DISABLED. We need this information to plan services for EVERYONE in Lambeth.

List Below EVERYONE, INCLUDING YOURSELF, living in this household.
Give the full name together with details for EVERYONE

1-5

6	NAME Write below Surname – Forename(s)	7 SEX Tick box Male (1) Female (2)	8-11 YEAR OF BIRTH Write Below	MARITAL STATUS Write below—Single, Married, Widowed, Divorced or Separated	12	13 CURRENTLY EMPLOYED? Tick box Yes(1) No(2)	14
0							
1							
2							
3							
4							
5							
6							
7							
8							
9							

15   16-18   19   20-21   22-27   80

SINCE WORK CAN AFFECT HEALTH, PLEASE COMPLETE FOR THE HEAD OF YOUR HOUSEHOLD ONLY
(Person with responsibility for supporting household or for rent/accommodation).

First Name and Age of HEAD OF HOUSEHOLD	What job does he/she do? (If Head is retired, unemployed, or not present, what was the job he/she held for most of his/her working life?)

Is (or was) the Head of the Household	☐ a manager working for an employer?	☐ a foreman or super-visor working for an employer?	☐ working for an employer?	☐ self-employed?
What qualifications, if any, were needed to obtain this job?				
What does the firm or organization do or make?				

WE APPRECIATE YOUR CO-OPERATION. THANK YOU.
Please check carefully that ALL questions on every page are answered.

Signature of person filling in form

Reproduced from Patrick DL, ed. Health and care of the physically disabled in Lambeth. Phase I report of The Longitudinal Disability Interview Survey. London: St Thomas's Hospital Medical School, Department of Community Medicine, 1981. With permission.

Exhibit 3.16 The Lambeth Disability Screening Questionnaire (Version 3)

Because of illness, accident or anything related to your health, do you have difficulty with any of the following? *Read out individually and code.*

    a. Walking without help
    b. Getting outside the house without help
    c. Crossing the road without help
    d. Travelling on a bus or train without help
    e. Getting in and out of bed or chair without help
    f. Dressing or undressing without help
    g. Kneeling or bending without help
    h. Going up or down stairs without help
    i. Having a bath or all over wash without help
    j. Holding or gripping (for example a comb or pen) without help
    k. Getting to and using the toilet without help
    l. Eating or drinking without help

Because of your health, do you have. . .

    m. Difficulty seeing newspaper print even with glasses
    n. Difficulty recognising people across the road even with glasses
    o. Difficulty in hearing a conversation even with a hearing aid
    p. Difficulty speaking

Because of your health, do you have difficulty. . .

    q. Preparing or cooking a hot meal without help
    r. Doing housework without help
    s. Visiting family or friends without help
    t. Doing any of your hobbies or spare time activities
    u. Doing paid work of any kind (if under 65)
    v. Doing paid work of your choice (if under 65)

Reproduced from Charlton JRH, Patrick DL, Peach H. Use of multivariate measures of disability in health surveys. J Epidemiol Community Health 1983;37:304. With permission.

Reliability

Sixty-eight people identified as disabled on the postal screening questionnaire were visited by an interviewer three to six months later. All were still classified as disabled in the follow-up interview, although there were discrepancies in replies to several individual items (1). No reliability information is available for versions 2 and 3 of the questionnaire.

Validity

Peach et al. showed low levels of agreement between self-ratings and ratings family physicians made of their patients. The low agreement was attributed primarily to the doctors' ignorance of the patients' disabilities (1).

In the Lambeth Health Survey, the version 2 screening questionnaire was followed by an interview survey of 892 respondents identified as disabled, and a comparison group of 346 nondisabled. The interval between the postal questionnaire and the interview ranged between 6 and 12 months (2). Comparison of the two assessments indicated a sensitivity of 87.7% and a specificity of 72.2% for the screening questionnaire (2, pp31–35). Because a change in health status may have occurred between the two assessments, these figures provide low estimates of the validity of the questionnaire.

Charlton et al. examined the concurrent validity of version 3 of the screening questionnaire by comparing it to the results of the Functional Limitations Profile (3). The 839 respondents were divided randomly into two groups. On 65% of these, regression analyses were used to assess how adequately the 22 screening questions predicted physical and psychosocial scores on the FLP. The predicted scores were then compared with the observed FLP results for the remaining 35% of the sample. The correlation of actual FLP scores and those predicted from the screening instrument was 0.79 for the physical and 0.50 for the psychosocial scales (3).

Commentary

The second version of the Lambeth questionnaire (Exhibit 3.15) is one of the very few validated postal screening instruments available. The method of using one person to record details about other family members is ingenious and apparently successful. The method is acceptable to respondents: after reminders a response rate of 86.6% was obtained in the Lambeth survey of 11,659 households. Of the remainder, only 5.2% refused, and 0.2% provided information too inadequate to analyze, while the rest could not be contacted (6). Locker et al. discussed methods for reducing the bias incurred in estimating prevalence due to nonresponse (5).

The authors of the screening instrument clearly have a considerable amount of data from which estimates of internal consistency and validity of each version could be derived. It is to be hoped that these results will be published, as at present we lack information on the reliability of the method. The questions are based on an established conceptual approach to disability, although the wording of the questions may not actually indicate performance as intended. Questions ask, "Do you have difficulty with . . . ?," a wording that seems to lie between performance and capacity: it does not tell us whether the person does or does not do the activity in question, or whether he cannot. Indeed, question phrasing is crucial: Patrick et al. attributed lower disability prevalence estimates obtained in previous surveys to their use of capacity question phrasing (6). This questionnaire is the best of the three survey methods that we review, although it should be more fully tested before being recommended for widespread use.

Address

Donald Patrick, PhD, MSPH, Department of Social and Administrative Medicine, Medical School, Wing D, Box 3, 208H, University of North Carolina, Chapel Hill, North Carolina, USA 27514

References

(1) Peach H, Green S, Locker D, Darby S, Patrick DL. Evaluation of a postal screening questionnaire to identify the physically disabled. Int Rehabil Med 1980;2: 189–193.

(2) Patrick DL, ed. Health and care of the physically disabled in Lambeth. Phase I report of The Longitudinal Disability Interview Survey. London: St Thomas's Hospital Medical School, Department of Community Medicine, 1981.

(3) Charlton JRH, Patrick DL, Peach H. Use of multivariate measures of disability in health surveys. J Epidemiol Community Health 1983;37:296–304.

(4) Patrick DL. Screening for disability in Lambeth: a progress report on health and care of the physically handicapped. London: St Thomas's Hospital Medical School, Department of Community Medicine, 1978.

(5) Locker D, Wiggins R, Sittampalam Y, Patrick DL. Estimating the prevalence of disability in the community: the influence of sample design and response bias. J Epidemiol Community Health 1981;35:208–212.

(6) Patrick DL, Darby SC, Green S, Horton G, Locker D, Wiggins RD. Screening for disability in the inner city. J Epidemiol Community Health 1981;35:65–70.

THE DISABILITY AND IMPAIRMENT INTERVIEW SCHEDULE
(A.E. Bennett and Jessie Garrad, 1970)

Purpose

This interview schedule was designed to measure the prevalence and severity of disability in epidemiological surveys; it also identifies associated impairment.

Conceptual Basis

The Disability and Impairment Interview Schedule follows the standard distinction between disability and impairment. Disability was defined as limitation of performance in "essential" activities of daily living, severe enough to entail dependence upon another person. Impairment was defined as an anatomical, pathological, or psychological disorder that may cause or be associated with disability (1).

Description

Bennett and Garrad's 1966 survey of the prevalence of disability in London, England, used a brief screening questionnaire that was followed by a 20-page interview schedule. The present review covers the disability section from the detailed schedule. Bennett has also described an 18-item and a 15-item disability screening questionnaire that are not reviewed here (2).

The schedule shown in Exhibit 3.17 is administered by interviewers trained to probe to identify actual levels of performance. The questions use performance rather than capacity wording, and the highest level of performance is recorded. If an answer falls between two defined levels, the less severe grade of limitation is recorded. Recognizing that there are reasons other than disability why people may not perform an activity, allowances are made in scoring the schedule, an example being men who do not perform domestic duties (1, 2). Details of the scoring system are not clear, although separate scores are provided for each topic, rather than a single score, which "masks different levels

Exhibit 3.17 The Disability and Impairment Interview Schedule. Section 1—Disability

SECTION I

MOBILITY

Walking Do you walk outdoors in the street (with crutch or stick if used)?

If 'Yes': one mile or more	☐	If 'No':		and:	
¼ mile	☐	Between rooms	☐•	Unaccompanied	☐
100 yds.	☐•	Within room	☐•	Accompanied	☐•
10 yds.	☐•	Unable to walk	☐•	Acc. + support	☐•

Stairs

Do you walk up stairs?

To 1st floor or above	☐	Unacc.	☐
5-8 steps or stairs	☐•	Acc.	☐•
2-4 steps or stairs	☐•	Acc. & Supp.	☐•
1 step	☐•	No need to mount stairs	☐
mount stairs other than by walking	☐•		
unable to mount stairs	☐•		

Do you walk down stairs?

From 1 floor to another	☐	Unacc.	☐
5-8 steps or stairs	☐•	Acc.	☐•
2-4 steps or stairs	☐•	Acc. & Supp.	☐•
1 step	☐•	No need to descend stairs	☐
goes down stairs other than by walking	☐•		
unable to descend stairs	☐•		

Transfer

	Yes	No		Yes	No
Do you need help to get into bed?	☐•	☐	Do you need help to sit down in a chair?	☐•	☐
Do you need help to get out of bed?	☐•	☐	Do you need help to stand up from a chair?	☐•	☐
Bedfast	☐•		Not applicable		☐

Travel

Do you drive yourself in a car?

Normal (unadapt.)	☐
Adapted	☐
Invacar	☐•
Self-propelled vehicle (outdoors)	☐•
Does not drive	☐

Do you travel by bus or train?

If 'Yes':		If 'No':	
Whenever necessary	☐	Unable to use bus and train	☐•
Only out of rush hour	☐•	Unable to use bus, train and car	☐•
and:			
Unaccompanied	☐	Does not travel by choice	☐
Accompanied	☐•	Uses private transport by choice	☐

Reproduced from an original obtained from Dr. A.E. Bennett. With permission.

SELF CARE

Are you able to feed yourself:	Are you able to dress yourself completely:	Are you able to undress yourself completely:	Are you able to use the lavatory:	Are you able to wash yourself:
Without any help ☐	Without any help ☐	Without any help ☐	Without any help ☐	Without any help ☐
With specially prepared food or containers ☐*	With help with fastenings ☐*	With help with fastenings ☐*	Receptacles without assistance ☐*	With assistance for shaving, combing hair, etc. ☐*
With assistance ☐*	With help other than fastenings ☐*	With help other than fastenings ☐*	Lavatory with assistance ☐*	With help for bodily washing ☐*
Not at all, must be fed ☐*	Does not dress ☐*	Not applicable ☐*	Receptacles with assistance ☐*	Not at all ☐*

DOMESTIC DUTIES

Do you do your own:

	all	part	none		preference	unable
Shopping	☐	☐	☐		☐	☐*
Cooking	☐	☐	☐		☐	☐*
Cleaning	☐	☐	☐		☐	☐*
Clothes washing	☐	☐	☐		☐	☐*
Men with no household duties	☐					

OCCUPATION

Do you have a paid job at present?

If 'Yes':		and:		If 'No':			
Full-time	☐	Normal working	☐	Males 65 Females 60 and over	Age retired	☐	
					Prem. retired	☐*	
Part-time	☐	Modified working	☐*		Non-employed	☐	
		Sheltered employment	☐*	Males 64 Females 59 and under	Unemployed	☐	
					Unfit	☐*	
					Non-employed	☐	

CROSS IN ANY BOX MARKED WITH AN ASTERISK INDICATES PRESENCE OF DISABILITY

of performance in different areas, results in loss of information, and can be misleading" (1, p101). Copies of the full schedule may be available at cost from Jessie van Dongen-Garrad.

The questionnaire discussed here was applied to a sample of 571 respondents aged 35 to 74 years, drawn from those identified as disabled and/or impaired by the screening questionnaire. The study sought primarily to provide information relevant to the planning of health and welfare services (2).

Reliability

Complete agreement was obtained on test-retest ratings for 80% of 153 subjects after a 12-month delay (1, p103). For 28 of the 31 respondents exhibiting some change on the questionnaire, medical records corroborated that there had been a change in impairment or disability status.

Guttman analyses of the questions gave a coefficient of reproducibility of 0.95 and a coefficient of scalability of 0.69 for females and 0.71 for males (4, p73). There were slight differences in the ordering of items in scales derived for males and for females (5, Tables I to III).

Validity

Data from medical and social work records of 52 outpatients were compared with information obtained with the interview schedule. The clinical records listed disability in a total of 118 areas, of which 108 (91.5%) were reflected in the interview schedule (1, p102).

Commentary

This survey method appears to provide data of similar quality to those of the OECD method. The format of the questionnaire is clear, but the method is old and there are no good studies of reliability and validity. Because of these limitations we would recommend using one of the other two screening instruments in preference.

Address

Jessie van Dongen-Garrad, Johan Wagenaarkade 38, 3533 TE Utrecht, The Netherlands

References

(1) Garrad J, Bennett AE. A validated interview schedule for use in population surveys of chronic disease and disability. Br J Prev Soc Med 1971;25:97–104.
(2) Bennett AE, Garrad J, Halil T. Chronic disease and disability in the community: a prevalence study. Br Med J 1970;3:762–764.
(3) Bennett AE, Ritchie K. Questionnaires in medicine: a guide to their design and use. London: Oxford University Press, 1975.
(4) Williams RGA, Johnston M, Willis LA, Bennett AE. Disability: a model and measurement technique. Br J Prev Soc Med 1976;30:71–78.
(5) St Thomas's health survey in Lambeth: disability survey. London: St Thomas's Hospital Medical School, Department of Clinical Epidemiology and Social Medicine, 1971.

CONCLUSION: IADL SCALES

The IADL scales reviewd in this section represent a bridge between the traditional, physical measurements represented by ADL scales and other indices such as social functioning scales. The broader approach of the IADL instruments is increasingly supplanting the older ADL methods, and it is clear that they have been more thoroughly tested and are more sensitive to minor variations in a patient's condition.

We criticized the ADL scales on several grounds: most were developed in relative isolation from other methods, and few were founded on a clear conceptual basis or critique of earlier work. The IADL scales show some signs of overcoming these weaknesses, although little work has yet been done to establish the formal correspondence among the various measurements, with the exception of the work of Jette. We regard research that compares different scales as a crucial stage in consolidating the discipline of measurement; this has been achieved in some fields such as that of psychological well-being (Chapter 4), but not yet in the field of functional disability measurement.

From our review of the IADL scales, however, several themes emerge. The content of the IADL scales stresses the patient's functioning within his particular environment, more closely reflecting handicap than impairment or disability. This theme is picked up and expanded in the indicators of social health, many of which define social health in terms of the ability to perform one's normal social roles. Perhaps because these topics require greater reliance on subjective data collected by self-report than do the more traditional indicators of physical functioning, more attention has been paid to establishing the validity and reliability of IADL scales than is the case with the older ADL methods. Because they are sensitive to lower levels of disablement, the IADL scales are more suited to use as survey methods for general population studies. It is also plausible that the IADL approach will come to rival, and perhaps replace, the traditional ADL scales in clinical studies. In their turn, the IADL scales may come to be replaced by the broader-ranging general measurement methods described in Chapter 8. There is no essential distinction between the IADL scales described above and the IADL component of several of the general health measurements covered in Chapter 8.

4
Psychological Well-Being

Of all the chapters in this book, the scope of the present one on psychological measurements has proved the most difficult to delimit. Unlike other fields of health measurement, the problem here is the embarrassment of riches: there are many well-tested measurements and it was not easy to set criteria for what should be included. It would be possible to fill an entire book with measurements of psychological morbidity: anxiety scales, depression inventories and psychiatric ratings. These we have not covered. Methods designed for assessing severe levels of mental or psychiatric disorder have also been omitted, as have scales that would only be used in clinical settings. In addition, there are many instruments that measure psychological health, or "subjective well-being," a theme commonly measured in surveys. There are large numbers of such instruments and our review cannot be exhaustive. We found it convenient to base our selection, and the way we have grouped psychological measurement scales in the book, on a classification of measurement methods proposed by Campbell (1). This noted that early measurements of psychological well-being viewed it largely as a cognitive process in which the individual compared his aspirations to his perception of his current situation: well-being was seen in terms of life satisfaction (1). Measurements of this first type are covered in Chapter 6, on life satisfaction and quality of life. A second category of well-being scales has recorded affective responses to experience—the feeling states inspired by daily experience. We include one example of this approach in the present chapter, represented by Bradburn's scale. A third approach to measuring psychological well-being is via questions that screen for psychological distress. This reflects a somewhat more clinical orientation, although the scales stop short of making diagnostic classifications; instead they screen for signs of general psychological distress. Psychological well-being would then be measured by exclusion, being inferred from the absence of symptoms of distress. The measurements reviewed in this chapter cover short-term psychological states rather than lasting traits, and describe human psychological responses in adapting to the environment, in a manner analogous to Selye's concept of stress, which covered the physiological process of adaptation.

There have been many attempts to clarify what is being measured—to distinguish, for example, between "distress" and "disorder," and between "psychological," "emotional" and "mental" well-being. The attempts have not always been successful, and the development of this field has been checkered by disputes over the intent and conceptual interpretation of the scales. Unfortunately, this was exacerbated by the tendency, in the earlier scales at least, for the author not to clarify conceptually what he was attempting to measure. Many of the earlier scales were developed empirically, by selecting questions that distinguished between well and emotionally distressed persons. This approach to constructing indices led to considerable dispute over the correct way to interpret the measurement, as seen with Langner's 22-item scale. The same set of questions has been said to indicate "mental health," "emotional adjustment," "psychological disturbance or disorder," "psychiatric or psychological symptoms," "mental illness," and has even been considered a "psychiatric case identification instrument." This disagreement indicates the disadvantage of the empirical approach, but it also reflects the complexity and uncertainty of establishing firm conceptual definitions—an uncertainty that we will witness again in Chapter 6 on life satisfaction and quality of life. Dohrenwend et al. have commented on this unhappy state of affairs in interpreting indicators of "non-specific psychological distress":

> As might be expected given the actuarial procedures and undifferentiated patient criterion groups used to construct them, none of the screening scales reflects a clearly specified conceptual domain. Thus, there is no ready correspondence between the content of the scales and conceptions of major dimensions or types of psychopathology such as mania, depression, hallucinations, or antisocial behavior. (2, p1229).

Dohrenwend also suggested that these scales provide general indications of distress, somewhat analogous to the measurement of body temperature in physical diagnosis: elevated scores tell you that something is wrong, but not what is wrong. In this chapter we refer to distress rather than disorder, and we use the broad term "psychological" to connote the relatively general level of discussion, which at times refers to mental and at times to emotional problems.

Perhaps because of these complexities, considerable attention has been paid to testing the validity of these methods—a far more active concern than exists in measurements of, say, physical disability. In many cases this critical attention has resulted in scales of very high quality, but there have been examples in which the critical interest in a scale has backfired. This most commonly occurs where a clear conceptual explanation of the purpose is lacking; this can have the unfortunate effect of encouraging critics to make piecemeal and uncoordinated modifications to scales. The most extreme case is Macmillan's Health Opinion Survey for which Exhibit 4.2 compares seven different, but widely used, versions. To add to the confusion, these versions all bear the same name. This problem is most acute with the older scales; the more recent methods reviewed in this chapter have somewhat clearer explanations of their purpose.

DESIGN OF PSYCHOLOGICAL INDICES

Two approaches have been used in constructing the measurements reviewed in this chapter: symptom checklists that include behavioral and somatic symptoms of distress, and questions that ask directly about positive and negative feelings of well-being. The common arguments in support of the symptom checklist hold that it is more objective and more adequately conceals the intent of the measurement; this is deemed necessary as respondents are expected to be reticent about reporting their true feelings. Indeed, it has been estimated that under-reporting of emotional problems in surveys may be as high as 60% (3). Thus, for example, Macmillan deliberately named his screening scale the "Health Opinion Survey" and designed it as a symptom checklist to obscure its intent. Conversely, symptom checklists almost certainly classify some physical disorders as psychological; they can also only detect more severe forms of disorder and they cannot identify emotional distress unless it is manifested somatically or behaviorally. Against these criticisms one must set the results of many validation studies that show that the symptom checklists can give high sensitivity and specificity rates when compared with psychiatric ratings. More recently, the argument that people will not respond honestly to direct questions about their emotional well-being has passed somewhat from favor. Influenced by the criticisms of the symptom checklist approach and by the growing awareness in the later 1950s of the potential accuracy of subjective reports, Gurin, and later Bradburn, led a movement towards surveying feelings of happiness and emotional well-being. This trend also reflected the theme of positive mental health, a concept that may be traced back, through Jahoda's work (5), to the WHO conception of health. The extensive recent work on social support, on coping and on health promotion emphasizes the need for questions on well-being as well as on symptoms of distress.

Later work suggested that the reaction against the symptom checklist approach may have been too strong, for they do succeed in detecting mental disorders even though, as Dohrenwend noted, they do not provide diagnostic information. Thus, the trend from symptom checklists towards direct questions on feelings has many of the characteristics of a dialectical process, and more recent methods represent a synthesis of the two approaches. Scales such as those developed by Dupuy and by Goldberg have combined the symptom checklist and questionnaire approaches to form a hybrid, a trend that marks the convergence of the screening methods of Langner and Macmillan with quality of life and life satisfaction scales. Perhaps these scales will offer the best of both worlds, and the coming years may see more use of them in studies of the protective impact of "positive mental health" (for example, in preventing cancer) and of the epidemiology of "wellness" in general. Questions on feelings are necessary to tap the positive end of the mental health spectrum, as they can be phrased to differentiate levels of health among asymptomatic individuals.

Several of the scales we review share questions in common. First, most of the symptom checklists originally drew items from the Army's neuropsychiatric screening instrument (4). This contained symptoms of adverse reactions to stressful situations, selected empirically as being capable of identifying recruits who subsequently performed poorly in military combat. Although these questions were originally designed for use with healthy, young adult males, they were adapted by Macmillan, and later by Langner, for more widespread use in community surveys, forming the first generation of psychological well-being scales. Despite widespread criticism of these scales, they still see occasional use: Langner's questions, for example, are quite frequently used in studies of the impact of life events, stress and social support on emotional health. We have reviewed the Macmillan and Langner scales for this reason and to provide a historical introduction to the field. More recent scales also share items in common: the Rand Mental Health Inventory incorporates many of Dupuy's questions from the General Well-Being Schedule, and these bear a strong family resemblance to items in Goldberg's General Health Questionnaire.

This chapter reviews six scales. All are suited for use in population surveys. The first two methods, the Health Opinion Survey and Langner's scale, are brief screening scales that use the symptom checklist approach. They do not cover positive well-being, which is a feature of the third method we review, Bradburn's Affect Balance Scale. This ten-item scale covers positive and negative emotional reactions to the stresses of daily living. The General Well-Being Schedule and the Mental Health Inventory that follow also cover both positive and negative feelings; they are somewhat longer scales (18 and 38 items) and are considerably newer. They also group their items more clearly into clinically definable symptom areas: anxiety, depression and so forth. This more clinical orientation is then pursued in Goldberg's General Health Questionnaire, the final scale in the chapter. This method is explicitly designed to detect acute, psychiatrically diagnosable disorders in population studies, and has seen widespread use in many parts of the world.

References

(1) Campbell A. Subjective measures of well-being. Am Psychol 1976;31:117–124.
(2) Dohrenwend BP, Shrout PE, Egri G, Mendelsohn FS. Nonspecific psychological distress and other dimensions of psychopathology. Arch Gen Psychiatry 1980; 37:1229–1236.
(3) United States Department of Health, Education and Welfare. Net differences in interview data on chronic conditions and information derived from medical records. Washington, DC: Government Printing Office, DHEW Publication No. (HSM)73-1331, 1973. (Vital and Health Statistics, Series 2, No. 57).
(4) Stouffer SA, Guttman L, Suchman EA, Lazarsfeld, PF, Star SA, Clausen JA. Measurement and prediction. Studies in social psychology in World War II. Volume IV. Princeton, New Jersey: Princeton University Press, 1950.
(5) Jahoda M. Current concepts of positive mental health. New York: Basic Books, 1958.

Table 4.1 Comparison of the Quality of Psychological Indices*

Measurement	Scale	Number of items	Application	Administered by (time)	Studies using method	Reliability		Validity	
						Testing thoroughness	Results	Testing thoroughness	Results
Health Opinion Survey (Macmillan)	ordinal	20	survey	self	many	+++	++	+++	++
Twenty-Two Item Screening Score of Psychiatric Symptoms (Langner)	ordinal	22	survey	self (5 min)	many	++	++	+++	+++
Affect Balance Scale (Bradburn)	ordinal	10	survey	self (few min)	many	++	++	++	++
General Well-Being Schedule (Dupuy)	ordinal	18	survey	self (10 min)	several	+++	+++	+++	++
Mental Health Inventory (Rand)	ordinal	38	survey	self	few	++	++	++	++
General Health Questionnaire (Goldberg)	ordinal	60	survey	self (6–8 min)	many	++	+++	+++	+++

*For an explanation of the categories used, see Chapter 1, pages 8–9.

THE HEALTH OPINION SURVEY
(Allister M. Macmillan; First Used in 1951, Published in 1957)

Purpose

Macmillan developed the Health Opinion Survey (HOS) as a "psychological screening test for adults in rural communities" (1). It was designed to identify "psychoneurotic and related types of disorder." Subsequently the HOS has been widely used in epidemiological studies, in estimating need for psychiatric services and in evaluating their impact.

Conceptual Basis

No information is available. Macmillan used the title "Health Opinion Survey" to disguise the purpose of the scale and to make respondents less reticent in reporting emotional problems (1, 2).

Description

The HOS comprises 20 items that were found to discriminate between 78 diagnosed neurotic cases and 559 community respondents in a pilot study in Nova Scotia, Canada (1, 3). The 20 items are shown in Exhibit 4.1 (1).

More than is the case with other instruments, the HOS has frequently been modified by those who have used it. Indeed, the original 20 items shown above were altered during the course of the studies in which Macmillan participated. Seven questions were deleted and replaced by questions on other topics, and nine were reworded. Subsequent users have not adhered strictly to either version; we present a comparison of the main variants in Exhibit 4.2, which gives Macmillan's original question topics and shows the variations made to his wording. This means that extreme caution is needed in interpreting results obtained with the scale, as it is seldom clear which version was used. Unfortunately, neither the results of the validation studies reported below nor the cutting points selected to distinguish sick from well respondents, will be strictly comparable among different studies.

The HOS may be self- or interviewer-administered. A three-point answer scale ("often," "sometimes," "hardly ever or never") was used originally; other versions have employed four- or five-point scales. Macmillan proposed a scoring system by which the questions may be weighted to maximally discriminate between neurotic and healthy respondents (1). Other users have reported high correlations between weighted and unweighted scores; the advantage of weighted scores seems slight (4). Macmillan suggested a cutting point of 60.0 for the weighted scoring system to distinguish between neurotic and non-neurotic populations; for the non-weighted score, 29.5 was optimal (4, p244).

Reliability

Leighton et al. reported a test-retest correlation of 0.87 "after a few weeks or months" (3, p208). Tousignant et al. obtained a coefficient of 0.78 for 387

Exhibit 4.1 The Original Version of the Health Opinion Survey

Note: The questions are not presented in the order as asked in the interview, but in decreasing rank order of their derived weights.

1. Do you have loss of appetite?
2. How often are you bothered by having an upset stomach?
3. Has any ill health affected the amount of work you do?
4. Have you ever felt that you were going to have a nervous breakdown?
5. Are you ever troubled by your hands sweating so that they feel damp and clammy?
6. Do you feel that you are bothered by all sorts (different kinds) of ailments in different parts of your body?
7. Do you ever have any trouble in getting to sleep and staying asleep?
8. Do your hands ever tremble enough to bother you?
9. Do you have any particular physical or health trouble?
10. Do you ever take weak turns?
11. Are you ever bothered by having nightmares? (Dreams that frighten or upset you very much?)
12. Do you smoke a lot?
13. Have you ever had spells of dizziness?
14. Have you ever been bothered by your heart beating hard?
15. Do you tend to lose weight when you have important things bothering you?
16. Are you ever bothered by nervousness?
17. Have you ever been bothered by shortness of breath when you were not exercising or working hard?
18. Do you tend to feel tired in the mornings?
19. For the most part, do you feel healthy enough to carry out the things that you would like to do?
20. Have you ever been troubled by "cold sweats"? (NOT a hot-sweat—you feel a chill, but you are sweating at the same time.)

Reproduced from Macmillan, AM. The Health Opinion Survey: technique for estimating prevalence of psychoneurotic and related types of disorder in communities. *Psychological Reports,* 1957, 3, 325–329, Table 1.

respondents after a ten-month delay (4, p243). Schwab et al. showed a high degree of stability between surveys in 1970 and 1973 for 517 respondents (5). There was no difference in the mean scores at the two times: 53.4% of the variance in 1973 scores was attributable to the 1970 score. When classified into normal and abnormal scores, 81.5% of respondents did not change their classification between the two surveys (5, p183).

Butler and Jones reported item-total correlations ranging from 0.20 to 0.62; the coefficient alpha for their 18-item version of the questionnaire was 0.84 (6, p557). Tousignant et al. reported item-total correlations ranging from 0.21 to 0.60 (4, p244).

Validity

There are many validation studies of the variants of the HOS and our review cannot be exhaustive. Macmillan reported a sensitivity of 92% (at a cutting point of 60.0 for the weighted scoring system), and specificity levels ranging from 75% to 88% according to the socioeconomic status of the presumed healthy population (1, p332). Leighton et al. reported correlations between clinical judgments of psychiatric status and the HOS, ranging from 0.37 to 0.57

Exhibit 4.2 Main Variants of the Health Opinion Survey

Note: A blank indicates that the question was omitted, " = " indicates identical wording, "V" indicates a minor variation in wording, "R" indicates the question was reworded.

Macmillan No. of items:	Leighton 20	Denis 18	Butler 18	Gunderson 20	Spiro 13	Gurin 20	Schwartz 20
1. Loss of appetite	R	=	R	R	R	=	=
2. Upset stomach	=	R	=	=	=	=	R
3. Ill health affected work		R	=	=	R	=	=
4. Nervous breakdown	V				=	=	=
5. Hands sweating	R	R	R	R	R	R	R
6. Bothered by ailments	V	=	R	R	R	R	R
7. Trouble sleeping	R	R	R	R	R	R	R
8. Hands tremble	=	R	=	=		=	=
9. Particular health trouble	R	R		R		R	R
10. Weak turns		R	R	R			
11. Nightmares	V	R	R	R		R	R
12. Smoke	R		R	R			
13. Spells of dizziness		R	R	R		=	=
14. Heart beating hard	=	=	=	=	R	=	=
15. Lose weight		R	R	R		V	V
16. Bothered by nervousness					R	R	R
17. Shortness of breath		R	R	R	R	=	=
18. Tired in mornings	=	=	=	V	R	R	R
19. Feel healthy enough		=	=	V	R	=	V
20. "Cold sweats"	V		V	V	R		

(3, pp208–210). The HOS discriminated adequately between the extremes of well and psychiatrically sick, but less adequately at intermediate stages of psychological distress (3).

Tousignant et al. administered the HOS to 88 psychiatric patients and to 88 matched community controls (4). All HOS items discriminated at $p < 0.001$; the sensitivity was 80.7%. A cutting point of 29.5 identified as sick 90% of the neurotic patients in the study, all the alcoholics, 70% of the 13 schizophrenics, 71% of 45 psychotics but only 30% of manic depressives (7, p391). Gunderson et al. evaluated the ability of the HOS to classify over 4,000 Navy personnel into the categories "fit" and "not fit for duty" (2). Thirteen items showed significant differences between the groups. Spiro et al. compared a sample of auto workers or their spouses who were receiving therapy for a psychiatric disorder with 888 undiagnosed workers and spouses. Eleven HOS questions were found to discriminate at the 0.001 level (8). Four questions were included in a discriminant function that provided a sensitivity of 63% and a specificity of 89% (8, p111). Whereas Macmillan's patients were hospitalized, none in Spiro's study was, and this may account for the lower sensitivity level.

Macmillan compared the HOS scores with the judgment of a psychiatrist; for 64 respondents he reported a 14% disagreement (1, p335). However, the disagreement may be much higher according to how the substantial number of cases rated "uncertain" by the psychiatrist are classified (4).

Tousignant et al. showed that replies to the HOS were associated with use of medications, psychological symptoms, reports of behavioral disturbances, and judgments of disorder made by interviewers (4, Table 3). Denis et al. showed highly significant variations in HOS scores by age, sex, occupation, marital status, education, income, language and geographical location (7). Butler and Jones obtained significant correlations with estimates of role conflict, family strain and frequency of illness (6). Schwartz et al. correlated the HOS with the New Haven Schizophrenia Index ($r = 0.39$) and with the Psychiatric Evaluation Form ($r = 0.55$) (9, p268). The HOS was found to cover neurotic traits only; it did not cover the range of psychotic symptoms exhibited by schizophrenics.

Three factor analyses have identified factors that were interpreted as representing physical and psychological problems (6, 8, 10). There was, however, no clear correspondence between the factor placement of those questions common to the three studies.

Alternative Forms

In addition to the variants noted above, Murphy used a questionnaire that included certain of the HOS items in a study in Vietnam (11). A French version was used in the Stirling County studies (3) and in Quebec by Tousignant et al. (4, 7).

Commentary

The HOS was extensively used during the 1960s and 1970s, including cross-cultural studies in Africa and North America (12, 13). There have also been a wide variety of validation studies and there is considerable evidence that it succeeds in its purpose as a screening test for neurotic disorders. Nonetheless, few would now recommend that the scale be used and, for the purposes of our review, there are several lessons to be learned from the history of the HOS.

The first comment illustrates our theme that indices should have a clear conceptual basis. Although the HOS can distinguish between neurotic patients and people without psychiatric diagnoses, it is not clear what a high score actually indicates: mental disorder or normal reactions to stress? Dohrenwend and

Dohrenwend suggested that the symptoms covered in indices such as the HOS may reflect normal processes of responding to temporary stressors, rather than neurotic disorders (14). Butler and Jones, indeed, commented that "continued use of the HOS and related mental health indices appears to offer greater potential if they are approached more as stress indicators than as general indices of mental health" (6). Empirically, however, the high test-retest reliability results obtained by Tousignant, Schwab and by Leighton suggest that the HOS is measuring a comparatively stable construct rather than a transient state.

Our second comment is that the empirical way in which the HOS was developed has further compounded the interpretation problem. The tactic of using physical symptoms to disguise the intent of the scale causes interpretation problems and may not have worked anyway: Tousignant et al. reported correlations between the HOS and a "lie scale" that indicated a tendency to avoid admitting to socially undesirable attributes (4, 7).* The studies that showed separate physical and psychological factors suggest that the HOS may reflect purely physical complaints as well as psychosomatic problems. Wells and Strickland have studied this bias and have suggested an approach to remove it from the scale (15). The unfortunate history of the development of so many versions of the HOS illustrates the confusion that can arise when health indices are modified piecemeal and without clear conceptual guidelines to define their content. Other more recent scales seem to have avoided this pitfall.

Ultimately, history may condemn the HOS, not because it does not work, but for reasons that relate to the uncertainty of exactly why it works and of how it should be interpreted. The problems with the HOS highlight the need for measurement methods to be founded on a secure conceptual basis that explains what they measure and how they should be interpreted. We cannot recommend further use of HOS for these reasons and because other scales, such as those of Goldberg and Dupuy, offer better alternatives.

Address

Alexander H. Leighton, MD, Department of Preventive Medicine, Faculty of Medicine, Dalhousie University, Halifax, Nova Scotia, Canada B3H 4H7

References

(1) Macmillan AM. The Health Opinion Survey: technique for estimating prevalence of psychoneurotic and related types of disorder in communities. Psychol Rep 1957;3:325–339.
(2) Gunderson EKE, Arthur RJ, Wilkins WL. A mental health survey instrument: the Health Opinion Survey. Milit Med 1968;133:306–311.

*On a humorous note, the principle of trying to obscure the intent of a question was carried to its logical conclusion in the No-Nonsense Personality Inventory (a spoof on the MMPI). Concealed among items such as "Sometimes I find it hard to conceal the fact that I am not angry," or "Weeping brings tears to my eyes" is question 69. Question 69 is entirely blank. In: Scherr GH, ed. The best of the Journal of Irreproducible Results. New York: Workman Publishing, 1983.

(3) Leighton DC, Harding JS, Macklin DB, Macmillan AM, Leighton AH. The character of danger: psychiatric symptoms in selected communities. Vol. III. New York: Basic Books, 1963.

(4) Tousignant M, Denis G, Lachapelle R. Some considerations concerning the validity and use of the Health Opinion Survey. J Health Soc Behav 1974;15:241–252.

(5) Schwab JJ, Bell RA, Warheit GJ, Schwab RB. Social order and mental health: the Florida Health Study. New York: Brunner/Mazel, 1979.

(6) Butler MC, Jones AP. The Health Opinion Survey reconsidered: dimensionality, reliability, and validity. J Clin Psychol 1979;35:554–559.

(7) Denis G, Tousignant M, Laforest L. Prévalence de cas d'intérêt psychiatrique dans une région du Québec. Can J Public Health 1973;64:387–397.

(8) Spiro HR, Siassi I, Crocetti GM. What gets surveyed in a psychiatric survey? A case study of the Macmillan index. J Nerv Ment Dis 1972;154:105–114.

(9) Schwartz CC, Myers JK, Astrachan BM. Comparing three measures of mental status: a note on the validity of estimates of psychological disorder in the community. J Health Soc Behav 1973;14:265–273.

(10) Gurin G, Veroff J, Feld S. Americans view their mental health: a nationwide interview survey. New York: Basic Books, 1960.

(11) Murphy JM. War stress and civilian Vietnamese: a study of psychological effects. Acta Psychiatr Scand 1977;56:92–108.

(12) Beiser M, Benfari RC, Collomb H, Ravel J-L. Measuring psychoneurotic behavior in cross-cultural surveys. J Nerv Ment Dis 1976;163:10–23.

(13) Jegede RO. Psychometric characteristics of the Health Opinion Survey. Psychol Rep 1977;40:1160–1162.

(14) Dohrenwend BP, Dohrenwend BS. The problem of validity in field studies of psychological disorder. J Abnorm Psychol 1965;70:52–69.

(15) Wells JA, Strickland DE. Physiogenic bias as invalidity in psychiatric symptom scales. J Health Soc Behav 1982;23:235–252.

THE TWENTY-TWO ITEM SCREENING SCORE OF PSYCHIATRIC SYMPTOMS
(Thomas S. Langner, 1962)

Purpose

The 22-item scale is a screening method to provide a "rough indication of where people lie on a continuum of impairment in life functioning due to very common types of psychiatric symptoms" (1, p269). The scale is intended to identify mental illness, but not to specify its type or degree; nor does it detect organic brain damage, mental retardation, or sociopathic traits (1).

Conceptual Basis

No information is available.

Description

The items were taken mainly from the United States Army's Neuropsychiatric Screening Adjunct and from the Minnesota Multiphasic Personality Inventory and was developed for the Midtown Manhattan Study of the social context of

mental disorder (2). Of 120 items originally tested, 22 were found to discriminate most adequately between "known well" people (as classified by a psychiatrist) and a group of psychiatric patients.

The scale consists of 22 closed-ended questions that cover somatic symptoms of anxiety, depression and other neurotic disturbances, and also records
subjective judgments of emotional states (3). Fabrega and McBee (4) and
Muller (5) concluded that the score assesses mild neurotic and psychosomatic
symptoms. In Langner's original work the questionnaire was administered by
an interviewer; self-completed (6, 7) and telephone versions (8, 9) have also
been used. The self-administered version requires few instructions and takes
less than five minutes to complete.

The items and response categories are shown in Exhibit 4.3. The score consists of the total number of responses that indicate sickness, termed "pathognomonic responses," designated by asterisks in the exhibit. Differential weights
were not used in the original. Haese and Meile proposed a scoring system that
provided a different weight for each item based on the conditional probability
of having a particular diagnosis with a certain symptom pattern (10). A comparison of this technique with the simpler, summative scoring system showed
few differences between their abilities to correctly classify patients and healthy
respondents. Logan recommended that four or more symptoms provided a
"convenient cutting point" for distinguishing well and sick groups (1). Twenty-
eight percent of nonpatients reported four or more symptoms, compared with
50% of expatients and 60% of outpatients. Other commentators have set scores
of 7 or 10 as cutting points (7, 8, 10).

Reliability

From a survey of over 11,000 respondents, Johnson and Meile obtained alpha
reliability coefficients of 0.77 and an Omega coefficient of 0.80 (this estimates
internal consistency where items fall on more than one factor) (9). They found
very little variation in these results across age, sex, and educational categories
(9, Table 1). Wheaton studied two samples (N = 613 and 250) over four years,
and reported path coefficients of 0.68 and 0.81 between the initial and subsequent scores for ten items that Crandell and Dohrenwend (11) recommended
be taken to form a psychological subscale (12, p399).

Validity

Using information obtained from an extensive interview that included the 22
items among 100 psychiatric symptoms, two psychiatrists independently rated
1,660 respondents on their degree of psychiatric impairment in the Midtown
Manhattan Study (1). Each of the 22 questions was then compared with this
rating; correlations ranged from 0.41 to 0.79, confirming that psychiatrists had
relied heavily on these items in forming their overall judgment (1, p273).

The data of Manis et al. yielded a sensitivity of 67% and a specificity of 63%
at a cutting point of four. A cutting point of ten gave a sensitivity of 20% and
a specificity of 96% (7, p111). These values are low and suggest the instrument
has limitations as a screening tool. The positive predictive value of the test in

Exhibit 4.3 Langner's Twenty-Two Item Screening Score of Psychiatric Symptoms

Note: An asterisk indicates the scored or pathognomonic responses. DK indicates Don't Know. NA indicates No Answer.

Item	Response
1. I feel weak all over much of the time.	*1. Yes 2. No 3. DK 4. NA
2. I have had periods of days, weeks, or months when I couldn't take care of things because I couldn't "get going."	*1. Yes 2. No 3. DK 4. NA
3. In general, would you say that most of the time you are in high (very good) spirits, good spirits, low spirits, or very low spirits?	1. High 2. Good *3. Low *4. Very Low 5. DK 6. NA
4. Every so often I suddenly feel hot all over.	*1. Yes 2. No 3. DK 4. NA
5. Have you ever been bothered by your heart beating hard? Would you say: often, sometimes, or never?	*1. Often 2. Sometimes 3. Never 4. DK 5. NA
6. Would you say your appetite is poor, fair, good or too good?	*1. Poor 2. Fair 3. Good 4. Too Good 5. DK 6. NA
7. I have periods of such great restlessness that I cannot sit long in a chair (cannot sit still very long).	*1. Yes 2. No 3. DK 4. NA
8. Are you the worrying type (a worrier)?	*1. Yes 2. No 3. DK 4. NA
9. Have you ever been bothered by shortness of breath when you were *not* exercising or working hard? Would you say: often, sometimes, or never?	*1. Often 2. Sometimes 3. Never 4. DK 5. NA
10. Are you ever bothered by nervousness (irritable, fidgety, tense)? Would you say: often, sometimes, or never?	*1. Often 2. Sometimes 3. Never 4. DK 5. NA

Item	Response
11. Have you ever had any fainting spells (lost consciousness)? Would you say: never, a few times, or more than a few times?	1. Never 2. A few times *3. More than a few times 4. DK 5. NA
12. Do you ever have any trouble in getting to sleep or staying asleep? Would you say: often, sometimes, or never?	*1. Often 2. Sometimes 3. Never 4. DK 5. NA
13. I am bothered by acid (sour) stomach several times a week.	*1. Yes 2. No 3. DK 4. NA
14. My memory seems to be all right (good).	1. Yes *2. No 3. DK 4. NA
15. Have you ever been bothered by "cold sweats"? Would you say: often, sometimes, or never?	*1. Often 2. Sometimes 3. Never 4. DK 5. NA
16. Do your hands ever tremble enough to bother you? Would you say: often, sometimes, or never?	*1. Often 2. Sometimes 3. Never 4. DK 5. NA
17. There seems to be a fullness (clogging) in my head or nose much of the time.	*1. Yes 2. No 3. DK 4. NA
18. I have personal worries that get me down physically (make me physically ill).	*1. Yes 2. No 3. DK 4. NA
19. Do you feel somewhat apart even among friends (apart, isolated, alone)?	*1. Yes 2. No 3. DK 4. NA
20. Nothing ever turns out for me the way I want it to (turns out, happens, comes about, i.e., my wishes aren't fulfilled).	*1. Yes 2. No 3. DK 4. NA

Exhibit 4.3 *(continued)*

Item	Response
21. Are you ever troubled with headaches or pains in the head? Would you say: often, sometimes, or never?	*1. Often 2. Sometimes 3. Never 4. DK 5. NA
22. You sometimes can't help wondering if anything is worthwhile anymore.	*1. Yes 2. No 3. DK 4. NA

Reproduced from Langner TS. A twenty-two item screening score of psychiatric symptoms indicating impairment. J Health Hum Behav 1962;3:271–273.

the Midtown study was also low: around 13% for the cutting point of four, 21% for the cutting point of seven. All 22 items in the scale discriminated between patients newly admitted to a mental hospital and samples drawn from the community (7, Table 1). A score derived from the nine most discriminative questions performed almost as well as the full scale (7). Manis reported a correlation of 0.65 with a 45-item scale of behavioral symptoms of mental health. Shader et al. reported a correlation of 0.77 between the scale and Taylor's Manifest Anxiety Scale (N = 566), and of 0.72 with a Minnesota Multiphasic Personality Inventory depression score, and of 0.72 with Eysenck's Neuroticism Scale (6, Table 8). Fabrega and McBee obtained correlations of 0.50 with psychiatrists' ratings of depression and anxiety, and 0.30 with scores indicating neuroticism (4).

Several studies have reviewed the meaning of the items in the 22-item scale. Crandell and Dohrenwend asked a sample of psychiatrists and internists to judge the content of each item. Ten items were judged to reflect psychological symptoms, five were psychophysiological, three were physical and four could not be classified. Responses to these four types of items reveal variations by age, sex and socioeconomic status (13, 14). A similar analysis was carried out by Seiler and Summers (15). Empirical studies of the structure of the scale have used cluster analysis (13, 14) and factor analysis (9). The cluster analysis identified five clusters that cut across the grouping made by psychiatrists in Crandell and Dohrenwend's study. Johnson and Meile factor analyzed the scale using data from a large community study. Three factors were identified, reflecting physical symptoms, psychological stress, and psychophysiological responses (9, Table 2). The authors concluded that the physical component in the scale did not act independently of the psychological or psychophysiological components, but rather contributed to the overall impression.

Commentary

Langner's scale has been widely used, but has also received considerable critical attention. These criticisms, although now old, will be reviewed to illustrate an important phase in the development of psychological indices.

As with the HOS, a debate has arisen over precisely what the 22-item scale measures; this again illustrates the need for a clear conceptual formulation of the aims of an index (see Chapter 2). The questions have been variously said to indicate "psychiatric or psychological symptoms," "psychological disturbance or disorder," "psychophysiological symptoms," "emotional adjustment," "mental health," or "mental illness" (3). The method has even been termed a "psychiatric case identification instrument" (10, p335). The debate is unlikely to be resolved, although Seiler's conclusion that the scale is partly an indicator of psychological stress and partly of physiological malaise (15) is supported by several commentators. Both the HOS and Langner scales may falsely interpret purely physical symptoms as reflecting psychological disorder (8, 9, 11, 13, 15). Somatic symptoms may also not provide a consistent indicator of psychological distress across different social groups: lower social class respondents may both suffer more physical illness and tend to express psychological disorders in physical, rather than psychological, terms (3, 8, 11). However, Meile has dissented and argued on the basis of large studies that the physical items did not provide evidence that diverged from that offered by the other questions in the scale (8, 9).

Several studies have shown a higher symptom response rate among women than men (14–16); this may reflect a reporting bias because women are less inhibited about reporting their symptoms (11). Clancy and Gove, however, showed that males and females did not differ in their bias towards acquiescing to the items and that the difference in responses seemed to reflect a true difference in symptoms experienced (16).

Seiler offered an extensive summary of the strengths and weaknesses of using the comparatively weak validation procedure of "known groups," and estimated that one third of the known mentally sick are not detected by the scale (3). Manis et al. commented that the scale holds some validity as a community survey technique, but cannot indicate the health of individuals (7). The interpretation of a high score may also not be clear: does this suggest an increasing probability of disorder or does it imply a more severe disorder? The scale contains no items covering positive mental health, so a low score will not distinguish between the absence of sickness and more positive states of well-being (3). As the 22-item scale does not claim to cover a number of important psychiatric problems, the low-scoring group may contain healthy people, plus various types of the mentally ill not identified by the items. These problems in interpreting the Langner scale have led to its virtual replacement by newer scales whose interpretation is clearer.

Unfortunately, this entry was not reviewed by Dr. Langner; it was reviewed by Dr. Seiler.

Address

Thomas S. Langner, Department of Epidemiology, Columbia University School of Public Health, 600 West 168th Street, New York, New York, USA 10032

References

(1) Langner TS. A twenty-two item screening score of psychiatric symptoms indicating impairment. J Health Hum Behav 1962;3:269–276.

(2) Srole L, Langner TS, Michael ST, Kirkpatrick P, Opler MK, Rennie TAC. Mental health in the metropolis: the Midtown Manhattan Study. New York: New York University Press, 1978.

(3) Seiler LH. The 22-item scale used in field studies of mental illness: a question of method, a question of substance, and a question of theory. J Health Soc Behav 1973;14:252–264.

(4) Fabrega H Jr, McBee G. Validity features of a mental health questionnaire. Soc Sci Med 1970;4:669–673.

(5) Muller DJ. Discussion of Langner's psychiatric impairment scale. Am J Psychiatry 1971;128:601.

(6) Shader RI, Ebert MH, Harmatz JS. Langner's psychiatric impairment scale: a short screening device. Am J Psychiatry 1971;128:596–601.

(7) Manis JG, Brawer MJ, Hunt CL, Kercher LC. Validating a mental health scale. Am Sociol Rev 1963;28:108–116.

(8) Meile RL. The 22-item index of psychophysiological disorder: psychological or organic symptoms? Soc Sci Med 1972;6:125–135.

(9) Johnson DR, Meile RL. Does dimensionality bias in Langner's 22-item index affect the validity of social status comparisons? An empirical investigation. J Health Soc Behav 1981;22:415–433.

(10) Haese PN, Meile RL. The relative effectiveness of two models for scoring the midtown psychological disorder index. Community Ment Health J 1967;3:335–342.

(11) Crandell DL, Dohrenwend BP. Some relations among psychiatric symptoms, organic illness, and social class. Am J Psychiatry 1967;123:1527–1537.

(12) Wheaton B. The sociogenesis of psychological disorder: reexamining the causal issues with longitudinal data. Am Sociol Rev 1978;43:383–403.

(13) Roberts RE, Forthofer RN, Fabrega H Jr. Further evidence on dimensionality of the index of psychophysiological stress. Soc Sci Med 1976;10:483–490.

(14) Roberts RF, Forthofer RN, Fabrega H Jr. The Langner items and acquiescence. Soc Sci Med 1976;10:69–75.

(15) Seiler LH, Summers GF. Toward an interpretation of items used in field studies of mental illness. Soc Sci Med 1974;8:459–467.

(16) Clancy K, Gove W. Sex differences in mental illness: an analysis of response bias in self-reports. Am J Sociol 1974;80:205–216.

THE AFFECT BALANCE SCALE
(Norman M. Bradburn, 1965, Revised 1969)

Purpose

The ten questions developed by Norman Bradburn were designed to indicate the psychological reactions (positive and negative) of people in the general population to events in their daily lives. Bradburn described his scale as an indicator of happiness or of general psychological well-being; these terms denote an individual's ability to cope with the stresses of everyday living. The scale is not concerned with detecting psychiatric or psychological *disorders,* which Bradburn viewed as reactions that persist after removal of the stressful conditions or that are out of proportion to the magnitude of the stress (1).

Conceptual Basis

From their early studies, Bradburn and Caplovitz suggested that subjective feelings of well-being could be indicated by a person's position on two independent dimensions, termed positive and negative affect (2). Overall well-being is expressed as the balance between these two, compensatory forces: an "individual will be high in psychological well-being in the degree to which he has an excess of positive over negative affect and will be low in well-being in the degree to which negative affect predominates over positive" (1, p9). Positive factors (e.g., being complimented) can compensate for the negative feelings to keep the overall sense of well-being at a constant level. The "affect balance score" represents this theme.

Beyond simply compensating for each other, positive and negative feelings were found empirically to be relatively independent of one another; they were not simply the opposite ends of a single dimension of well-being. Bradburn commented that this did not imply that positive and negative feelings

> can occur simultaneously or that people move from positive to negative feelings and back again in a cyclical fashion. We mean that within a given period of time, such as a week or two, one may experience many different emotions, both positive and negative, and that in general there is no tendency for the two types to be experienced in any particular relation to one another. (1, p225).

To indicate the independence of the dimensions, Bradburn cited the example of a man who has an argument with his wife, which may increase their negative feelings without changing their positive feelings. Different circumstances were found to contribute to the presence of positive and negative affects.

Description

Bradburn's research formed part of the National Opinion Research Center's investigations into mental health at about the same time that Macmillan, Leighton, Gurin and Langner were working on similar themes. The original scale developed by Bradburn consisted of 12 questions, seven measuring positive and five measuring negative affect. Responses were coded on a frequency scale ("once," "sometimes," "often"). Four questions were deleted and two others added to give the ten questions (five positive, five negative) that have been widely used. They are shown in Exhibit 4.4.

The wording of the questions has remained constant in most studies, but the wording of the question stem has varied. Bradburn specified a time referent (originally "the past week," subsequently, "the past few weeks"); some users have changed this to "the past few months" (3), while others have asked "How often do you feel each of these ways?" (4, 5).

The scale is self-administered, and replies may use a dichotomous yes/no reply or a scale of three, four, or five points representing the frequency of expe-

Exhibit 4.4 The Affect Balance Scale

During the past few weeks, did you ever feel _____ (Yes/No)

A. Particularly excited or interested in something?
B. Did you ever feel so restless that you couldn't sit long in a chair?
C. Proud because someone complimented you on something you had done?
D. Very lonely or remote from other people?
E. Pleased about having accomplished something?
F. Bored?
G. On top of the world?
H. Depressed or very unhappy?
I. That things were going your way?
J. Upset because someone criticized you?

Reproduced from Bradburn NM. The structure of psychological well-being. Chicago: Aldine, 1969:267. With permission.

riencing the feelings; a three-point scale ("often," "sometimes," "never") has been most commonly used. Differential weights were tested, but did not significantly alter the results and so are not used (6). The affect balance score is calculated as the positive score minus the negative. The resulting balance scale has occasionally been collapsed into one with fewer categories (4, 5).

Reliability

Bradburn reported test-retest reliability results over three days for 174 respondents. The resulting test-retest associations (Yule's Q) exceeded 0.90 for nine of the items, while the question "excited or interested" had a reliability of 0.86 (1).

Internal consistency results from a number of subsamples ranged from 0.55 to 0.73 for the positive scale and from 0.61 to 0.73 for the negative scale (7, p196). Warr obtained median item-total correlations for the positive scale of 0.47 and 0.48 for the negative scale (8, p114). Correlations among the items in the two scales were modest, in the range of 0.24 to 0.26 (8). Warr also summarized the response patterns to the questions from five studies; although the absolute rates of affirmative replies varied between studies, the rank ordering of the questions by response rates was remarkably consistent.

Validity

Bradburn provided extensive evidence of agreement between the questions and other indices of self-reported well-being. He gave evidence of discriminant validity by showing contrasts in response patterns between employed and unemployed, rich and poor, and between different occupational levels (1). Positive affect was shown to be related to social participation, satisfaction with social life and engaging in novel activities. Several of these findings have been confirmed in subsequent studies. The independence of positive and negative affect scores and their lack of association with age have been widely replicated (7–12). Similarly, correlations have frequently been reported with ratings of overall happiness (10, 11), employment status (8, 13), and social participation (3, 7, 11, 13). Kushman and Lane reported significant associations with minority status and the sex of the respondent (13).

Berkman used eight of the questions in the Alameda County survey and reported a correlation of 0.48 with a 20-item Index of Neurotic Traits (5). Warr reported significant correlations between the affect scales and an anxiety rating and a scale of feelings about one's present life among steel workers who had been laid off (8). Beiser obtained a correlation of 0.42 between negative affect and a psychiatrist's rating of "psychiatric caseness" (11).

Cherlin and Reeder reported results of a factor analysis of the ten items; these formed two clearly distinct factorial groups, although the authors questioned whether these measured affect (see "Commentary").

Alternative Forms

A translation into French was made in Canada (14); a German version has been published (15).

Reference Standards

Reference standards for the Canadian population are available from the 1978–1979 Canada Health Survey (sample size 23,000) (14, 16).

Commentary

There are several important strengths in Bradburn's scale. The questions have been widely and consistently used in many, large surveys, so that it is possible to compare findings across studies; reference standards are available. The clear conceptual description of the purpose of the scale seems to have prevented some of the misconceptions and disputes over interpretation that have characterized the HOS and Langner scales. The fact that the question wording has remained virtually unchanged also constitutes a major advantage to this method. Bradburn's scale was also innovative in its inclusion of both positive and negative questions. This has permitted empirical examination of the concept of "positive mental health."

At the same time, detailed criticisms have been made of the method by Cherlin and Reeder (7), Beiser (3, 11), and Brenner (12). The Bradburn scale is brief and covers a broad scope, so it inevitably suffers some resulting psychometric weaknesses: the internal consistency, for example, is low compared with that of the HOS or Langner scales. The interpretation of several questions has been challenged; Cherlin and Reeder argued that the theme covered by the questions is broader than that implied by Bradburn's term "affect": the positive dimension includes activation or participation (7). Beiser implied a similar criticism when he altered the term "positive affect" to "pleasurable involvement" to reflect the item content more adequately; he also discarded the item "On top of the world" (3, 11).

Behind criticisms of individual questions lies the general issue of the adequacy of Bradburn's two-component model of emotional well-being. Reality appears to be more complex (7), and the somewhat surprising finding of statistical independence between positive and negative affect may be an artifact of the question phrasing, a possibility that Bradburn had recognized (1). Five questions refer to specific events (e.g., "Upset because someone criticized you") and these do, indeed, seem to be independent of one another (7). The positive and negative questions covering more general feelings tend, however, to show a comparatively strong inverse relationship (12). Because of these criticisms, Cherlin and Reeder questioned the affect balance score as the summary statistic because it may entail a loss of information compared with reporting positive and negative scores separately (7). Kammann et al. (17) recently commented on the continuing debate over the independence of positive and negative affect; the theme will be discussed further in our review of the Rand Mental Health Inventory.

The Bradburn scale was instrumental in stimulating research in the measurement of subjective well-being and happiness. It served to demonstrate that these qualities can be measured, a claim that was disputed when the scale was introduced.† Nonetheless, the scale is 20 years old, and despite its historic significance, users should seriously consider applying a more recent alternative, such as the General Well-Being Schedule or the Mental Health Inventory.

Address

Norman M. Bradburn, PhD, Director, National Opinion Research Center, 6030 South Ellis, Chicago, Illinois, USA 60637

References

(1) Bradburn NM. The structure of psychological well-being. Chicago: Aldine, 1969.
(2) Bradburn NM, Caplovitz D. Reports on happiness: a pilot study of behavior related to mental health. Chicago: Aldine, 1965.
(3) Beiser M, Feldman JJ, Egelhoff CJ. Assets and affects: a study of positive mental health. Arch Gen Psychiatry 1972;27:545–549.
(4) Berkman PL. Life stress and psychological well-being: a replication of Langner's analysis in the Midtown Manhattan Study. J Health Soc Behav 1971;12:35–45.
(5) Berkman PL. Measurement of mental health in a general population survey. Am J Epidemiol 1971;94:105–111.
(6) Bradburn NM, Miles C. Vague quantifiers. Public Opinion Q 1979;43:92–101.
(7) Cherlin A, Reeder LG. The dimensions of psychological well-being: a critical review. Sociol Methods Res 1975;4:189–214.
(8) Warr P. A study of psychological well-being. Br J Psychol 1978;69:111–121.
(9) Phillips DL. Social participation and happiness. Am J Sociol 1967;72:479–488.
(10) Gaitz CM, Scott J. Age and the measurement of mental health. J Health Soc Behav 1972;13:55–67.

†Such research appears very prevalent. In one of Unger's Herman cartoons a Martian survey researcher, his flying saucer parked nearby, is inquiring whether the bemused simpleton Herman is "'extremely happy,' 'happy,' 'average,' or 'bored stiff'?"

(11) Beiser M. Components and correlates of mental well-being. J Health Soc Behav 1974;15:320–327.
(12) Brenner B. Quality of affect and self-evaluated happiness. Soc Indicat Res 1975; 2:315–331.
(13) Kushman J, Lane S. A multivariate analysis of factors affecting perceived life satisfaction and psychological well-being among the elderly. Soc Sci Q 1980; 61:264–277.
(14) Health and Welfare Canada. The health of Canadians: report of the Canada Health Survey. Ottawa, Canada: Ministry of Supply and Services, 1981. (Catalogue No. 82-538E).
(15) Noelle-Neumann E. Politik und Glück. In: Baier H, ed. Freiheit und Sachzwang Beiträge zu Ehren Helmut Schelskys. Opladen: West Deutscher Verlag, 1977:207–262.
(16) McDowell I, Praught E. On the measurement of happiness: an examination of the Bradburn scale in the Canada Health Survey. Am J Epidemiol 1982;116:949–958.
(17) Kammann R, Farry M, Herbison P. The analysis and measurement of happiness as a sense of well-being. Soc Indicat Res 1984;15:91–115.

THE GENERAL WELL-BEING SCHEDULE
(Harold J. Dupuy, 1977)

Purpose

The General Well-Being Schedule (GWB) offers a brief but broad-ranging indicator of subjective feelings of psychological well-being and distress for use in community surveys.

Conceptual Basis

The only conceptual description of the content of the GWB is contained in an unpublished paper by Dupuy (1). Reflecting the theories of Kurt Lewin, the scale assesses how the individual feels about his "inner personal state," rather than about external conditions such as income, work environment, or neighborhood (1). The scale reflects both positive and negative feelings: six dimensions cover anxiety, depression, general health, positive well-being, self-control and vitality.

Description

The GWB is a self-administered questionnaire that was developed for the U.S. Health and Nutrition Examination Survey (HANES I) (2). A draft instrument contained 68 items, 18 of which were used in the HANES study and form the usual set of questions referred to as the GWB. They are shown in Exhibit 4.5.

The GWB includes both positive and negative questions. Each item has the time frame "during the last month" and the first 14 questions use six-point response scales representing intensity or frequency. The ordinal qualities of

Exhibit 4.5 The General Well-Being Schedule

a. Name *(Last, first, middle)*	b. Deck No.	c. Sample No.	d. Sex	e. Age
	171	_ _ _ _ _	1 ☐ Male 2 ☐ Female	_ _

READ — This section of the examination contains questions about how you feel and how things have been going with you. For each question, mark (X) the answer which best applies to you.

1. How have you been feeling in general? *(DURING THE PAST MONTH)*	1. (001) 1 ☐ In excellent spirits 2 ☐ In very good spirits 3 ☐ In good spirits mostly 4 ☐ I have been up and down in spirits a lot 5 ☐ In low spirits mostly 6 ☐ In very low spirits
2. Have you been bothered by nervousness or your "nerves"? *(DURING THE PAST MONTH)*	2. (002) 1 ☐ Extremely so -- to the point where I could not work or take care of things 2 ☐ Very much so 3 ☐ Quite a bit 4 ☐ Some -- enough to bother me 5 ☐ A little 6 ☐ Not at all
3. Have you been in firm control of your behavior, thoughts, emotions OR feelings? *(DURING THE PAST MONTH)*	3. (003) 1 ☐ Yes, definitely so 2 ☐ Yes, for the most part 3 ☐ Generally so 4 ☐ Not too well 5 ☐ No, and I am somewhat disturbed 6 ☐ No, and I am very disturbed
4. Have you felt so sad, discouraged, hopeless, or had so many problems that you wondered if anything was worthwhile? *(DURING THE PAST MONTH)*	4. (004) 1 ☐ Extremely so -- to the point that I have just about given up 2 ☐ Very much so 3 ☐ Quite a bit 4 ☐ Some -- enough to bother me 5 ☐ A little bit 6 ☐ Not at all
5. Have you been under or felt you were under any strain, stress, or pressure? *(DURING THE PAST MONTH)*	5. (005) 1 ☐ Yes -- almost more than I could bear or stand 2 ☐ Yes -- quite a bit of pressure 3 ☐ Yes -- some - more than usual 4 ☐ Yes -- some - but about usual 5 ☐ Yes - a little 6 ☐ Not at all

these response options were checked empirically (1). The remaining four questions use 0 to 10 rating scales defined by adjectives at each end. In coding replies, the polarity of certain questions is reversed, so that a low score represents more severe distress. Dupuy used a total score running from 0 to 110 and for this, 14 is subtracted from the score derived from the codes shown in Exhibit 4.5. Dupuy proposed cutting points to represent three levels of disorder: scores of 0 to 60 reflect "severe distress," 61 to 72 "moderate distress," while 73 to 110 represent "positive well-being" (1). Six subscores may be formed as we show in Exhibit 4.6. Using the labels proposed by Brook et al. (4), the subscores measure anxiety, depression, positive well-being, self-control, vitality and general health.

6. How happy, satisfied, or pleased have you been with your personal life? *(DURING THE PAST MONTH)*	6.	(006) 1 ☐ Extremely happy – could not have been more satisfied or pleased 2 ☐ Very happy 3 ☐ Fairly happy 4 ☐ Satisfied -- pleased 5 ☐ Somewhat dissatisfied 6 ☐ Very dissatisfied
7. Have you had any reason to wonder if you were losing your mind, or losing control over the way you act, talk, think, feel, or of your memory? *(DURING THE PAST MONTH)*	7.	(007) 1 ☐ Not at all 2 ☐ Only a little 3 ☐ Some -- but not enough to be concerned or worried about 4 ☐ Some and I have been a little concerned 5 ☐ Some and I am quite concerned 6 ☐ Yes, very much so and I am very concerned
8. Have you been anxious, worried, or upset? *(DURING THE PAST MONTH)*	8.	(008) 1 ☐ Extremely so -- to the point of being sick or almost sick 2 ☐ Very much so 3 ☐ Quite a bit 4 ☐ Some -- enough to bother me 5 ☐ A little bit 6 ☐ Not at all
9. Have you been waking up fresh and rested? *(DURING THE PAST MONTH)*	9.	(009) 1 ☐ Every day 2 ☐ Most every day 3 ☐ Fairly often 4 ☐ Less than half the time 5 ☐ Rarely 6 ☐ None of the time
10. Have you been bothered by any illness, bodily disorder, pains, or fears about your health? *(DURING THE PAST MONTH)*	10.	(010) 1 ☐ All the time 2 ☐ Most of the time 3 ☐ A good bit of the time 4 ☐ Some of the time 5 ☐ A little of the time 6 ☐ None of the time
11. Has your daily life been full of things that were interesting to you? *(DURING THE PAST MONTH)*	11.	(011) 1 ☐ All the time 2 ☐ Most of the time 3 ☐ A good bit of the time 4 ☐ Some of the time 5 ☐ A little of the time 6 ☐ None of the time
12. Have you felt down-hearted and blue? *(DURING THE PAST MONTH)*	12.	(012) 1 ☐ All of the time 2 ☐ Most of the time 3 ☐ A good bit of the time 4 ☐ Some of the time 5 ☐ A little of the time 6 ☐ None of the time

Reliability

Using the HANES data, Monk reported test–retest reliability coefficients (after three months) of 0.68 and 0.85 for "two different groups" (2, p183). Fazio reported a retest coefficient of 0.85 after three months for 195 college students (3, p10). Edwards et al. obtained a retest coefficient of 0.68 for 98 college graduates (see 5, p26).

Exhibit 4.5 (*continued*)

13. Have you been feeling emotionally stable and sure of yourself? *(DURING THE PAST MONTH)*	13.	(013) 1 ☐ All of the time 2 ☐ Most of the time 3 ☐ A good bit of the time 4 ☐ Some of the time 5 ☐ A little of the time 6 ☐ None of the time
14. Have you felt tired, worn out, used-up, or exhausted? *(DURING THE PAST MONTH)*	14.	(014) 1 ☐ All of the time 2 ☐ Most of the time 3 ☐ A good bit of the time 4 ☐ Some of the time 5 ☐ A little of the time 6 ☐ None of the time
		For each of the four scales below, note that the words at each end of the 0 to 10 scale describe opposite feelings. Circle any number along the bar which seems closest to how you have generally felt DURING THE PAST MONTH.
15. How concerned or worried about your **HEALTH** have you been? *(DURING THE PAST MONTH)*	15.	(015) 0 1 2 3 4 5 6 7 8 9 10 Not concerned at all ... Very concerned
16. How **RELAXED** or **TENSE** have you been? *(DURING THE PAST MONTH)*	16.	(016) 0 1 2 3 4 5 6 7 8 9 10 Very relaxed ... Very tense
17. How much **ENERGY, PEP, VITALITY** have you felt? *(DURING THE PAST MONTH)*	17.	(017) 0 1 2 3 4 5 6 7 8 9 10 No energy AT ALL, listless ... Very ENERGETIC, dynamic
18. How **DEPRESSED** or **CHEERFUL** have you been? *(DURING THE PAST MONTH)*	18.	(018) 0 1 2 3 4 5 6 7 8 9 10 Very depressed ... Very cheerful

Reproduced from Fazio AF. A concurrent validational study of the NCHS General Well-Being Schedule. Hyattsville, Maryland: U.S. Department of Health, Education and Welfare, National Center for Health Statistics, 1977:34–36. With permission.

The internal consistency of the GWB is very high: in Fazio's study the coefficients were 0.91 for 79 males and 0.95 for 116 females (3, p11). Ware et al. reviewed three other studies that reported internal consistency; all provided coefficients over 0.90 (5). The HANES data provided an internal consistency of 0.93 (N = 6,913) (1, p7). Fazio reported correlations among the subscores ranging from 0.16 to 0.72 (3, Table 6).

Validity

There is considerable evidence for the correlational validity of the GWB. In Fazio's validation study, the GWB total score correlated 0.47 with an interviewer's rating of depression, 0.66 with the Zung Depression Scale and 0.78

Exhibit 4.6 The General Well-Being Schedule: Subscore Labels and Question Topics

Subscore labels	Question topics
Anxiety	2. nervousness 5. strain, stress, or pressure 8. anxious, worried, upset 16. relaxed—tense
Depression	4. sad, discouraged, hopeless 12. down-hearted, blue 18. depressed
Positive well-being	1. feeling in general 6. happy, satisfied with life 11. interesting daily life
Self-control	3. firm control of behavior, emotions 7. afraid losing mind, or losing control 13. emotionally stable, sure of self
Vitality	9. waking fresh, rested 14. feeling tired, worn-out 17. energy level
General health	10. bothered by bodily disorders 15. concerned, worried about health

with the Personal Feelings Inventory (3, Table B). The average correlation of the GWB and six independent depression scales was 0.69; the average correlation was 0.64 with three anxiety scales (3, p10). Simpkins and Burke obtained correlations of 0.70 with a 10-item depression score, 0.58 with the Lubin Depression Adjective Checklist, and 0.80 with the Self-Rating Depression Scale (N = 198). For 63 respondents, the correlation between the GWB total score and the Langner scale was 0.41 (5, 6). Brook et al. reported correlations between the GWB subscales and reports of stress at home and at work ranging from 0.17 to 0.59 (4, Table 12).

Correlations between individual GWB subscales and criterion ratings were reported by Fazio (3) and by Ware et al. (5). In the main, such correlations were high, frequently falling between 0.65 and 0.90. Using an interviewer's rating as the criterion, Fazio noted:

> three very short subscales of the GWB correlated with the criterion about as well or better than the many other scales that had many more items (3, p8 and Table A).

Correlations with use of services were summarized by Ware et al. and fell in the range of 0.09 to 0.48 (5, pp48–49). The draft version of the GWB contained a validation question: "Have you had severe enough personal, emotional, behavior or mental problems that you felt you needed help DURING THE PAST YEAR?" Dupuy showed a correlation of 0.53 between the GWB total score and this question (N = 2,007 from the HANES survey); Simpkins and Burke reported a correlation of 0.67 (5, Table 9).

Using the HANES data, Dupuy constructed a sociodemographic index (reflecting social class and size of household), a somatic index (which covered use of medications, self-report of symptoms of anxiety and a self-rating of general health), and a psychological problem index. The multiple correlation between the GWB overall score and the last two of these indices was 0.73 (1, p9). The GWB was only weakly related to sociodemographic status ($r = 0.25$), and this association disappeared when the somatic and the psychological problem indices were controlled (1). Fifty-five questions covering clinical symptoms and self-perceptions of health in the HANES study explained 31% of the variance in GWB scores (7).

Edwards showed a modest but significant contrast between psychiatric day patients and national norms (5). He also showed the GWB capable of detecting progress made by 21 psychiatric day patients following two weeks of treatment. Simpkins and Burke's comparison of community and psychiatric patient samples yielded a point biserial correlation of 0.56 (5, p38).

From the HANES data, Dupuy and Wan and Livieratos reported factor analyses of the GWB items, providing three factors that explained 51% of the variance (7). The first factor included items suggesting anxiety, tension and depression, and accounted for 18% of total variance. The second contained items on health and energy and the third comprised positive well-being or life satisfaction items.

Reference Standards

Dupuy derived United States national reference standards from the HANES data (5). Seventy-one percent of the adult population fell into the "positive well-being" category (scores 73 to 110), 15.5% showed moderate distress (scores 61 to 72), and 13.5% were classified as experiencing "severe distress" (scores 0 to 60) (1). About 60% of the population were both free of severe problems over the past year and in a state of positive well-being during the past month.

Alternative Forms

The GWB items shown in Exhibit 4.5 were incorporated with modifications in the draft version of the Rand Mental Health Inventory and extensive scaling, reliability, and validity tests were carried out. Despite the modifications, the considerable overlap between the GWB and the Rand draft instrument (which they termed the "HIS-GWB") has led us to include some of the Rand findings here as suggestive of the quality of the GWB questions.

The validity of Dupuy's hypothesized grouping of items into six subscales was evaluated empirically on 1,209 respondents using multitrait and factor analyses (5). A six-factor solution provided results that agreed closely with the structure hypothesized by Dupuy, providing scores indicating anxiety, depression, self-control, positive well-being, general health, and vitality (5). Internal consistency coefficients for the six subscales ranged from 0.72 to 0.88 (5, Table 20). One-week test–retest reliability estimates were made for the anxiety and positive well-being scales, and were 0.70 and 0.74, respectively (N = 437) (5, Table 20). Test–retest reliability declined to 0.50 when the interval exceeded one month (5). Validity was examined by correlating GWB subscales and over-all scores with 24 validating variables covering stress, recognition of mental problems, life satisfaction and use of mental health care. Of 192 correlations, 158 were statistically significant ($p < 0.01$) in the hypothesized direction. The nonsignificant associations pertained to stressful life events, which occurred rarely in the sample under study (5). Fifteen of the GWB items were retained for use in the final version of the Rand Mental Health Inventory, which we describe in a separate review (5, p94; 8).

A ten-item version of the GWB has been developed, called the Psychological Mental Health Index (9). Four subscales are included: positive well-being (items 1 and 6 from Exhibit 4.5), depressed mood (items 4, 12), behavioral-emotional control (items 3, 7, and 13) and tension-anxiety (items 2, 5, and 8). Administered to chronic psychotic patients, a retest coefficient of 0.27 was obtained; internal consistency alpha scores ranged from 0.69 to 0.85. The item total correlations were low, ranging from 0.38 to 0.64 (9, p233). The ten-item scale correlated 0.45 with a therapist-rated symptom score. In the light of these low coefficients, Ulin concluded that further research is needed to test this abbreviation of the GWB before it can be recommended for general use.

Commentary

The General Well-Being Schedule improves upon the older methods reviewed in this chapter in several respects. Like the Bradburn scale, it includes positive well-being but, reflecting a criticism of the Bradburn scale, it divides the posi-tive questions into separate dimensions. It avoids reference to physical symp-toms of emotional distress and so avoids the interpretation problems seen with the HOS and Langner scales. The available reliability and validity tests show extremely good results—the internal consistency is higher than for other scales and there is wide evidence of agreement with other, purpose-built depression and anxiety scales. A possible weakness in the performance of the scale was noted by Edwards et al., who showed that, while the internal consistency of the scale exceeded 0.94, the test–retest reliability is low, at 0.69 (10). A measure-ment that contains fluctuations over time may be of little use in assessing indi-viduals, although it may be adequate for groups.

Given the quality of the General Well-Being Schedule, it is unfortunate that so many of the validation studies remain unpublished. Analyses of the psycho-metric properties of the scale could be produced from the HANES data, for example. The most useful document summarizing the unpublished material is the Rand review by Ware et al. (5). Fazio's study indicated that the GWB per-formed as well as several other leading scales in assessing emotional distress in a student sample. He concluded " . . . the GWB emerged as the single most useful instrument in measuring depression" (3). Although Dupuy's description of the conceptual structure of the GWB is vague, the results of a large factor analytic study provided data that support the dimensions originally built into the scale. This consistency is rare indeed.

Some debate has arisen over the most useful way to score the GWB. The internal consistency of the 18 items is very high, so that forming subscores may be redundant. Wan and Livieratos argued that the three factors obtained from the HANES data did not offer a suitable approach to scoring; inclusion of all 18 items in a single score may be the most appropriate method. Having very few items, subscales would inevitably provide only crude measurements; Fazio's results did, indeed, show lower internal consistency for the subscales than for the instrument as a whole.

Because of its outstanding reliability and validity results, we recommend that the General Well-Being Schedule be seriously considered for use where a general population indicator of subjective well-being is required. We know less about its adequacy as a case-detection instrument, for which the General Health Questionnaire is recommended.

This entry was not reviewed by Dr. Dupuy; it was, however, checked by Dr. Fazio.

Address

Harold J. Dupuy, PhD, Psychological Advisor, National Center for Health Statistics, Health, Education and Welfare, Hyattsville, Maryland, USA

References

(1) Dupuy HJ. Self-representations of general psychological well-being of American adults. Paper presented at American Public Health Association Meeting, Los Angeles, California, October 17, 1978.
(2) Monk M. Blood pressure awareness and psychological well-being in the Health and Nutrition Examination Survey. Clin Invest Med 1981;4:183–189.
(3) Fazio AF. A concurrent validational study of the NCHS General Well-Being Schedule. Hyattsville, Maryland: U.S. Department of Health, Education and Welfare, National Center for Health Statistics, 1977. (Vital and Health Statistics Series 2, No. 73. DHEW Publication No. (HRA) 78-1347).
(4) Brook RH, Ware JE Jr, Davies-Avery A, Stewart AL, Donald CA et al. Overview of adult health status measures fielded in Rand's Health Insurance Study. Med Care 1979;17:1–131.
(5) Ware JE Jr, Johnston SA, Davies-Avery A, Brook RH. Conceptualization and measurement of health for adults in the Health Insurance Study. Vol. III, Mental health. Santa Monica, California: Rand Corporation, 1979. (Publication No. R-1987/3-HEW).
(6) Simpkins C, Burke FF. Comparative analyses of the NCHS General Well-Being Schedule: response distributions, community vs. patient status discriminations, and content relationships. Nashville, Tennessee: Center for Community Studies, George Peabody College, 1974. (Contract No. HRA 106-74-13).
(7) Wan TTH, Livieratos B. A validation of the General Well-Being Index: a two-stage multivariate approach. Paper presented at American Public Health Association Meeting, Washington, DC, October 30–November 3, 1977.
(8) Veit CT, Ware JE. The structure of psychological distress and well-being in general populations. J Consult Clin Psychol 1983;51:730–742.

(9) Ulin PR. Measuring adjustment in chronically ill clients in community mental health care: an assessment of the Psychological Mental Health Index. Nurs Res 1981;30:229–235.

(10) Edwards DW, Yarvis RM, Mueller DP, Zingale HC, Wagman WJ. Test-taking and the stability of adjustment scales: can we assess patient deterioration? Evaluation Q 1978;2:275–291.

THE MENTAL HEALTH INVENTORY
(Rand Corporation and John E. Ware, 1979)

Purpose

The Mental Health Inventory (MHI) is a measurement of psychological distress and well-being, developed for use in population surveys.

Conceptual Basis

Veit and Ware discussed the limitations of early screening tests such as the HOS and the Langner scale. Because of their physical orientation, such methods may not be able to distinguish changes in mental health from changes in physical health, and many of the symptoms they include are rarely encountered in the general population (1). Veit and Ware noted:

> a substantial proportion of people in a general population rarely or never report occurrences of even the most prevalent psychological distress symptoms. To increase measurement precision, it may be necessary to extend the definition of mental health . . . to include characteristics of psychological well-being (e.g., feeling cheerful, interest in and enjoyment of life). Psychological well-being items have the potential to improve the precision of mental health measurement by distinguishing among persons who receive perfect scores on measures of psychological distress. (1, p730).

As well as being developed as a screening instrument, the MHI was also used to examine the structure of mental health: are distress and positive well-being separate dimensions (as argued by Bradburn), and are these concepts themselves multidimensional, implying that they should be further subdivided (1)? To develop an instrument that could reflect the multidimensional nature of psychological well-being, Ware et al. incorporated four factors hypothesized by Dupuy—anxiety, depression, loss of behavioral/emotional control, and general positive affect—and added a fifth factor, emotional ties, to form the basis for the MHI (1).

Description

The MHI was designed as the primary mental health measurement in the Rand Health Insurance Experiment. It focuses on psychological symptoms of mood and anxiety and of loss of control over feelings, thoughts and behavior (2). The MHI uses 15 items from Dupuy's General Well-Being Schedule: the GWB items covering general health and vitality were discarded because they failed discriminant tests of validity (1). Twenty items were drawn from other scales to cover anxiety, depression, general positive affect and loss of behavioral or emotional control; three items were written to cover the fifth hypothesized factor, emotional ties. To these 38 items, another eight may be added to assess a socially desirable response set (2). Details of the development of the MHI and the origin of the questions are given in several sources (1, 2). The questions and response scales are shown in Exhibit 4.7 along with the factor placement of each item.

The questionnaire is self-administered and items refer to mental health during the past month. Most of the response scales have six options. To ensure comparability, the response options were kept close to those used in the questionnaires from which the items were originally drawn. The subscales can be scored and interpreted separately or scores can be aggregated into an overall measure known as the Mental Health Index (1). When combining all the scores it is necessary to reverse the scoring of the positive section. This may be done by subtracting the raw score from 67.

Reliability

The MHI was tested on a representative population sample of 5,089 respondents in the Rand Health Insurance Experiment. One-year test–retest results were based on 3,525 respondents, and coefficients ranged from 0.56 (for the depression scale) to 0.63 (for anxiety). Test–retest reliability of the overall score was 0.64 (1). Internal consistency coefficients ranged from 0.83 to 0.92 for the five scales, and 0.96 for the overall score (1, Table 6).

Validity

Veit and Ware presented an extensive discussion of the factorial structure of the MHI, from which they derived a hierarchical model of the structure of the scores it provides. The items were found to fall into the five factors indicated in Exhibit 4.7. Correlations among the factors ranged from −0.39 to 0.77 and the five factors were, in turn, grouped into two higher-order factors termed psychological distress (incorporating the negative items) and psychological well-being. These factors correlated −0.75, and may be regarded as forming a bipolar distress versus well-being measurement of general mental health. This result supported the multidimensional model of emotional well-being that was hypothesized, although a strong, general factor underlies the instrument (1).

Ware et al. showed a strong association between MHI scores and the use of ambulatory mental health services in a prospective study (3). The results lent added support to the inclusion of items covering positive psychological well-being. Correlations between the MHI and criterion measurements are shown by Ware et al. (4). The correlations between the various sections of the MHI and a life events scale ranged from 0.12 to 0.26; correlations with life satisfaction ran from 0.40 to 0.51, and correlations with an indicator of severe emotional problems ranged from 0.48 to 0.58 (4, Table 4).

Exhibit 4.7 The Mental Health Inventory, Showing Response Scales and Factor Placement of Each Item

Note: The answer scales vary from question to question and are shown at the foot of the table. Letters to the right of each question indicate the response scale that is applicable: T refers to the answer scale indicating time or frequency, AN indicates the scale running from always to never, and U indicates a unique answer category. The factor placement of each item is shown in the right hand column: Anx = anxiety, Dep = depression, Behav = behavioral/emotional control, Pos = general positive affect and Emotion = emotional ties.

Question	Response scale	Factor
How happy, satisfied, or pleased have you been with your personal life during the past month?	U1	Pos
How much of the time have you felt lonely during the past month?	T	Emotion
How often did you become nervous or jumpy when faced with excitement or unexpected situations during the past month?	AN	Anx
During the past month, how much of the time have you felt that the future looks hopeful and promising?	T	Pos
How much of the time, during the past month, has your daily life been full of things that were interesting to you?	T	Pos
How much of the time, during the past month, did you feel relaxed and free of tension?	T	Pos
During the past month, how much of the time have you generally enjoyed the things you do?	T	Pos
During the past month, have you had any reason to wonder if you were losing your mind, or losing control over the way you act, talk, think, feel, or of your memory?	U2	Behav
Did you feel depressed during the past month?	U3	Dep
During the past month, how much of the time have you felt loved and wanted?	T	Emotion
How much of the time, during the past month, have you been a very nervous person?	T	Anx
When you got up in the morning, this past month, about how often did you expect to have an interesting day?	AN	Pos
During the past month, how much of the time have you felt tense or "high-strung"?	T	Anx
During the past month, have you been in firm control of your behavior, thoughts, emotions, feelings?	U4	Behav
During the past month, how often did your hands shake when you tried to do something?	AN	Anx
During the past month, how often did you feel that you had nothing to look forward to?	AN	Behav
How much of the time, during the past month, have you felt calm and peaceful?	T	Pos
How much of the time, during the past month, have you felt emotionally stable?	T	Behav
How much of the time, during the past month, have you felt downhearted and blue?	T	Dep
How often have you felt like crying, during the past month?	AN	Behav
During the past month, how often did you feel that others would be better off if you were dead?	AN	Behav
How much of the time, during the past month, were you able to relax without difficulty?	T	Anx
During the past month, how much of the time did you feel that your love relationships, loving and being loved, were full and complete?	T	Emotion

135

Exhibit 4.7 (*continued*)

Question	Response scale	Factor
How often, during the past month, did you feel that nothing turned out for you the way you wanted it to?	AN	Behav
How much have you been bothered by nervousness, or your "nerves," during the past month?	U5	Anx
During the past month, how much of the time has living been a wonderful adventure for you?	T	Pos
How often, during the past month, have you felt so down in the dumps that nothing could cheer you up?	AN	Behav
During the past month, did you ever think about taking your own life?	U6	Behav
During the past month, how much of the time have you felt restless, fidgety, or impatient?	T	Anx
During the past month, how much of the time have you been moody or brooded about things?	T	Dep
How much of the time, during the past month, have you felt cheerful, lighthearted?	T	Pos
During the past month, how often did you get rattled, upset, or flustered?	AN	Anx
During the past month, have you been anxious or worried?	U7	Anx
During the past month, how much of the time were you a happy person?	T	Pos
How often during the past month did you find yourself having difficulty trying to calm down?	AN	Anx
During the past month, how much of the time have you been in low or very low spirits?	T	Dep
How often, during the past month, have you been waking up feeling fresh and rested?	U8	Pos
During the past month, have you been under or felt you were under any strain, stress, or pressure?	U9	Dep

Response scales and scores:

T

    (1) All of the time   (4) Some of the time
    (2) Most of the time   (5) A little of the time
    (3) A good bit of the time   (6) None of the time

AN

    (1) Always   (4) Sometimes
    (2) Very often   (5) Almost never
    (3) Fairly often   (6) Never

U1

    (1) Extremely happy, could not have been more satisfied or pleased
    (2) Very happy most of the time
    (3) Generally satisfied, pleased
    (4) Sometimes fairly satisfied, sometimes fairly unhappy
    (5) Generally dissatisfied, unhappy
    (6) Very dissatisfied, unhappy most of the time

U2

    (1) No, not at all
    (2) Maybe a little
    (3) Yes, but not enough to be concerned or worried about it
    (4) Yes, and I have been a little concerned
    (5) Yes, and I am quite concerned
    (6) Yes, and I am very much concerned about it

U3

    (1) Yes, to the point that I did not care about anything for days at a time

    (2) Yes, very depressed almost every day

    (3) Yes, quite depressed several times

    (4) Yes, a little depressed now and then

    (5) No, never felt depressed at all

U4

    (1) Yes, very definitely

    (2) Yes, for the most part

    (3) Yes, I guess so

    (4) No, not too well

    (5) No, and I am somewhat disturbed

    (6) No, and I am very disturbed

U5

    (1) Extremely so, to the point where I could not take care of things

    (2) Very much bothered

    (3) Bothered quite a bit by nerves

    (4) Bothered some, enough to notice

    (5) Bothered just a little by nerves

    (6) Not bothered at all by this

U6

    (1) Yes, very often

    (2) Yes, fairly often

    (3) Yes, a couple of times

    (4) Yes, at one time

    (5) No, never

U7

    (1) Yes, extremely so, to the point of being sick or almost sick

    (2) Yes, very much so

    (3) Yes, quite a bit

    (4) Yes, some, enough to bother me

    (5) Yes, a little bit

    (6) No, not at all

U8

    (1) Always, every day

    (2) Almost every day

    (3) Most days

    (4) Some days, but usually not

    (5) Hardly ever

    (6) Never wake up feeling rested

U9

    (1) Yes, almost more than I could stand or bear

    (2) Yes, quite a bit of pressure

    (3) Yes, some, more than usual

    (4) Yes, some, about normal

    (5) Yes, a little bit

    (6) No, not at all

Adapted from Veit CT, Ware JE Jr. The structure of psychological distress and well-being in general populations. J Consult Clin Psychol 1983;51:733,Table 1. Also from Ware JE Jr, Johnston SA, Davies-Avery A, Brook RH. Conceptualization and measurement of health for adults in the Health Insurance Study: Vol. III, Mental Health. Santa Monica, California: Rand Corporation, 1979, Table 27 and Appendix E.

Reference Standards

Veit and Ware presented mean scores for each section of the MHI, although these figures are based on slightly different numbers of items from those shown in Exhibit 4.7 (1, Table 6).

Commentary

As well as its use in the Rand Health Insurance Experiment, the MHI has been used in other studies to predict the use of services (1). The inventory incorporates the most adequate questions from some of the leading mental health scales; it has been carefully constructed and appears to have been used without alterations to the wording of the questions. Perhaps because the MHI was originally applied in conjunction with other scales of physical and social health, it does not use items reflecting somatic symptoms and therefore avoids the problems that beset the earlier scales such as the HOS and the Langner scale. Fuller results from the Rand study will shortly be available, and these will provide further evidence on validity and reliability of the scale. Factor analyses supported the hypothesized distinction between mental and physical factors; this would appear to indicate the desirability of presenting separate scores for distress and well-being (1). From the early results obtained using this scale, we recommend that it be seriously considered as an alternative to the General Well-Being Schedule in general population surveys because more published material is available and because it appears to have extended the scope of Dupuy's scale. A direct comparison of the sensitivity and specificity of the two methods would be beneficial.

Address

John E. Ware, Jr, The Rand Corporation, 1700 Main Street, Santa Monica, California, USA 90406

References

(1) Veit CT, Ware JE Jr. The structure of psychological distress and well-being in general populations. J Consult Clin Psychol 1983;51:730–742.
(2) Ware JE Jr, Johnston SA, Davies-Avery A, Brook RH. Conceptualization and measurement of health for adults in the Health Insurance Study: Vol. III, Mental Health. Santa Monica, California: Rand Corporation, 1979. (R-1987/3-HEW).
(3) Ware JE Jr, Manning WG Jr, Duan N, Wells KB, Newhouse JP. Health status and the use of ambulatory mental health services. Am Psychol 1984;39:1090–1100.
(4) Ware JE Jr, Davies-Avery A, Brook RH. Conceptualization and measurement of health for adults in the Health Insurance Study: Vol. VI, Analysis of relationships among health status measures. Santa Monica, California: Rand Corporation, 1980. (R-1987/6-HEW).

THE GENERAL HEALTH QUESTIONNAIRE
(David Goldberg, 1972)

Purpose

The General Health Questionnaire (GHQ) is a self-administered screening instrument designed to detect current, diagnosable psychiatric disorders. The method may be used in surveys or clinical settings to identify potential cases, leaving the task of diagnosing actual disorder to a psychiatric interview (1).

Conceptual Basis

The GHQ is designed to identify two main classes of problem: "inability to carry out one's normal 'healthy' functions, and the appearance of new phenomena of a distressing nature" (2). It focuses on breaks in normal functioning rather than on life-long traits; therefore it only covers personality disorders or patterns of adjustment (such as homosexuality) where these are associated with distress. The GHQ was not intended to detect severe illness such as schizophrenia or psychotic depression, although subsequent experience with the scale suggests that these conditions are detected (3).

The GHQ was designed to cover four identifiable elements of distress: depression, anxiety, social impairment and hypochondriasis (chiefly indicated by organic symptoms) (1). Subsequent empirical analyses of the factor structure of the GHQ have largely confirmed this coverage (4). Goldberg suggests that his approach to psychiatric disorder is close to the lowest level of the hierarchy of mental illness outlined by Foulds and Bedford, which they term "dysthymic states." "An individual falling into any of these states might be said to be *disturbed,* emotionally stirred up, altered in this respect from his normal self" (3). Such individuals will be prone to minor somatic symptoms and may show outwardly observable changes in social behaviors.

Although the GHQ does cover separate types of distress, it is not intended to distinguish among psychiatric disorders or to be used in making diagnoses. No assumptions were made concerning a hierarchy among the symptoms included in the questionnaire: probable cases are identified on the basis of checking any 12 or more of the 60 symptoms included, and the results express the likelihood of psychiatric disorder.

Description

The GHQ was designed for use in general population surveys, in primary medical care settings or among general medical outpatients (3). It was meant to be a first-stage screening instrument for psychiatric illness that could then be verified and diagnosed. The questions ask whether the respondent has recently experienced a particular symptom (like abnormal feelings or thoughts) or type of behavior. Emphasis is on changes in condition, not on the absolute level of the problem, so items compare the present state to the person's normal situation with responses ranging from "less than usual" to "much more than usual" (3). The questionnaire begins with relatively neutral questions, and leads to the more overtly psychiatric items towards the end. The questions were drawn from existing instruments or were written especially, and those that discriminated between severely ill, mildly ill psychiatric patients and healthy people were retained. Details of the item selection procedure are given by Goldberg (1, 3). The GHQ is normally completed by the patient; Goldberg reports that more than 95% of respondents could do this and were "remarkably frank about admitting symptoms."

The main version of the GHQ, shown in Exhibit 4.8, contains 60 items, and Goldberg recommends using this version where possible because of its superior validity. However, from the outset Goldberg proposed alternative, shorter versions for use where all 60 questions could not be asked. These include 30-, 20- and 12-item abbreviations, and the GHQ-28 or "Scaled GHQ" that contains items selected via factor analyses (2). We show the items included in the abbreviated versions in Exhibit 4.9. Note that the exhibits give the original wording of the items; some may be rephrased using an American idiom and these are shown under the heading "Alternative Forms." The GHQ-28 provides four scores, measuring somatic symptoms, anxiety and insomnia, social dysfunction, and severe depression, and is intended for studies in which an investigator requires more information than is provided by a single severity score (2). There is only a partial overlap between the GHQ-28 and the GHQ-30, which share just 14 items. The 30-, 20- and 12-item versions are balanced in terms of "agreement sets"—that is, in each version half of the questions are worded to indicate illness if answered "yes" and half indicate illness if answered "no." The shortened versions also discard 12 questions that were answered positively by physically ill patients (1). It takes 6 to 8 minutes to complete the GHQ-60, and 3 to 4 minutes for the GHQ-30 (3).

Items may be scored using conventional 0-1-2-3 Likert scores for the response categories shown in Exhibit 4.8. Alternatively, a two-point score rates problems as present or absent, ignoring frequency (3). In the latter approach, known as "the GHQ score," replies are coded 0-0-1-1. Comparing the two scoring methods, Goldberg found little advantage to the Likert approach and recommended the simpler system (2). Correlations between the two scoring methods lie between 0.92 and 0.94 (5, Table 3). Individual item discriminant weights were tried but held little advantage, so were discarded in the interests of simplicity. Scores can be interpreted as indicating the severity of psychological disturbance on a continuum; as a screening test the score expresses the probability of being a psychiatric case. Any 12 positive answers on the GHQ-60 identify a probable case. Cutting points for the other versions are as follows: 4/5 for the GHQ-30 and GHQ-28, and 3/4 for the GHQ-20. At the cutting point the probability of being a case is 0.5. A cutting point of 2/3 has been tested for the GHQ-12 (5). These threshold scores may have to be altered depending on the expected prevalence of disorder and according to the purpose of the study: prevalence surveys versus detection of severe disorders, for example. Cutting points of 9/10, 10/11 or 11/12 have been used for the GHQ-60 (3).

Exhibit 4.8 The General Health Questionnaire (60-Item Version)

Please read this carefully:

We should like to know if you have had any medical complaints, and how your health has been in general, *over the past few weeks.* Please answer ALL the questions on the following pages simply by underlining the answer which you think most nearly applies to you. Remember that we want to know about present and recent complaints, not those that you had in the past.

It is important that you try to answer ALL the questions.

Thank you very much for your co-operation.

HAVE YOU RECENTLY:

1. — *been feeling perfectly well and in good health?*	Better than usual	Same as usual	Worse than usual	Much worse than usual
2. — *been feeling in need of a good tonic?*	Not at all	No more than usual	Rather more than usual	Much more than usual
3. — *been feeling run-down and out of sorts?*	Not at all	No more than usual	Rather more than usual	Much more than usual
4. — *felt that you are ill?*	Not at all	No more than usual	Rather more than usual	Much more than usual
5. — *been getting any pains in your head?*	Not at all	No more than usual	Rather more than usual	Much more than usual
6. — *been getting a feeling of tightness or pressure in your head?*	Not at all	No more than usual	Rather more than usual	Much more than usual
7. — *been able to concentrate on whatever you're doing?*	Better than usual	Same as usual	Less than usual	Much less than usual
8. — *been afraid that you were going to collapse in a public place?*	Not at all	No more than usual	Rather more than usual	Much more than usual
9. — *been having hot or cold spells?*	Not at all	No more than usual	Rather more than usual	Much more than usual
10. — *been perspiring (sweating) a lot?*	Not at all	No more than usual	Rather more than usual	Much more than usual
11. — *found yourself waking early and unable to get back to sleep?*	Not at all	No more than usual	Rather more than usual	Much more than usual
12. — *been getting up feeling your sleep hasn't refreshed you?*	Not at all	No more than usual	Rather more than usual	Much more than usual
13. — *been feeling too tired and exhausted even to eat?*	Not at all	No more than usual	Rather more than usual	Much more than usual

Exhibit 4.8 (continued)

HAVE YOU RECENTLY:

14. — *lost much sleep over worry?*	Not at all	No more than usual	Rather more than usual	Much more than usual
15. — *been feeling mentally alert and wide awake?*	Better than usual	Same as usual	Less alert than usual	Much less alert
16. — *been feeling full of energy?*	Better than usual	Same as usual	Less energy than usual	Much less energetic
17. — *had difficulty in getting off to sleep?*	Not at all	No more than usual	Rather more than usual	Much more than usual
18. — *had difficulty in staying asleep once you are off?*	Not at all	No more than usual	Rather more than usual	Much more than usual
19. — *been having frightening or unpleasant dreams?*	Not at all	No more than usual	Rather more than usual	Much more than usual
20. — *been having restless, disturbed nights?*	Not at all	No more than usual	Rather more than usual	Much more than usual
21. — *been managing to keep yourself busy and occupied?*	More so than usual	Same as usual	Rather less than usual	Much less than usual
22. — *been taking longer over the things you do?*	Quicker than usual	Same as usual	Longer than usual	Much longer than usual
23. — *tended to lose interest in your ordinary activities?*	Not at all	No more than usual	Rather more than usual	Much more than usual
24. — *been losing interest in your personal appearance?*	Not at all	No more than usual	Rather more than usual	Much more than usual
25. — *been taking less trouble with your clothes?*	More trouble than usual	About same as usual	Less trouble than usual	Much less trouble
26. — *been getting out of the house as much as usual?*	More than usual	Same as usual	Less than usual	Much less than usual
27. — *been managing as well as most people would in your shoes?*	Better than most	About the same	Rather less well	Much less well
28. — *felt on the whole you were doing things well?*	Better than usual	About the same	Less well than usual	Much less well
29. — *been late getting to work, or getting started on your housework?*	Not at all	No later than usual	Rather later than usual	Much later than usual

30. — *been satisfied with the way you've carried out your task?*	More satisfied	About same as usual	Less satisfied than usual	Much less satisfied
31. — *been able to feel warmth and affection for those near to you?*	Better than usual	About same as usual	Less well than usual	Much less well
32. — *been finding it easy to get on with other people?*	Better than usual	About same as usual	Less well than usual	Much less well
33. — *spent much time chatting with people?*	More time than usual	About same as usual	Less than usual	Much less than usual
34. — *kept feeling afraid to say anything to people in case you made a fool of yourself?*	Not at all	No more than usual	Rather more than usual	Much more than usual
35. — *felt that you are playing a useful part in things?*	More so than usual	Same as usual	Less useful than usual	Much less useful
36. — *felt capable of making decisions about things?*	More so than usual	Same as usual	Less so than usual	Much less capable
37. — *felt you're just not able to make a start on anything?*	Not at all	No more than usual	Rather more than usual	Much more than usual
38. — *felt yourself dreading everything that you have to do?*	Not at all	No more than usual	Rather more than usual	Much more than usual
39. — *felt constantly under strain?*	Not at all	No more than usual	Rather more than usual	Much more than usual
40. — *felt you couldn't overcome your difficulties?*	Not at all	No more than usual	Rather more than usual	Much more than usual
41. — *been finding life a struggle all the time?*	Not at all	No more than usual	Rather more than usual	Much more than usual
42. — *been able to enjoy your normal day-to-day activities?*	More so than usual	Same as usual	Less so than usual	Much less than usual
43. — *been taking things hard?*	Not at all	No more than usual	Rather more than usual	Much more than usual
44. — *been getting edgy and bad-tempered?*	Not at all	No more than usual	Rather more than usual	Much more than usual
45. — *been getting scared or panicky for no good reason?*	Not at all	No more than usual	Rather more than usual	Much more than usual

143

Exhibit 4.8 *(continued)*

HAVE YOU RECENTLY:

46. — *been able to face up to your problems?*	More so than usual	Same as usual	Less able than usual	Much less able
47. — *found everything getting on top of you?*	Not at all	No more than usual	Rather more than usual	Much more than usual
48. — *had the feeling that people were looking at you?*	Not at all	No more than usual	Rather more than usual	Much more than usual
49. — *been feeling unhappy and depressed?*	Not at all	No more than usual	Rather more than usual	Much more than usual
50. — *been losing confidence in yourself?*	Not at all	No more than usual	Rather more than usual	Much more than usual
51. — *been thinking of yourself as a worthless person?*	Not at all	No more than usual	Rather more than usual	Much more than usual
52. — *felt that life is entirely hopeless?*	Not at all	No more than usual	Rather more than usual	Much more than usual
53. — *been feeling hopeful about your own future?*	More so than usual	About same as usual	Less so than usual	Much less hopeful
54. — *been feeling reasonably happy, all things considered?*	More so than usual	About same as usual	Less so than usual	Much less than usual
55. — *been feeling nervous and strung-up all the time?*	Not at all	No more than usual	Rather more than usual	Much more than usual
56. — *felt that life isn't worth living?*	Not at all	No more than usual	Rather more than usual	Much more than usual
57. — *thought of the possibility that you might make away with yourself?*	Definitely not	I don't think so	Has crossed my mind	Definitely have
58. — *found at times you couldn't do anything because your nerves were too bad?*	Not at all	No more than usual	Rather more than usual	Much more than usual
59. — *found yourself wishing you were dead and away from it all?*	Not at all	No more than usual	Rather more than usual	Much more than usual
60. — *found that the idea of taking your own life kept coming into your mind?*	Definitely not	I don't think so	Has crossed my mind	Definitely has

Copyright © General Practice Research Unit 1968
(de Crespigny Park, London, S.E. 5)

Reproduced from Goldberg DP. The detection of psychiatric illness by questionnaire. London: Oxford University Press, 1972, Appendix 8. With permission.

144

Exhibit 4.9 Abbreviated Versions of the General Health Questionnaire

Note: Using the item numbers from Exhibit 4.8, the contents of the shortened versions are as follows:

GHQ-12

7. able to concentrate
14. lost sleep over worry
35. playing a useful part
36. capable of making decisions
39. constantly under strain
40. couldn't overcome difficulties

42. enjoy normal activities
46. face up to problems
49. unhappy and depressed
50. losing confidence in yourself
51. thinking of yourself as worthless
54. feeling reasonably happy

GHQ-20

In addition to the 12 items above, the 20-item version includes:

21. busy and occupied
26. getting out of house as usual
28. doing things well
30. satisfied with carrying out task

43. taking things hard
47. everything on top of you
55. nervous and strung-up
58. nerves too bad

Note: Item 30 is replaced by item 15 for use in the United States (3, p19).

GHQ-30

In addition to the 20 items above, the 30-item version includes:

20. restless, disturbed nights
27. managing as well as most people
31. feel warmth and affection
32. easy to get on with others
33. much time chatting

41. life a struggle all the time
45. scared or panicky
52. life entirely hopeless
53. hopeful about your future
56. life not worth living

Note: Item 33 is replaced by item 16 for use in the United States (3, p19).

GHQ-28

The 28-item version is as follows:

Scale A Somatic Symptoms	Scale B Anxiety and Insomnia
1. feeling perfectly well	14. lost sleep over worry
2. in need of a good tonic	18. difficulty staying asleep
3. run down	39. constantly under strain
4. felt that you are ill	44. edgy and bad-tempered
5. pains in head	45. scared or panicky
6. pressure in your head	47. everything on top of you
9. hot or cold spells	55. nervous and strung-up

Scale C Social Dysfunction	Scale D Severe Depression
21. busy and occupied	51. thinking of yourself as worthless
22. taking longer over things	52. life entirely hopeless
28. doing things well	56. life not worth living
30. satisfied with carrying out task	57. make away with yourself
35. playing a useful part	58. nerves too bad
36. capable of making decisions	59. dead and away from it all
42. enjoy normal activities	60. idea of taking your life

Adapted from Goldberg DP. The detection of psychiatric illness by questionnaire. London: Oxford University Press, 1972, Appendix 6.

Reliability

The test–retest coefficient after six months was 0.90 (N = 20) when the stability of the patient's condition was confirmed by repeating a standard psychiatric examination (3, p15). For another 65 patients who judged their own condition as having remained "about the same," the retest coefficient was 0.75 (3).

Split-half reliability on the 60-item version was 0.95 for 853 respondents (3). The equivalent value for the GHQ-30 was 0.92, for the GHQ-20, 0.90 and for the GHQ-12, 0.83 (1, Table 27). Chan and Chan reported an alpha of 0.85 for a clinical version of the GHQ-30 (6, Table 1).

Inter-rater reliability for 12 interviews showed a disagreement on only 4% of symptom scores (7, p 410).

Validity

The General Health Questionnaire is probably the most thoroughly tested of the methods that we review in this book. Validation studies have been undertaken in many different countries and most have used directly comparable procedures.

Goldberg provided a table summarizing five studies that compared the GHQ-60 with a standardized psychiatric interview that he developed, the Clinical Interview Schedule (3, 8). Results from studies in England, Australia and Spain were very consistent, with correlations between the two scales ranging from 0.76 to 0.81. Sensitivity values ranged from 81% to 91%; specificity results in four of the studies ranged between 88% and 94%, while in the remaining study it was 73% (3, Table 4.1). Subsequent studies have also given comparable results: Hobbs et al. reported a correlation of 0.72 with the Clinical Interview Schedule, and sensitivity results between 84% and 96% at specificities from 70% to 91% (9, Table IV). Slightly lower figures were obtained by Nott and Cutts with postpartum women (7).

Somewhat less adequate results were obtained by Benjamin et al., who applied the GHQ-60 to 92 women aged 40 to 49 years (10). They obtained a sensitivity of 54.5% at a specificity of 91.5%, and a Spearman correlation of 0.63 with the Clinical Interview Schedule (10). On further examination, the false negatives proved to be those who had long-standing disorders (see "Commentary"). Comparisons of the GHQ and the Present State Examination were made in England and India, giving correlations between 0.71 and 0.88 (3, Table 4.1).

Turning to the abbreviated versions of the GHQ, four studies of the 30-item scale have shown sensitivity values between 71% and 91%, at specificities in the same range (3, 11). Sensitivity for the GHQ-28 was 85.6% at a specificity of 86.8% (3, p22). We present comparative data on the sensitivity and specificity of four versions of the GHQ in Table 4.2 (from 1, Table 27). The same analysis was repeated for 120 general practice patients in Sydney, Australia, by Tennant with sensitivities ranging from 86.6% to 90%, and specificities ranging from 90% to 94.4% (12, Table 1). Rather lower figures were obtained comparing GHQ-30 scores with the Schedule for Affective Disorders and Schizophre-

Table 4.2 A Comparison of the Sensitivity and Specificity Results for Four Versions of the General Health Questionnaire

Note: The patients completed the GHQ-60. Validity estimates for the shortened versions were calculated by analyzing subsets of questions from the 60-item version.

	General practice patients		Hospital outpatients	
	Sensitivity %	Specificity %	Sensitivity %	Specificity %
GHQ-60	95.7	87.8	80.6	93.3
GHQ-30	91.4	87.0	64.5	91.6
GHQ-20	88.2	86.0	64.5	96.7
GHQ-12	93.5	78.5	74.2	95.0

nia with a sensitivity of 68% and a specificity of 81% (13, Table 3). A comparison of the GHQ-28, 30 and 12 with young respondents showed the GHQ-28 was superior when compared with the Present State Examination (5). Correlations among the three abbreviated GHQ scales fell between 0.85 and 0.97 (5, Table 3).

Tarnopolovsky et al. examined the sensitivity and specificity of the 30-item GHQ as compared with the Clinical Interview Schedule, producing results that appear to be at odds with those reviewed above. The sensitivity results varied according to the prevalence of the disorder in the study population. When half of the population scored above the cutting point, the sensitivity was 78%. Using statistical manipulations, Tarnopolovsky estimated that the sensitivity would fall to 54% as the ratio of high to low scoring cases falls to 22%. Kendall's tau correlations with the interview schedule ranged from 0.34 to 0.45 (11, Table V).

The validity results of the GHQ may be compared with those obtained using rival screening tests. Goldberg provided a table summarizing the results from which we drew the comparisons shown in Table 4.3 (1, Table 32).

The correlation of the GHQ-30 with the Hopkins Symptom Checklist of physical and psychological symptoms was 0.78 (14, p65); the GHQ showed slightly higher sensitivity and specificity values (3).

Table 4.3 Comparison of the Validity of the General Health Questionnaire with that of Other Scales

	Sensitivity %	Specificity %	Overall misclassification %
GHQ-60	95.7	87.8	10.3
GHQ-30	85.0	79.5	19.1
Cornell Index	73.5	81.7	17.8
HOS (Macmillan)	75–84	54–68	22–40
22-Item Scale (Langner)	73.5	81.7	17.8

The validity of the GHQ-28 was reviewed by Goldberg and Hillier. The correlation of the overall score with the Clinical Interview Schedule was 0.76 (2, Table 5). A correlation of 0.73 was obtained with the clinical depression rating, and of 0.67 with the anxiety rating. Using a cutting point of 4/5, the sensitivity was 88%, the specificity 84.2%, and the overall misclassification rate was 14.5% (2).

Goldberg summarized data on the association between the GHQ and demographic variables. Females tended to show higher scores; there was little clear association between age and GHQ scores, although there was a significant tendency for lower social class respondents to have higher scores (3).

The factor structure of the GHQ was studied by Goldberg and used as a basis for abbreviating the scale. Several analyses produced relatively consistent factors: somatic symptoms, sleep disturbance (sometimes combined with anxiety), social dysfunction and severe depression (3; 4, Table 5). In subsequent studies Hobbs extracted three factors, covering debility (failure to cope), depression and somatic symptoms (9).

A factor analysis of the 30-item version identified factors covering depression and anxiety, insomnia and lack of energy, social functioning and anhedonia (unhappiness) (14). Cleary et al. reported similar findings from analyses of 1,072 respondents in Wisconsin (13). A Chinese study identified five factors: anxiety, inadequate coping, depression, insomnia and social dysfunction (6). Scales in the GHQ-28 (selected via factor analysis) measure somatic symptoms, anxiety and insomnia, social dysfunction and severe depression. These scales are not independent of each other: correlations range from 0.33 to 0.58 (2, Table 9). A factor analysis of the GHQ-12 from an Australian sample provided three factors: anhedonia and sleep disturbance, social performance, and loss of confidence (4). The evidence available suggests that several of the GHQ factors are stable across samples and among different versions of the questionnaire.

Alternative Forms

The GHQ was developed in England, but with the clear objective of making comparative studies of psychiatric illness in England and the United States. Several of the items are rephrased for American use (1, 3):

2. ____ been feeling in need of some medicine to pick you up?
18. ____ had difficulty staying asleep?
27. ____ been managing as well as most people would in your place?
47. ____ found everything getting too much for you?
55. ____ been feeling nervous and uptight (or hung up) all the time?
57. ____ thought of the possibility that you might do away with yourself?

Commentary

The General Health Questionnaire offers a leading example of how a health measurement method should be developed. It was well founded on a clear conceptual approach, the initial item selection and item analyses are fully documented, and the questions have not been revised by subsequent users. The validation studies have been thorough and extensive; they have used comparable approaches and have consistently indicated a high degree of validity, markedly higher than that of rival methods. The scale has been tested in numerous countries and shows remarkably consistent validity results. Goldberg's book (1) is a model of clarity and thoroughness; unfortunately, the manual of the GHQ does not contain copies of the questionnaire (3).

Most of the criticisms that have been raised over the GHQ reflect limitations imposed by the deliberate design of the instrument. The response categories ask whether each symptom is worse than usual, and if a person has suffered a symptom for a long time and has come to consider it "usual," the scale will not identify this as a problem. Benjamin et al. viewed this as a limitation of the scale, although Goldberg developed the GHQ to measure changes in a person's condition and not the absolute level of the problem (10). It screens, therefore, for acute rather than chronic conditions. There has also been some dispute over the suitability of the items in the GHQ-60 that reflect physical symptoms ("feeling of tightness or pressure in your head," "perspiring a lot"). The physical items were excluded from the abbreviated versions of the GHQ as they produced a number of false positive responses, although the problem seems to be far less serious than it is with Macmillan's HOS. Tennant, however, noted that "all false positives were subjects with substantial physical illness" (12): the difficulty of using somatic questions to screen for psychiatric disorders may still not have been resolved. The main dissonant note in the validation studies comes from Tarnopolovsky's study, which suggests that sensitivity rates may be lower than those obtained by Goldberg (11). However, Tarnopolovsky's study was small, and used estimation procedures to model changes in sensitivity rather than actual empirical evidence, so it should be replicated before we accept that its results are valid. The GHQ is most useful as part of a medical consultation, and has seen widespread use in general practice for screening for mental disorders. We highly recommend it for these applications.

Address

David Goldberg, Professor, Department of Psychiatry, University Hospital of South Manchester, West Didsbury, Manchester, England M20 8LR

References

(1) Goldberg DP. The detection of psychiatric illness by questionnaire. London: Oxford University Press, 1972. (Maudsley Monograph No. 21).

(2) Goldberg DP, Hillier VF. A scaled version of the General Health Questionnaire. Psychol Med 1979;9:139–145.

(3) Goldberg D. Manual of the General Health Questionnaire. Windsor, England: NFER Publishing, 1978.

(4) Worsley A, Gribbin CC. A factor analytic study of the twelve item General Health Questionnaire. Aust NZ J Psychiatry 1977;11:269–272.

(5) Banks MH. Validation of the General Health Questionnaire in a young community sample. Psychol Med 1983;13:340–353.

(6) Chan DW, Chan TSC. Reliability, validity and the structure of the General Health Questionnaire in a Chinese context. Psychol Med 1983;13:363–371.

(7) Nott PN, Cutts S. Validation of the 30-item General Health Questionnaire in postpartum women. Psychol Med 1982;12:409–413.

(8) Goldberg DP, Cooper B, Eastwood MR, Kedward HB, Shepherd M. A standardized psychiatric interview for use in community surveys. Br J Prev Soc Med 1970;24:18–23.

(9) Hobbs P, Ballinger CB, Smith AHW. Factor analysis and validation of the General Health Questionnaire in women: a general practice survey. Br J Psychiatry 1983; 142:257–264.

(10) Benjamin S, Decalmer P, Haran D. Community screening for mental illness: a validity study of the General Health Questionnaire. Br J Psychiatry 1982; 140:174–180.

(11) Tarnopolovsky A, Hand DJ, McLean EK, Roberts H, Wiggins RD. Validity and uses of a screening questionnaire (GHQ) in the community. Br J Psychiatry 1979;134:508–515.

(12) Tennant C. The General Health Questionnaire: a valid index of psychological impairment in Australian populations. Med J Aust 1977;2:392–394.

(13) Cleary PD, Goldberg ID, Kessler LG, Nycz GR. Screening for mental disorder among primary care patients. Arch Gen Psychiatry 1982;39:837–840.

(14) Goldberg DP, Rickels K, Downing R, Hesbacher P. A comparison of two psychiatric screening tests. Br J Psychiatry 1976;129:61–67.

CONCLUSION

The more recent measurements presented in this chapter show evidence of considerable refinement in a field that was initially beset by unclear objectives and methodological disputes. The conceptual basis of the more recent scales, their statement of purpose and their interpretation are all far more clearly spelled out than was the case for the early methods. The newer methods have generally been used without changes to the question wording, thus enhancing the comparability of results across different studies.

The major lessons to be learned relate to the conceptual formulation of an index. This area of measurement is inherently less specific than that of physical disability, and immense effort has been expended on debating what the scales measure. While the results of validation studies show the HOS or the Langner scale capable of screening for clinically identifiable disorders, they do not offer differential diagnoses in the traditional way that psychiatrists classify mental disorders. As we noted above, they represent the psychological counterpart of Selye's notion of stress, the nonspecific element common to a variety of disorders that warn the observer that something is wrong but do not specify what. This idea may have been clear to the originators of the early scales, but if so, it was not sufficiently explained to prevent subsequent users from misinterpreting or overinterpreting the scales. Newer measurements have provided more explicit definitions of how they should and should not be interpreted, and of what high scores do and do not indicate.

We have also seen that there are serious disadvantages to making piecemeal alterations to the questions in a scale. If changes become necessary, it would be well to indicate this by altering the title, perhaps by adding a version number, similar to the approach used by Goldberg. We would also wish to discourage premature publication of draft questionnaires. Because of the pressure to publish in academic circles, draft forms of a measurement are frequently published and it then becomes difficult to ensure that users apply the final, definitive version.

The current status of this area of general psychological measurement is best summarized in terms of the individual measurement methods. The Goldberg scale provides a good method for screening for general psychological and psychiatric disorder. It has been used internationally, and many validation studies have demonstrated its psychometric qualities. The field of more subjective feelings of well-being is currently represented by Dupuy's scale, although the Bradburn questions continue to see some use. This may be because of the unfortunate lack of published validation studies on Dupuy's scale. It is disappointing that a scale of the potential of the General Well-Being Schedule does not benefit from a manual such as that produced by Goldberg for the General Health Questionnaire. The gap in the field of subjective well-being covered for so many years by the Bradburn scale was only partially covered by the Goldberg and Dupuy methods. More recently, this gap has been filled by the Rand scale, which expands the scope of the General Well-Being Schedule by adding a number of positive items. This provides a good example of the planned and systematic development of a measurement method that reflects the current state of conceptual development and builds deliberately on existing measurements.

5
Social Health

The theme of social health is less familiar to us and is less frequently discussed, measured and researched than the topics of physical and psychological health. Being less familiar, several potential misconceptions about social health must be addressed at the outset. As the word "social" does not refer to a characteristic of individuals, it is not immediately clear how a person can be rated in terms of social health. And, indeed, there is an important tradition of regarding social health as a characteristic of society rather than of individuals:

> A society is healthy when there is equal opportunity for all and access by all to the goods and services essential to full functioning as a citizen. (1, p75).

Indicators of social health in this sense might include the distribution of economic wealth, the public accessibility of the decision-making process, or the accountability of public officials. In keeping with our approach in this book, however, we will not discuss indicators of the health of a society, but will consider only measurements of the rather less intuitively obvious concept of the social health of individuals. A representative definition of this theme would be:

> Social health is that dimension of an individual's well-being that concerns how he gets along with other people, how other people react to him, and how he interacts with social institutions and societal mores. (1, p75).

The definition is broad; it incorporates elements of personality and social skills and it also in part reflects the norms of the society in which the individual finds himself. In fact, most measurements of the social health of individuals do not employ the word "healthy," but speak instead of "well-being," "adjustment," "performance" or "social functioning." Why, then, should we regard this sphere of human interaction as a part of health at all?

Since the WHO definition of health, the emphasis on treating patients as social beings who live in a complex social context has permeated many branches of medicine. This approach holds that the ultimate aim of medical care should be to reintegrate the individual into a normal, productive life in society, rather than merely to treat his medical symptoms. This philosophy created a demand for new measurement scales to assess need for care and to evaluate outcomes. But aside from the philosophical appeal of considering social adjustment as a component of health, there are strictly practical reasons for measuring an individual's social well-being and social adjustment. The expense of institutional care and the resulting emphasis on discharging patients as early as possible implies a need to assess the ability of patients to live independently in the community. The movement away from institutional care in the mental health field, which has been responsible for partially emptying and sometimes closing large mental hospitals, has fostered studies of the quality of adjustment to community living or social functioning, especially among older patients (2). Studies of this type are equally relevant in the area of physical rehabilitation, and indices of social functioning can be used to evaluate the outcomes of rehabilitation in terms of social restoration: has the individual returned to a productive and stable position in society (3)? A further reason to measure social health, albeit in a slightly different sense, is to examine the influence of social support and social ties on a person's physical and psychological well-being. This treats the social adjustment not as a dependent, but as an independent, variable. Reviews of this field are given by Antonovsky (4), Berkman and Breslow (5), and Murawski et al. (6).

These contrasting ways of defining social health—in terms of adjustment, social support or the ability to perform normal roles in society—and the measurements that have been developed for each are further examined in the following sections.

SOCIAL ADJUSTMENT AND SOCIAL ROLES

The approach to social health that views it in terms of social or community adjustment derived primarily from the work of sociologists and, in the health field, of psychiatrists. Psychiatric interest in social health arose because problems in personal or social relationships and communication represent the commonest reason for seeking care for nonpsychotic mental disorders. The adequacy of a person's social interaction and adjustment may therefore serve to indicate need for care and to measure outcomes, especially for psychotherapy. The development of scales to measure adjustment also coincided with a gradual shift in psychiatry away from medical concepts of mental illness, emphasizing disease or deviance, towards a concern with mental distress viewed in terms of inadequate social integration and adjustment: can the individual function adequately in his personal relationships? This is most commonly expressed as social adjustment, broadly definable in terms of the interplay between the individual and his social environment (7). Linn has viewed adjustment in a dynamic sense, covering the person's equilibrium or success in reducing tensions and in satisfying needs (2). Interest in social adjustment is, of course, not peculiar to psychiatry: schools do more than teach a child to read and write, for they stress the importance of learning to function as a social being.

Social adjustment may be measured either by considering a person's satisfaction with his relationships, or by studying his performance of various social roles. The subjective approach to measuring social adjustment records affective responses such as discontent, unhappiness (as measured, for example, by Linn's Social Dysfunction Rating Scale), and anxiety. This area of measurement is diffuse, and there are no clear boundaries between measurements of social health in this sense and measurements of life satisfaction, happiness or quality of life. These scales are therefore often subsumed under the general heading of "subjective well-being," but we have attempted to form a finer classification. Measurement of happiness and general affective well-being that are not specifically related to social relationships, such as the Bradburn scale, are included in Chapter 4 on psychological well-being. Measurements of affective responses that focus on social relationships in particular are included in the present chapter (e.g., Linn's scale). Measurements of related themes such as life satisfaction, quality of life and adjustment are included in Chapter 6 on life satisfaction.

One of the major problems with measurements of social adjustment is that of selecting an appropriate standard against which to evaluate adjustment. Standards of social adjustment vary greatly from one culture to another, ranging from an emphasis on "oneness with nature" and rejection of worldly values in oriental cultures to an emphasis on material possessions in certain sectors of contemporary Western society (3). Expectations also vary among social classes within a culture, making it difficult to compare adjustment across different times and places. The most common way to avoid these problems is to focus the measurement on specific social roles for which there is some agreement about appropriate behavior.

The social role approach to assessing adjustment is based loosely on sociological role theory and implies a valuation: how adequately is the person performing compared to normal social expectations? A person who cannot function in a way that meets the normal demands of his situation may be considered as socially disabled (8). Although this does not eliminate the problem of defining what is normal, there are, at least, recognized norms for many defined roles. These may be formally couched in the law, or in less formal regulations, traditions, or agreements among individuals. Although approaches based on norms seem to offer promise, they are not sufficiently refined to indicate what should be included in a social health questionnaire. Ultimately the selection of topics appears to be a more or less arbitrary process. Most operational definitions of social roles consider housework, occupation, community involvement, marital and parental roles, and leisure activities. It will be noted that most of these topics are also covered in the IADL scales (see Chapter 3), so that the role approach to measuring social health brings it conceptually very close to indices of physical handicap. A social role approach is used in the measurement methods of Weissman and of Gurland, reviewed in this chapter.

There are several conceptual problems with using role theory as an approach to measuring social health. Assumptions have to be made over how to evaluate performance: should it be compared to some ideal, to the person's own aspirations or to other peoples' expectations of his performance? The first tends to be insufficient: while there are recognized norms for much behavior, there is little consensus over what constitutes a socially "correct" definition of the marital role, for example. Norms vary between social strata, and there is little agreement over the relative importance of different roles. Alternative approaches also suffer problems: comparing a person's performance against the aspirations of their spouse, for example, makes it hard to evaluate pathology, as the partner may have unrealistically high or low expectations. The role approach has been criticized as being rigid and conservative; it may be impractical to evaluate the legitimacy of individual reasons for not behaving in a "normal" way. Platt argued that the role approach implies viewing the "ideal individual as an object which passively shapes itself to the culture and the external environment. He should be satisfied with his situation and if he is not, then he is not fully adjusted" (9, p103). Pursuing this criterion further, one might argue that the world of the socially healthy is "characterized by harmony, happiness and consensus, and is inhabited by men and women who are consistently interested, active, friendly, adequate, guilt-free, nondistressed and so on. If they show anything less than interest in their work they are maladjusted." (9, p106).

Recognizing these potential problems, several scales such as that of Remington and Tyrer avoid imposing fixed definitions of what constitutes normal or adequate performance. The Katz Adjustment Scales use another approach which combines the objective assessments of the role approach with subjective evaluations of satisfaction made by the respondent: to evaluate how important it is that the individual does or does not fulfill his social role requires information as to how he views that role. This is close to the concept of the Person-Environment Fit; rather than stressing adherence to somewhat arbitrary principles of behavior, the socially healthy person would be one who has found a comfortable niche in which to operate to the best of his capacities, and to the satisfaction of those around him.

SOCIAL SUPPORT

Many studies in the field of social epidemiology have highlighted the importance of social support in attenuating the effects of stressful events and thereby reducing the incidence of disease (10–12). In addition, social support contributes to positive adjustment in the child and adult, and encourages personal growth. Because of the recognition of the importance of social integration and social support, we review some social support scales in this chapter.

Social support is generally defined in terms of the availability of people whom the individual trusts, on whom he can rely, and who make him feel cared for and valued as a person. Social support may be distinguished from the related concept of social networks, which refers to the roles and ties that link individuals along definable paths of kinship, friendship or acquaintance. Social networks may be seen as the structure through which support is provided (13).

An early scale that covered aspects of social support was the Berle Index, published in 1952 (14). Aside from this, there were until recently few formal measurements of social support, and many studies relied on indirect indicators such as marital status or other sociodemographic variables (13). The field has, however, become an important area of growth in sociomedical indices, and several new scales are currently in various stages of testing and refinement. Important stimuli for the development of more formal measurement indices came from conceptual discussions of support, including Bowlby's theories of attachment (15), and from Weiss's work (16). Weiss saw social support as performing both instrumental and expressive functions for the individual: it provides for social integration, nurturance, alliance and guidance, and also fosters feelings of worth and intimacy. Issues in the measurement of social support have included the debate over whether it is the number of social contacts a person has or their quality that is important, and over how to compare the value of formal affiliations and informal friendships. In general, the emphasis now lies with assessing the quality of relationships rather than their number or type.

In this chapter the theme of social support is represented by the scales of Henderson, Sarason and McFarlane, and social support is also covered to some extent in the scale developed by Linn. References to other, more recent scales that are still in the process of development, are given at the end of the chapter. There are also relevant scales in other chapters in the book, such as the Functional Assessment Inventory of Crewe and Athelstan in Chapter 8, which review the resources that may assist a patient in coping with physical handicaps.

SCOPE OF THE CHAPTER

As with other chapters, we have presented the measurements in order of increasing sophistication and complexity. The majority of scales measuring social health assess social adjustment, and this orientation is clearly seen in the selection we present in this chapter. We review two major social adjustment scales: Gurland's Structured and Scaled Interview to Assess Maladjustment and Weissman's Social Adjustment Scale, which was derived from the former. In addition, we review the Social Dysfunction Rating Scale of Linn and the Social Functioning Schedule of Remington and Tyrer which have seen less intensive development than the Gurland or Weissman scales. We present brief reviews of Clare's Social Maladjustment Schedule and of the older but widely used Katz Adjustment Scales covering social performance and satisfaction with this. The theme of social support is represented here by McFarlane's Social Relationship Scale, by the Interview Schedule for Social Interaction of Henderson et al., and by Sarason's Social Support Questionnaire. Finally, the more recent Rand Social Health Battery is included as an approach to measuring social interaction, conceptually close to social support, but concentrating more on the extent of interaction than on its supportive qualities. Table 5.1 provides a quick reference comparison of the format and quality of these scales. The conclusion to the chapter mentions other scales that we considered

Table 5.1 Comparison of the Quality of Social Health Measurements*

Measurement	Scale	Number of items	Application	Administered by (time)	Studies using method	Reliability		Validity	
						Testing thoroughness	Results	Testing thoroughness	Results
Social Relationship Scale (McFarlane)	ordinal	6	research	self (interviewer assisted)	few	+	++	+	0
Social Support Questionnaire (Sarason)	ordinal	27	research	self	several	++	++	++	++
Social Maladjustment Schedule (Clare)	ordinal	42 ratings	clinical, survey	interviewer (45 min)	few	+	+	++	+
Katz Adjustment Scales (Katz)	ordinal	205†	clinical, survey	self	many	+	+	+	?
Social Health Battery (Rand Corporation)	ordinal	11	survey	self	few	++	+	++	+
Social Dysfunction Rating Scale (Linn)	ordinal	21	research	expert	several	+	++	++	++
Social Functioning Schedule (Remington and Tyrer)	ordinal	121	clinical	expert (10–20 min)	few	+	+	++	++
Interview Schedule for Social Interaction (Henderson)	ordinal	52	research, clinical	interviewer (45 min)	few	++	++	+++	++
Structured and Scaled Interview to Assess Maladjustment (SSIAM) (Gurland)	ordinal	60	clinical, research	interviewer (30 min)	several	+	++	++	++
Social Adjustment Scale—SR (Weissman)	ordinal	42	clinical, survey	self (15–20 min)	many	+++	++	+++	+++

*For an explanation of the categories used, see Chapter 1, pages 8–9.
†There are 205 items in the 5 sections of this instrument. The questions can be answered twice, once by the patient and once by a relative.

157

for inclusion, and which may be of value to researchers unable to find what they require in the main review section.

References

(1) Russell RD. Social health: an attempt to clarify this dimension of well-being. Int J Health Educ 1973;16:74–82.

(2) Linn MW. Assessing community adjustment in the elderly. In: Raskin A, Jervik LF, eds. Assessment of psychiatric symptoms and cognitive loss in the elderly. Washington, DC: Hemisphere Press, 1979:187–204.

(3) Berger DG, Rice CE, Sewall LG, Lemkau PV. Posthospital evaluation of psychiatric patients: the Social Adjustment Inventory Method. Psychiatric Studies and Projects 1964;2:2–30.

(4) Antonovsky A. Health, stress, and coping. San Francisco: Jossey-Bass, 1980.

(5) Berkman LF, Breslow L. Health and ways of living: the Alameda County Study. New York: Oxford University Press, 1983.

(6) Murawski BJ, Penman D, Schmitt M. Social support in health and illness: the concept and its measurement. Cancer Nursing 1978;1:365–371.

(7) Weissman MM, Sholomskas D, John K. The assessment of social adjustment: an update. Arch Gen Psychiatry 1981;38:1250–1258.

(8) Ruesch J, Brodsky CM. The concept of social disability. Arch Gen Psychiatry 1968;19:394–403.

(9) Platt S. Social adjustment as a criterion of treatment success: just what are we measuring? Psychiatry 1981;44:95–112.

(10) Broadhead WE, Kaplan BH, James SA, Wagner EH, Schoenbach VJ, Grimson R, Heyden S, Tibblin G, Gehlbach SH. The epidemiologic evidence for a relationship between social support and health. Am J Epidemiol 1983;117:521–537.

(11) Mitchell RE, Billings AG, Moos RH. Social support and well-being: implications for prevention programs. J Primary Prev 1982;3:77–98.

(12) Bruhn JG, Philips BU. Measuring social support: a synthesis of current approaches. J Behav Med 1984;7:151–169.

(13) Lin N, Dean A, Ensel WM. Social support scales: a methodological note. Schizophr Bull 1981;7:73–89.

(14) Berle BB, Pinsky RH, Wolf S, Wolff HG. A clinical guide to prognosis in stress diseases. JAMA 1952;149:1624–1628.

(15) Bowlby J. Attachment and loss. Vol. I, Attachment. London: Hogarth, 1969.

(16) Weiss RS. The provisions of social relationships. In: Rubin Z, ed. Doing unto others. Englewood Cliffs, New Jersey: Prentice-Hall, 1974:17–26.

THE SOCIAL RELATIONSHIP SCALE
(Allan H. McFarlane, 1981)

Purpose

The Social Relationship Scale (SRS) was developed to measure the extent of an individual's network of social relationships and its perceived helpfulness in cushioning the effects of life stresses on health (1). This social support scale was intended primarily as a research instrument for use in studies of life events.

Conceptual Basis

The notion that social support is a buffer against disease formed the stimulus for the development of this scale: social bonds are considered necessary for the individual to cope with adverse events. The scale was designed to summarize the qualitative and quantitative aspects of a person's network of relationships that help him to deal with stresses (1).

Description

The SRS is a self-administered scale that is introduced by a trained interviewer who orients the respondent and who prompts the respondent at the end to review possible relationships that may have been forgotten. The scale originally formed one section in a larger questionnaire concerned with the impact of life changes on emotional well-being (2). The respondent was asked to identify the people who supported him in each of six areas in which he had experienced life changes. The SRS can, however, be used as a social support indicator on its own (Dr. McFarlane, personal communication, 1985).

The scale covers six areas of life change and the question stem and response scale are standard for each. The six areas of life change include: work-related events, monetary and financial events, home and family events, personal health events, personal and social events, and society in general. The format of the scale is shown in Exhibit 5.1. The scale shown in the exhibit is applied six times, referring to each of the six topics listed above. Respondents are asked to give the initials of the person they talked to; the type of relationship (spouse, close family, distant family, friend, fellow worker, professional); the helpfulness of the discussion on a seven-point scale; and whether that person would come to them to discuss similar problems, as an indication of reciprocity in the relationship (2).

Three scores may be calculated. The quality of the network is estimated from the average of the seven-point helpfulness ratings, while the extent of the network is estimated from a count of the total number of different individuals whom the respondent mentions (3). A score reflecting the degree of reciprocity is established by counting the number of people named who the respondent thinks would come to him to discuss similar problems. McFarlane designated a relationship as multiplex if a support person was named in three separate problem areas (2).

Reliability

Test-retest reliability was assessed on 73 students after a one-week interval. Correlations for the numbers of individuals in the person's network ranged from 0.62 to 0.99, with a median of 0.91 (1, p92). Correlations for the helpful-

Exhibit 5.1 Format of the Social Relationship Scale

Example 1: Home and family

Please list the people with whom you generally discuss home and family, using the first name or initials only. After each name or set of initials fill in a one- or two-word description of the relation each person has to you. Then go on to check the circle which indicates the degree of helpfulness or unhelpfulness of your discussions with each person, and lastly, check off yes or no if you feel this person would come to you to discuss home and family. Don't feel you have to fill up all the spaces provided. If you find you need more spaces, please inform the interviewer.

I discuss home and family with:

Name or initials	**Relation**	**Helpfulness of discussion** *(Check one circle)*				**Would this person come to you to discuss home and family?** Yes	No
________	________	makes things a lot worse	makes things a bit worse	helps things a bit	helps things a lot	( )1	( )2
________	________	makes things a lot worse	makes things a bit worse	helps things a bit	helps things a lot	( )1	( )2
________	________	makes things a lot worse	makes things a bit worse	helps things a bit	helps things a lot	( )1	( )2
________	________	makes things a lot worse	makes things a bit worse	helps things a bit	helps things a lot	( )1	( )2
________	________	makes things a lot worse	makes things a bit worse	helps things a bit	helps things a lot	( )1	( )2
________	________	makes things a lot worse	makes things a bit worse	helps things a bit	helps things a lot	( )1	( )2
________	________	makes things a lot worse	makes things a bit worse	helps things a bit	helps things a lot	( )1	( )2
________	________	makes things a lot worse	makes things a bit worse	helps things a bit	helps things a lot	( )1	( )2

Reproduced from McFarlane AH, Neale KA, Norman GR, Roy RJ, Streiner DL. Methodological issues in developing a scale to measure social support. Schizophr Bull 1981;7:91. With permission.

ness score were lower, ranging from 0.54 to 0.94, giving a median of 0.78 (1, p93).

Validity

Content validity was assessed by submitting the preliminary version of the scale to four psychiatrists who made recommendations for improvements that were subsequently incorporated in the scale. Discriminal validity was assessed by comparing 15 couples with known marital or family problems with 18 couples who were judged, in the process of being selected as "parent therapists," to be able to communicate effectively with each other. The scale showed significant differences in its ratings of the marital relationship between these groups. Response bias was also examined, to ascertain whether respondents tended to give socially desirable replies. This was tested on a sample of 19 postgraduate students by altering the question stem so as to deliberately encourage a biased response, and then assessing how far this differed from the responses given with the standard question stem. The results suggested that the standard wording showed significantly less bias towards a socially desirable response in all areas (1).

Reference Standards

McFarlane et al. provided descriptive statistics by sex and marital status for the SRS scores, derived from a sample of 518 general population respondents (1, Table 5).

Commentary

This brief rating scale covers both the quantity of social contacts and their supportive quality, in a manner similar to Sarason's Social Support Questionnaire. The structure of the questionnaire is similar to that used in Part I of the Personal Resource Questionnaire developed by Brandt and Weinert (4). The SRS can be quickly administered; it provides information on both helpful and unhelpful network members, but it does not specify the type of support that is given. McFarlane et al. have used the scale in a study of reactions to life events and have drawn several conclusions concerning the role of social support. For example, the quality of social supports, that is, the helpfulness of relationships, had greater impact than quantity (2). Those who felt least helped by their social networks had larger networks, made more contact with them, and reported more stressful events in their current, as well as their past life (2). The early results of its use appear promising, but before we can fully recommend the SRS, further reliability and validity tests on larger samples and in other centers are necessary.

Address

Allan McFarlane, MD, Department of Psychiatry, McMaster University, 1200 Main Street West, Hamilton, Ontario, Canada L8S 3Z5

References

(1) McFarlane AH, Neale KA, Norman GR, Roy RJ, Streiner DL. Methodological issues in developing a scale to measure social support. Schizophr Bull 1981;7:90–100.

(2) McFarlane AH, Norman GR, Streiner DL, Roy RG. Characteristics and correlates of effective and ineffective social supports. J Psychosom Res 1984;28:501–510.

(3) McFarlane AH, Norman GR, Streiner DL, Roy RG. The process of social stress: stable, reciprocal, and mediating relationships. J Health Soc Behav 1983;24:160–173.

(4) Brandt PA, Weinert C. The PRQ—a social support measure. Nurs Res 1981;30:277–280.

THE SOCIAL SUPPORT QUESTIONNAIRE
(Irwin G. Sarason, 1983)

Purpose

The Social Support Questionnaire (SSQ) is intended to quantify the availability of, and satisfaction with, social support (1). It was designed primarily as a research instrument.

Conceptual Basis

As with McFarlane's scale, the development of this instrument was stimulated by the many studies that link social support with health. Sarason et al. noted that social support contributes to positive adjustment and personal development and provides a buffer against the effects of stress (1). After reviewing alternative conceptual approaches to social support, Sarason et al. focused on two central elements in the concept: the perception that there is a sufficient number of available others to whom a person can turn in times of need and a degree of satisfaction with the support available (1,2).

Description

The SSQ is a 27-item self-administered scale. Each question requires a two-part answer: respondents are asked to list the people to whom they could turn and on whom they could rely in specified sets of circumstances (availability), and to rate how satisfied they are with the available support (satisfaction). A maximum of nine persons can be listed as supports for each item, their identity being indicated by their initials and relationship to the respondent. The satisfaction rating is the same for each item, and uses a six-point scale running from "very satsified" to "very dissatisfied." The instructions and answer categories for the scale are shown in Exhibit 5.2; the 27 items are shown in Exhibit 5.3.

The 27 items were drawn from a larger pool by discarding those with low intercorrelations (1). A support score for each item is the number of support persons listed (the "number score"). The mean of these scores across the 27 items gives an overall support score (SSQN). A satisfaction score (SSQS) is based on the mean of the 27 satisfaction scores.

Exhibit 5.2 The Social Support Questionnaire: Instructions

The following questions ask about people in your environment who provide you with help or support. Each question has two parts. For the first part, list all the people you know, excluding yourself, whom you can count on for help or support in the manner described. Give the person's initials and their relationship to you (see example). Do not list more than one person next to each of the letters beneath the question.

For the second part, circle how satisfied you are with the overall support you have.

If you have no support for a question, check the words "No one," but still rate your level of satisfaction. Do not list more than nine persons per question.

Please answer all questions as best you can. All your responses will be kept confidential.

EXAMPLE

Who do you know whom you can trust with information that could get you in trouble?

No one

1) T.N. (brother)	4) T.N. (father)	7)
2) L.M. (friend)	5) L.N. (employer)	8)
3) R.S. (friend)	6)	9)

How satisfied?

6—very satisfied	5—fairly satisfied	4—a little satisfied	3—a little dissatisfied	2—fairly dissatisfied	1—very dissatisfied

Reproduced from the Social Support Questionnaire obtained from Dr. Irwin G. Sarason. With permission.

Reliability

For the number scores, inter-item correlations ranged from 0.35 to 0.71, with a mean of 0.54. The correlations of each item with the total score (omitting that item from the total score) ranged from 0.51 to 0.79; the alpha coefficient of internal reliability was 0.97. For the satisfaction scores, the inter-item correlations ranged from 0.21 to 0.74, with a coefficient alpha of 0.94 (N = 602) (1, p130).

Test-retest correlations of 0.90 for the overall number score and 0.83 for the satisfaction score were obtained from 105 students after a four-week interval (1, p130).

Validity

Separate factor analyses were performed for the two types of score. In both cases a strong first factor was identified, accounting for 82% of the variance in the numbers score and 72% in the satisfaction score (1). Sarason concluded that the two scores represent different dimensions of social support. The correlation between the number and satisfaction scores have been studied in several samples, and ranged from 0.21 to 0.34 (1, pp130–131).

Criterion validity was studied on samples of psychology students. Significant negative correlations were obtained between the SSQ and a depression scale (correlations ranged from -0.22 to -0.43) (1, Table 2). For females only, both

Exhibit 5.3 The Social Support Questionnaire: Question Stems

Note: The answer categories and the satisfaction question are the same for all questions and are therefore shown only for the first question in the exhibit.

1. Whom can you really count on to listen to you when you need to talk?

No one	1)	4)	7)
	2)	5)	8)
	3)	6)	9)

How satisfied?

| 6—very satisfied | 5—fairly satisfied | 4—a little satisfied | 3—a little dissatisfied | 2—fairly dissatisfied | 1—very dissatisfied |

2. Whom could you really count on to help you if a person whom you thought was a good friend insulted you and told you that he/she didn't want to see you again?
3. Whose lives do you feel that you are an important part of?
4. Whom do you feel would help you if you were married and had just separated from your spouse?
5. Whom could you really count on to help you out in a crisis situation, even though they would have to go out of their way to do so?
6. Whom can you talk with frankly, without having to watch what you say?
7. Who helps you feel that you truly have something positive to contribute to others?
8. Whom can you really count on to distract you from your worries when you feel under stress?
9. Whom can you really count on to be dependable when you need help?
10. Whom could you really count on to help you out if you had just been fired from your job or expelled from school?
11. With whom can you totally be yourself?
12. Whom do you feel really appreciates you as a person?
13. Whom can you really count on to give you useful suggestions that help you to avoid making mistakes?
14. Whom can you count on to listen openly and uncritically to your innermost feelings?
15. Who will comfort you when you need it by holding you in their arms?
16. Whom do you feel would help if a good friend of yours had been in a car accident and was hospitalized in serious condition?
17. Whom can you really count on to help you feel more relaxed when you are under pressure or tense?
18. Whom do you feel would help if a family member very close to you died?
19. Who accepts you totally, including both your worst and your best points?
20. Whom can you really count on to care about you, regardless of what is happening to you?
21. Whom can you really count on to listen to you when you are very angry at someone else?
22. Whom can you really count on to tell you, in a thoughtful manner, when you need to improve in some way?
23. Whom can you really count on to help you feel better when you are feeling generally down-in-the-dumps?
24. Whom do you feel truly loves you deeply?
25. Whom can you count on to console you when you are very upset?
26. Whom can you really count on to support you in major decisions you make?
27. Whom can you really count on to help you feel better when you are very irritable, ready to get angry at almost anything?

Reproduced from the Social Support Questionnaire obtained from Dr. Irwin G. Sarason. With permission.

scales of the SSQ correlated negatively with hostility and lack of protection scales; for both sexes there was a slight, but not significant, correlation between the satisfaction score and a social desirability scale (coefficients ranged from 0.16 to 0.24) (1, Table 2). A correlation of 0.57 was obtained between the satisfaction score and an optimism scale, while the number score correlated 0.34 (1, p132).

With 295 students, a significant association was found between the numbers of positive life events and the number score on the SSQ, with more positive events reported among those with higher SSQ scores (1). Those with more social support also felt more able to control the occurrence of life events (1, Table 3). In a study of 163 men in military training, respondents who had many negative life events and less support showed a higher frequency of chronic illness than other groups (2). From this study, Sarason et al. showed significant agreement between an experimenter's rating of the social competence of the respondent and the number score; those in high and low support groups differed significantly in their scores on a loneliness questionnaire and a social competence questionnaire (3).

Commentary

Of the several social support scales that we reviewed, this appears to be one of the most adequate. Like the alternative scales, however, it is new and therefore requires further evidence for validity and reliability. A great reliance, for example, has been placed on psychology students in the validity studies, and it will be important to assess how the scale performs with other samples, and how it correlates with other social support scales. Nonetheless, we recommend that this scale be considered for use as a social support instrument, and more recent evidence for its validity may be obtainable from Dr. Sarason.

Address

Irwin G. Sarason, PhD, Department of Psychology, University of Washington, Seattle, Washington, USA 98195

References

(1) Sarason IG, Levine HM, Basham RB, Sarason BR. Assessing social support: the Social Support Questionnaire. J Pers Soc Psychol 1983;44:127–139.

(2) Sarason IG, Sarason BR, Potter EH, Antoni MH. Life events, social support, and illness. Psychosom Med 1985;47:156–163.

(3) Sarason BR, Sarason IG, Hacker TA, Basham RB. Concomitants of social support: social skills, physical attractiveness, and gender. J Pers Soc Psychol 1985;49:469–480.

THE SOCIAL MALADJUSTMENT SCHEDULE
(Anthony W. Clare, 1978)

Purpose

This rating form was designed to measure social maladjustment among adults
with chronic neurotic disorders. It was initially intended for use in psychiatric
research, but has also been used in studies in family practice and with general
population samples.

Conceptual Basis

Clare and Cairns argued that scales measuring social adjustment in terms of
conformity to social roles and norms will not permit comparisons across social
groups in which norms and social expectations differ. They designed their scale
to combine an interviewer's objective assessment of the patient's material circumstances and performance with the patient's own ratings of satisfaction. The
topics covered in the scale were derived from a review of previous
measurements.

Description

The Social Maladjustment Schedule is a 26-page interview that covers six
domains: housing, occupation and social role, economic situation, leisure and
social activities, family relationships, and marriage. Questions in each domain
cover three themes that were described by Clare and Cairns as follows:

> the social schedule examines each individual's life from 3 main standpoints: first,
> it attempts to assess what the individual *has,* in terms of his living conditions,
> money, social opportunities in a number of areas; secondly, it measures what he
> *does* with his life, what use he makes of his opportunities, how well he copes;
> finally, it measures what he *feels* about it, that is to say how satisfied he is with
> various aspects of his social situation. (1, p592).

A trained interviewer administers the semi-structured interview in the respondent's home; the interviewer may also incorporate information collected from
the spouse. The interview requires about 45 minutes; the schedule is available,
with a training manual, at cost from Dr. Clare. The content of the schedule is
summarized in Exhibit 5.4.

From the individual's responses the interviewer makes a total of 42 ratings
on four-point scales that describe the extent of maladjustment in each area.
Ten ratings cover material conditions, 14 refer to management of social oppor-
tunities and activities and 18 cover satisfaction (2). The ratings concentrate on
levels of maladjustment; no differentiation is made between degrees of satisfactory functioning, all of which are scored equally. An overall score may also
be used, with higher scores indicating poorer adjustment.

Exhibit 5.4 Structure and Content of the Social Maladjustment Schedule

| Subject area | Rating category with each item rated shown below the appropriate category | | |
	Material conditions	Social management	Satisfaction
Housing	Housing conditions	Household care	Satisfaction with housing
	Residential stability	Management of housekeeping	
Occupation/social role	Occupational stability	Quality of personal interaction with workmates	Satisfaction with occupation/social role (includes housewives, unemployed, disabled, retired)
	Opportunities for interaction with workmates*		Satisfaction with personal inter-action with workmates
Economic situation	Family income	Management of income	Satisfaction with income
Leisure/social activities	Opportunities for leisure and social activities*	Extent of leisure and social activities	Satisfaction with leisure and social activities
	Opportunities for interaction with neighbours	Quality of interaction with neighbours	Satisfaction with interaction with neighbours
			Satisfaction with heterosexual role
Family and domestic relationships	Opportunities for interaction with relatives*	Quality of interaction with relatives	Satisfaction with interaction with relatives
		Quality of solitary living	Satisfaction with solitary living
	Opportunities for domestic interaction (i.e., with unrelated others or adult offspring in household)	Quality of domestic interaction (i.e., with unrelated others or adult offspring in household)	Satisfaction with domestic interaction
	Situational handicaps to child management*	Child management	Satisfaction with parental role
Marital		Fertility and family planning	
		Sharing of responsibilities and decision-making	Satisfaction with marital harmony
		Sharing of interests and activities	Satisfaction with sex-ual compatibility

*This group of items rates objective restrictions which might be expected to impair functioning in the appropriate area. "Situational handicaps to child management" assesses difficulties likely to exacerbate normal problems of child-rearing, e.g., inadequate living space, an absent parent. Objective restrictions on leisure activities include extreme age, physical disabilities, heavy domestic or work commitments, isolated situation of the home, etc.

Reproduced with permission from Clare AW, Cairns VE. Design, development and use of a standardized interview to assess social maladjustment and dysfunction in community studies. Psychol Med 1978;8:592,Table 1. Copyright Cambridge University Press.

Reliability

Inter-rater reliability was assessed using analyses of variance; agreement was close with the exception of 3 of the 25 items tested, for which significant differences were obtained (1, Table 3). Weighted kappas ranged from 0.55 to 0.94 with most coefficients falling above 0.70 (1, Table 4).

Validity

Factor analyses were applied to various samples, but the results did not clearly replicate the dimensions around which the schedule was constructed, and from this Clare and Cairns inferred the need to calculate an overall score. This overall maladjustment score was associated (at $p < 0.05$) with a rating made using Goldberg's standardized psychiatric interview. From Clare's data, a sensitivity of 30% and a specificity of 80% may be calculated, compared with the Goldberg rating (1, Table 7).

Alternative Forms

A 41-item self-report Social Problem Questionnaire has been derived from the Social Maladjustment Schedule (3).

Commentary

Clare and Cairns offer a thorough conceptual discussion of the development of indices of social health, reviewing the problems of comparing social behavior across cultural groups and discussing the balance to be set between recording objective life circumstances and personal satisfaction. Although their scale was explicitly designed to reflect this distinction, empirical data from factor analyses did not confirm the intended conceptual structure.

The scale seems well designed, but has not seen widespread use other than by its original authors (3–5) and beyond the initial development work little further evidence for the reliability and validity of the scale has been published. The scale covers only the negative aspects of social adjustment; for assessing social support or the positive indications of integration a different scale, such as that of Henderson or McFarlane, would be needed. The Social Maladjustment Schedule may find a role in studies that require detailed information on social maladjustment and that have the resources to carry out home interviews, but the decision to use the instrument should be taken in the light of future evidence on its validity and reliability.

Address

Anthony W. Clare, MD, Department of Psychological Medicine, St. Bartholomew's Hospital Medical School, West Smithfield, London, England EC1A 7BE

References

(1) Clare AW, Cairns VE. Design, development and use of a standardized interview to assess social maladjustment and dysfunction in community studies. Psychol Med 1978;8:589–604.

(2) A manual for use in conjunction with the General Practice Research Unit's standardized social interview schedule. London: Institute of Psychiatry, 1979.

(3) Corney RH, Clare AW, Fry J. The development of a self-report questionnaire to identify social problems: a pilot study. Psychol Med 1982;12:903–909.

(4) Clare AW. Psychiatric and social aspects of pre-menstrual complaint. Psychol Med 1983;13(suppl 4):1–58.

(5) Corney RH. Social work effectiveness in the management of depressed women: a clinical trial. Psychol Med 1981;11:417–423.

THE KATZ ADJUSTMENT SCALES
(Martin M. Katz, 1963)

Purpose

This set of scales was originally intended to measure the social adjustment of psychiatric patients following treatment; the scales incorporate judgments made by the patient and by a relative. The assessments cover psychiatric symptoms, social behavior, home and leisure activities. The scales have also been used in population surveys.

Conceptual Basis

Katz and Lyerly viewed the aims of psychiatric treatment in terms of increasing the patient's adjustment to living in the community. Adjustment was defined as a balance between the individual and his environment, freedom from symptoms of psychopathology, absence of personal distress, suitable patterns of social interaction, and adequate performance in social roles (1). This conceptual approach brings the adjustment scales close to indices of positive mental well-being. In addition to the individual's own feelings of well-being and satisfaction, the assessment of social adjustment must reflect the view of others in his milieu: "the extent to which persons in the patient's social environment are satisfied with his type and level of functioning" (1). This led to the approach of basing the measurement on judgments made by the individual and by those close to him.

Description

Two sets of scales are used, one completed by the patient (S scales) and the other by a relative (R scales). The scales are introduced by an interviewer but are completed by the patient and a relative; the questions use nontechnical language. The patient reports on his somatic symptoms, mood, level of activities and personal satisfaction. A relative who has been in close contact with the patient reports on the patient's behavior and indicates the extent to which other people are satisfied with his functioning. The scales need not be administered as a set.

On form R1 (127 items) the relative rates the patient's psychiatric symptoms (e.g., "looks worn out," "laughs or cries for no reason"). Form R1 also covers social behavior (e.g., "dependable" or "gets into fights with people"). Four-point scales indicate the frequency of each symptom and these may be summed into an overall score. Form R2 contains 16 items on the individual's performance of socially expected activities: social responsibilities, self-care, community activities. Three-point frequency response scales are used. The items and response scales on form R3 are identical to those on R2, save that the relative now indicates his expectation of the patient's level of performance in these activities following discharge. A score indicating the relative's satisfaction with the patient's performance may be derived from the discrepancy between expectations (form R3) and actual performance (form R2) (1). In a similar manner, a pair of 23-item forms (R4 and R5) cover the relative's ratings of the patient's level of free-time activities and the relative's expectations for this. Items cover hobbies and social, community, and self-improvement activities.

The patient also completes five forms. Form S1 contains 55 items derived from the Hopkins Symptom Checklist on somatic symptoms and mood from which a total score may be calculated. The other four forms are equivalent to the relative's rating forms R2 to R5, and include the same items with minor changes to the wording. Because the wording of the fourth set of forms is identical, Katz refers to these as RS4.

The forms are too long to reproduce here; a summary of the items is given in Katz and Lyerly's article (1, Tables 1–3). As the questions in form R2 cover social health, we include a summary of them in Exhibit 5.5.

Exhibit 5.5 The Katz Adjustment Scale Form R2 (Level of Performance of Socially Expected Activities) and Form R3 (Level of Expectations for Performance of Social Activities)

Note: The two forms are used to derive separate measures and in combination, to provide a "level of satisfaction" measure.

1. Helps with household chores	9. Goes to parties and other social activities
2. Visits his friends	10. Gets along with neighbors
3. Visits his relatives	11. Helps with family shopping
4. Entertains friends at home	12. Helps in the care and training of children
5. Dresses and takes care of himself	13. Goes to church
6. Helps with the family budgeting	14. Takes up hobbies
7. Remembers to do important things on time	15. Works
8. Gets along with family members	16. Supports the family

The response scales for form R2 include three categories: "is not doing," "is doing some," and "is doing regularly." For form R3, the responses are: "did not expect him to be doing," "expected him to be doing some" and "expected him to be doing regularly."

Reproduced with permission from Katz, M. M., and Lyerley, S. B. Methods for measuring adjustment and social behavior in the community: I. Rationale, description, discriminative validity and scale development. *Psychological Reports*, 1963, 13, 503–535, Table 2.

Reliability

Kuder-Richardson internal consistency coefficients for eleven subscores on form R1 were calculated on two samples of patients. Coefficients ranged from 0.41 to 0.87, with a median coefficient of 0.72 (N = 315) (1, Table 7).

Validity

The relative's forms discriminated significantly between patients judged on clinical grounds to be well adjusted and those who were poorly adjusted. The data published by Hogarty and Katz indicate consistent contrasts in responses between psychiatric patients and a sample from the general population (2). Scores for the 127 items in form R1 were factor analyzed and found to fall on 13 factors.

Reference Standards

Hogarty and Katz reported reference standards for the 13 factor scores on form R1, derived from a sample of 450 community respondents aged 15 years and over. The standards are presented by age, sex, social class, and marital status (2, Table 1).

Commentary

The Katz Adjustment Scales were taken for some time as the standard approach to measuring social adjustment, but they are now very old and lack evidence of validity. A Science Citation Index search reveals that several dozen studies have used the scales, but a closer examination reveals that virtually none presents data from which conclusions may be drawn concerning reliability and validity of the measurements. We cannot, therefore, agree with the conclusion of Chen and Bryant, who claimed that "extensive efforts were made to establish the different forms of reliabilities and validities, all of which were found satisfactory" (3). The Katz scales have had, nonetheless, a considerable impact on the design of subsequent methods. For example, the approach of combining ratings by a patient and a relative was innovative and has been followed in subsequent scales, such as that of Clare and Cairns. Considering the age of the Katz scales and the scant evidence for reliability and validity, we recommend their use only if none of the other scales we describe applies.

Address

Martin M. Katz, PhD, Department of Psychiatry, Albert Einstein College of Medicine, Bronx Municipal Hospital, Pelham & Eastchester Boulevard, Bronx, New York, USA 10461

References

(1) Katz MM, Lyerly SB. Methods for measuring adjustment and social behavior in the community. I. Rationale, description, discriminative validity and scale development. Psychol Rep 1963;13:503–535.

(2) Hogarty GE, Katz MM. Norms of adjustment and social behavior. Arch Gen Psychiatry 1971;25:470–480.

(3) Chen MK, Bryant BE. The measurement of health—a critical and selective overview. Int J Epidemiol 1976;4:257–264.

THE SOCIAL HEALTH BATTERY
(Rand Corporation, 1978)

Purpose

The Social Health Battery provides objective indications of levels of social resources and social interaction. It is intended for use in general population surveys.

Conceptual Basis

The questionnaire was intended to measure social well-being or support, terms that are used interchangeably by Donald and Ware (1, 2). The social circumstances of the individual are measured on two distinct dimensions: the numbers of social resources a person has and the frequency with which he is in contact with friends and relatives (1, 2). "Conceptual confusion between mental health and the more qualitative aspects of social support led us . . . to focus on more objective behavioral approaches to the measurement of social support" (1, p362). Donald and Ware view social support as conceptually distinct from the physical and mental components of health status, but as an external factor that affects the level of health.

Description

This self-administered scale was developed along with the Rand physical and psychological scales as an outcome measurement for the Health Insurance Experiment involving adults aged 14 to 61 years. The scale has not yet been tested on the elderly. The 11-items include predominantly objective indicators of two kinds: those that define social resources (e.g., number of friends) and those that define contacts (e.g., the frequency of seeing friends or involvement in group activities). The scale covers home and family, friendships, social and community life; it specifically excludes work-related performance and items that do not necessarily involve interaction, such as attending sports events (2). Nor does the scale cover satisfaction with relationships. The development of the questionnaire is described by Donald and Ware (2), and it is shown in Exhibit 5.6.

Forced choice and open-ended responses are used. A scoring format devel-

Exhibit 5.6 The Social Health Battery

1. About how many families in your neighborhood are you well enough aquainted with, that you visit each other in your homes?
   _____families

2. About how many *close* friends do you have—people you feel at ease with and can talk with about what is on your mind? (You may include relatives.) (Enter number on line)
   _____close friends

3. Over a year's time, about how often do you get together with friends or relatives, like going out together or visiting in each other's homes? (Circle one)

Every day	1
Several days a week	2
About once a week	3
2 or 3 times a month	4
About once a month	5
5 to 10 times a year	6
Less than 5 times a year	7

4. During the *past month*, about how often have you had friends over to your home? (Do *not* count relatives.) (Circle one)

Every day	1
Several days a week	2
About once a week	3
2 or 3 times in past month	4
Once in past month	5
Not at all in past month	6

5. About how often have you visited with friends at *their* homes during the *past month?* (Do not count relatives.) (Circle one)

Every day	1
Several days a week	2
About once a week	3
2 or 3 times in past month	4
Once in past month	5
Not at all in past month	6

6. About how often were you on the telephone with close friends or relatives during the *past month?* (Circle one)

Every day	1
Several times a week	2
About once a week	3
2 or 3 times	4
Once	5
Not at all	6

7. About how often did you write a letter to a friend or relative during the *past month?* (Circle one)

Every day	1
Several times a week	2
About once a week	3
2 or 3 times in past month	4
Once in past month	5
Not at all in past month	6

Exhibit 5.6 (*continued*)

8. In general, how well are you getting along with other people these days—would you say better than usual, about the same, or not as well as usual? (Circle One)

Better than usual	1
About the same	2
Not as well as usual	3

9. How often have you attended a religious service during the *past month?* (Circle one)

Every day	1
More than once a week	2
Once a week	3
2 or 3 times in past month	4
Once in past month	5
Not at all in past month	6

10. About how many voluntary groups or organizations do you belong to—like church groups, clubs or lodges, parent groups, etc. ("Voluntary" means because you want to.)

_____groups or organizations   (Write in number. If none, enter "0.")

11. How active are you in the affairs of these groups or clubs you belong to? (If you belong to a great many, just count those you feel closest to. If you don't belong to any, circle 4.)

(Circle one)

Very active, attend most meetings	1
Fairly active, attend fairly often	2
Not active, belong but hardly every go	3
Do not belong to any groups or clubs	4

Reproduced from Donald CA, Ware JE Jr. The measurement of social support. Res Commun Ment Health 1984;4:334–335. With permission.

oped by Donald and Ware is used to recode the printed response options: this is shown in Exhibit 5.7. High scores indicate a more favorable social score, although the authors give no guidance about critical scores that might differentiate good from poor adjustment. On the basis of factor analyses, the items may be grouped to form two subscales and an overall score (1). Item 7 (writing letters) was dropped from analyses of scale results because few people answered affirmatively and because it did not correlate with the total score. The Rand group recommends deleting the question from the instrument (Cathy Donald Sherbourne, personal communication, 1985). The first subscale, social contacts, includes items 3, 4 and 5 from Exhibit 5.6; a group participation scale includes items 10 and 11. An overall social support score uses all the items except for numbers 7 (writing letters) and 8 (getting along with others). The authors recommend using scores for individual items and subscales rather than the overall score, pending additional validity studies (1). They also recommend standardizing items to a mean of zero and a standard deviation of one before forming subscores (2).

Reliability

The inter-item correlations are in general low, with only five of 45 correlations exceeding 0.40 (1, Table 8). Internal consistency coefficients for the three subscores were 0.72 for social contacts, 0.84 for group participation, and 0.68 for

Exhibit 5.7 Scoring Method for the Social Health Battery

Abbreviated item content	Recoding rule
Neighborhood family acquaintances	$(0 = 0)(1 = 1)(2 = 2)(3 = 3)(4 = 4)$ (5 thru 10 = 5) (11 or higher = 6)
Close friends and relatives	$(0 = 0)(1 = 1)(2 = 2)(3 = 3)(4 = 4)$ (5 thru 9 = 5) (10 thru 20 = 6) (21 thru 25 = 7) (26 thru 35 = 8) (36 or higher = 9)
Visits with friends/relatives	(1 thru 3 = 4) (4 = 3) (5,6 = 2) (7 = 1)
Home visits by friends	(1 thru 4 = 3) (5 = 2) (6 = 1)
Visits to homes of friends	(1 thru 3 = 3) (4,5 =2) (6 = 1)
Telephone contacts	$(1 = 5)(2 = 4)(3,4 = 3)(5 = 2)(6 = 1)$
Getting along	$(1 = 3)(2 = 2)(3 = 1)$
Attendance at religious services	$(1,2 = 5)(3 = 4)(4 = 3)(5 = 2)(6 = 1)$
Voluntary group membership	$(0 =0)(1 = 1)(2 = 2)(3 = 3)(4 = 4)$ (5 or higher = 5)
Level of group activity	$(1 = 4)(2 = 3)(3 = 2)(4 = 1)$

Reproduced from Donald CA, Ware JE Jr. The measurement of social support. Res Commun Ment Health 1984;4:350,Table 6. With permission.

the social support index (1, Table 11). The corresponding one-year test-retest coefficients were 0.55, 0.68, and 0.68 while coefficients for individual items ranged from 0.23 to 0.80.

Validity

Preliminary validation results were drawn from 4,603 interviews in the Health Insurance Experiment. Correlations were calculated between each of the 11 items and three criterion scores: a 9-item self-rating of health in general, a 3-item measure of emotional ties, and a 9-item psychological well-being scale. The correlations were low, with only three of 33 Pearson correlations equal to or above 0.20 (1, Table 4). Correlations for the three aggregated indices were somewhat higher: the social support index correlated 0.32 with the psychological well-being scale and 0.20 with emotional ties (1, Table 13). The social support score was found to predict variations in mental health, as measured by the Rand Mental Health Inventory, explaining 12% of the variance (3). The question on writing letters was found not to correlate with two of the criterion scores, and was not used in calculating overall scores nor in further analyses of the scale.

Reference Standards

Table 7 in Donald and Ware's report shows the response patterns for ten items for 4,603 respondents from the Rand study (1).

Commentary

This scale was based on an extensive review of social health measurements and was designed to reflect areas identified by current literature as being important

(4). It is one of the few scales we review that was not designed for use with patients, and the authors have made some interesting observations on the point beyond which an increase in social contacts does not bring additional benefits to a person's well-being.

The preliminary testing of the method has the advantage of using a large, representative sample, but the design of the scale complicates the validation process. That is, items were deliberately chosen to represent a concept of social health independent of physical and psychological well-being, so that the low intercorrelations obtained in the validation studies may be expected. This is a dilemma of discriminant validity: showing that a scale does not correlate with something it is supposed to differ from does not imply it would correlate with another scale closer in meaning. The results so far published do not suggest high levels of validity or reliability, and further studies are required to indicate how the instrument compares with alternative social health measurements, and how well it agrees with assessments made by independent observers. Given the currently slender evidence for validity and reliability, we recommend that potential users of the scale first check to see whether additional evidence on its quality has been published.

Address

Cathy A. Donald Sherbourne, The Rand Corporation, 1700 Main Street, PO Box 2138, Santa Monica, California, USA 90406

References

(1) Donald CA, Ware JE Jr. The measurement of social support. Res Commun Ment Health 1984;4:325–370.
(2) Donald CA, Ware JE Jr. The quantification of social contacts and resources. Santa Monica, California: Rand Corporation, 1982. (R-2937-HHS).
(3) Williams AW, Ware JE Jr, Donald CA. A model of mental health, life events, and social supports applicable to general populations. J Health Soc Behav 1981;22:324–336.
(4) Donald CA, Ware JE Jr, Brook RH, Davies-Avery A. Conceptualization and measurement of health for adults in the Health Insurance Study. Vol. IV, Social Health. Santa Monica, California: Rand Corporation, 1978.

THE SOCIAL DYSFUNCTION RATING SCALE
(Margaret W. Linn, 1969)

Purpose

The Social Dysfunction Rating Scale (SDRS) assesses the negative aspects of a person's social adjustment. This rating scale is applied by a clinician and is intended as a research instrument.

Conceptual Basis

Effective social functioning, in Linn's conceptual formulation,

> would suggest equilibrium within the person and in his interaction with his environment. . . . Dysfunction, on the other hand, implies discontent and unhappiness, accompanied by negative self-regarding attitudes. It furthermore suggests handicapping anxiety and other pathological interpersonal functions that reduce flexibility in coping with stressful situations or achieving self-actualization in what is to that person a significant role. . . . From this standpoint, dysfunction is seen as coping with either personal, interpersonal, or geographic environment in a maladaptive manner. In this respect, the SDRS seeks to quantify the objective observations of man's dysfunctional interaction with his environment. (1, p299).

Linn's scale concentrates on symptoms of low morale and reduced social participation; it does not assess the positive elements in a person's adjustment.

Description

The Social Dysfunction Rating Scale is applied by an interviewer, generally a social worker or other therapist familiar with the patient. The questions are semi-structured and combine the interviewer's evaluations with the respondent's own self-evaluation (1, p301). For instance, the interviewer rates the availability of friends and social contacts, after which the respondent is asked if he feels a need for more friends. The scale, shown in Exhibit 5.8, includes 21 symptoms of social and emotional problems, each judged on a six-point severity scale. The ratings are grouped into three classes: four items refer to the respondent's view of himself, six refer to his interpersonal relationships, and eleven concern his lack of success and dissatisfaction in social situations.

Linn et al. provide definitions of the items and instructions for completing the scale. As an example, comments on item 4 read as follows:

> 4. *Self-health concern.* The frequency and severity of complaints of body illness are rated. Evaluation is based on degree to which the person believes that physical symptoms are an important factor in his total well-being. No consideration is given for actual organic basis of illness. Only the frequency and severity of complaints are rated. (1, p301).

Higher scores on the scale reflect greater dysfunction. Items are not weighted differently, although Linn et al. have considered using discriminant function coefficients as item weights (1, p305).

Reliability

The agreement between two raters in scoring 40 subjects was measured; intraclass correlations for the 21 items ranged from 0.54 to 0.86 (1, Table 1). The agreement between seven raters, who independently rated ten schizophrenics in group interviews, yielded a Kendall's index of concordance of 0.91 (1, p303).

Exhibit 5.8 The Social Dysfunction Rating Scale

Directions: Score each of the items as follows:

1. Not Present	3. Mild	5. Severe
2. Very Mild	4. Moderate	6. Very severe

Self system

1. _____ Low self concept (feelings of inadequacy, not measuring up to self ideal)
2. _____ Goallessness (lack of inner motivation and sense of future orientation)
3. _____ Lack of a satisfying philosophy or meaning of life (a conceptual framework for integrating past and present experiences)
4. _____ Self-health concern (preoccupation with physical health, somatic concerns)

Interpersonal system

5. _____ Emotional withdrawal (degree of deficiency in relating to others)
6. _____ Hostility (degree of aggression toward others)
7. _____ Manipulation (exploiting of environment, controlling at other's expense)
8. _____ Over-dependency (degree of parasitic attachment to others)
9. _____ Anxiety (degree of feeling of uneasiness, impending doom)
10. _____ Suspiciousness (degree of distrust or paranoid ideation)

Performance system

11. _____ Lack of satisfying relationships with significant persons (spouse, children, kin, significant persons serving in a family role)
12. _____ Lack of friends, social contacts
13. _____ Expressed need for more friends, social contacts
14. _____ Lack of work (remunerative or non-remunerative, productive work activities which normally give a sense of usefulness, status, confidence)
15. _____ Lack of satisfaction from work
16. _____ Lack of leisure time activities
17. _____ Expressed need for more leisure, self-enhancing and satisfying activities
18. _____ Lack of participation in community activities
19. _____ Lack of interest in community affairs and activities which influence others
20. _____ Financial insecurity
21. _____ Adaptive rigidity (lack of complex coping patterns to stress)

Patient:_____Rater:_____Date:_____

Reproduced from Linn MW, Sculthorpe WB, Evje M, Slater PH, Goodman SP. A Social Dysfunction Rating Scale. J Psychiatr Res 1969;6:300. Copyright Pergamon Press Ltd. With permission.

Validity

The scale was applied to schizophrenic outpatients and nonpsychiatric respondents. A discriminant function analysis correctly classified 92% of the 80 respondents (1, Table 2). In the same study, a correlation of 0.89 was obtained between the total scale scores and a global judgment of adjustment made by a social worker who interviewed the respondents (1, p305). The data were factor analyzed, producing five factors, termed apathetic-detachment, dissatisfaction, hostility, health-finance concern, and manipulative-dependency (1).

Commentary

The Social Dysfunction Rating Scale covering the negative aspects of social functioning was based on considerable conceptual work on the theme of social adjustment among the elderly (1–3). The inter-rater reliability can be high for overall scores, although agreement over individual scales shows a wide variation. A major concern with the scale is its lack of validation. Although it was first described in 1969 and has been used in several studies (4–7), the only validity results come from a single study of 80 subjects. The question of how best to score the scale also requires further investigation, especially as the empirical factor analysis results do not match the three subdivisions built into the scale (self-perceptions, interpersonal relations and social performance). It is not clear whether a total score or various subscores offer the best way to summarize the results of the index. Compared with other scales in this chapter, the Social Dysfunction Rating Scale is brief, covers a broad range of low-level symptoms of maladjustment, and has the advantage that its author continues to work actively in this field.

Address

Margaret W. Linn, PhD, Director, Social Science Research, Veterans Administration Medical Center, 1201 Northwest 16th Street, Miami, Florida, USA 33125

References

(1) Linn MW, Sculthorpe WB, Evje M, Slater PH, Goodman SP. A Social Dysfunction Rating Scale. J Psychiatr Res 1969;6:299–306.
(2) Linn MW. Studies in rating the physical, mental, and social dysfunction of the chronically ill aged. Med Care 1976;14(suppl 5):119–125.
(3) Linn MW. Assessing community adjustment in the elderly. In: Raskin A, Jervik LF, eds. Assessment of psychiatric symptoms and cognitive loss in the elderly. Washington, DC: Hemisphere Press, 1979:187–204.
(4) Linn MW, Caffey EM Jr. Foster placement for the older psychiatric patient. J Gerontol 1977;32:340–345.
(5) Linn MW, Caffey EM Jr, Klett CJ, Hogarty G. Hospital vs community (foster) care for psychiatric patients. Arch Gen Psychiatry 1977;34:78–83.
(6) Linn MW, Klett CJ, Caffey EM Jr. Foster home characteristics and psychiatric patient outcome: the wisdom of Gheel confirmed. Arch Gen Psychiatry 1980;37:129–132.
(7) Linn MW, Caffey EM, Klett CJ, Hogarty GE, Lamb HR. Day treatment and psychotropic drugs in the aftercare of schizophrenic patients. Arch Gen Psychiatry 1979;36:1055–1066.

THE SOCIAL FUNCTIONING SCHEDULE
(Marina Remington and P.J. Tyrer, 1979)

Purpose

The Social Functioning Schedule (SFS) is a semi-structured interview designed to assess the problems a person experiences in various aspects of social functioning. The scale was designed for evaluating treatment of neurotic outpatients.

Conceptual Basis

The SFS uses a role performance approach to assess functioning, but does not impose external standards to define adequate performance. Instead, the patient is asked to record difficulties experienced, in effect comparing behavior with his own expectations. The questions are phrased in terms of difficulties; they do not specify what form the difficulties may take (1).

Description

The SFS includes 12 sections: employment, household chores, contribution to household, money, self-care, marital relationship, care of children, patient-child relationships, patient-parent and household relationships, social contacts, hobbies and spare time activities. The first two, the fourth and the last sections are subdivided into problems in managing activities in that area and the feelings of distress that result. Sections that are irrelevant for a particular respondent may be omitted.

The SFS is intended for use by a psychologist or physician in clinical practice settings. It is a rating scale based on "a number of suggested questions designed to encompass the range of difficulty encountered with neurotic out-patients. The examiner is free to adapt and add questions where this is necessary to gain sufficient information." (2, p1). The schedule includes a total of 121 questions, not all of which would be relevant to every respondent. After asking the questions in each section, the interviewer rates the level of problems in that area on a visual analogue scale running from "none" to "severe difficulties." The ratings cover only difficulties reported by the patient; the rater avoids making normative judgments. Ratings refer to the past four weeks with the exception of six months for the employment questions, and the interview takes 10 to 20 minutes. Numerical scores are derived from the analogue scales by measurement, and an overall score is calculated as the average of the relevant subsections; lower scores represent better adjustment.

The SFS is too long to reproduce here; as an illustration, the section on work problems is shown in Exhibit 5.9. Note that the version shown is a slight revision of that originally described by Remington and Tyrer (1). Copies of the complete instrument may be obtained from Dr. Tyrer.

Reliability

Inter-rater reliability was assessed using the intraclass correlation. Results ranged from 0.45 to 0.81 for different sections (average, 0.62) (1, p153). Ratings made by patients were compared with those made by spouses; correlations ranged from 0.45 to 0.80 (1, Table 1).

Exhibit 5.9 Example of a Section from the Social Functioning Schedule

1. Work problems—behaviour

    1a Performance: As far as you know, how has S [the Subject] been coping with work? Does S have any difficulties? (Rate performance at work tasks.)

	0	1	2
Not known	no problems	reduced output/given	unable to perform his
Not applicable		easier job	job/others have
			taken over

    1b Time keeping: Does S usually get to work on time?

	0	1	2
Not known	usually arrives at a	has occasionally	has been more than 1
Not applicable	reasonable time	missed ½–1 hour, or	hour late on more
		been more than 1	than two occasions
		hour late	in last 4 weeks

    1c Overactivity: Does S take on too much? (Is he rushed? Does he miss breaks or work late a lot?)

	0	1	2
Not known	does a day's work	rushes to complete	work frequently
Not applicable	but no more—	jobs, on a tight	occupies evenings
	work does not	schedule and/or	and weekends
	intrude on	occasionally works	
	personal time	late or brings work	
		home	

    Other problems (specify) _____

      _____

1. Rate work problems—behaviour

      none   severe difficulties

      ├──┤

2. Work problems—Stress

    Does S talk about work? Has S complained about work recently? Has S seemed upset about work or under strain because of work?

    2a Interest and satisfaction: Does S say that he likes his work? Has S complained that he is bored or fed up with work?

	0	1	2
Not known	S seems	S reports that he is	S indicates that he is
Not applicable	reasonably	disinterested or	utterly bored or
	satisfied with work	somewhat	dissatisfied with
	situation	dissatisfied with	work
		work	

    2b Distress: Does S seem to take work in his stride, or does work get him down? Does he appear troubled when he gets home from work? Does S complain that he has lost confidence? (Exclude boredom and dissatisfaction; include worry, strain, anxiety and anger).

	0	1	2
Not known	no noticeable	some degree of	S reports extreme
Not applicable	discomfort due to	distress occasionally	distress or informant
	work	reported or observed	observes this most of
			the time

Exhibit 5.9 (*continued*)

2c Work relationships—friction: Has S talked about other people at work? In general how
    does he get on with them? Has S mentioned any quarrels or friction recently? (Include
    overt interpersonal difficulty with both clients and colleagues regardless of degree of
    associated distress).

	0	1	2
Not known	generally, smooth	some friction or	friction or quarrelling
Not applicable	easy relationships	quarrelling during	is a constant feature
		each week	of work situation

2d Work relationships—exploitation: Has S complained that he is treated unfairly at work?
    Has he complained that he feels put upon or dominated?

	0	1	2
Not known	S reports no	S reports occasional	S complains of
Not applicable	exploitation	injustices or	extreme exploitation
		exploitation	

Other problems (specify) _____

1. Rate work problems—stress

   none   severe difficulties

   |———————————————————————————————————————|

Reproduced from the Social Functioning Schedule obtained from Dr. P.J. Tyrer. With permission.

Validity

Discriminant ability was tested by comparing ratings of three groups: patients
with personality disorders, other psychiatric outpatients (mainly psychotic
patients on maintenance therapy) and the spouses of patients. The scale distinguished between the personality-disordered patients and the other groups, but
not between normals and other psychiatric cases.

In a study of 171 general practice patients referred for psychiatric consultation, the SFS showed significant differences between patients rated with different levels of certainty as psychiatric cases by a psychiatrist (3). The scale was
not, however, able to differentiate among clinically defined categories of personality disorder. In another study, the SFS score correlated strongly with the
total score of the Present State Examination ($r = 0.69$) (3, p7). A correlation
of 0.65 was obtained with a five-point indicator of level of alcohol consumption used as the outcome of an alcohol detoxification program for 27 patients
(4, Table 1).

Commentary

The Social Functioning Schedule covers problems in social interaction and
role performance and the patient's satisfaction with this, in a manner similar
to that of Weissman's and Gurland's scales. It does not indicate the level of
social support available to the patient, nor does it cover positive levels of functioning: the highest rating in each section is expressed in terms of the absence
of identifiable problems. This is comparable to the approach used in several of
the scales we review, as is the use of a semi-structured interview format. The

scale is being used in current research and preliminary validity and reliability analyses are available.

Potential criticisms of the SFS include the possibility of interviewer bias in translating responses into the visual analogue ratings. This may have caused the relatively low interrater reliability results, although the intraclass correlations used here normally give a coefficient as much as 0.20 lower than a Pearson correlation computed on the same data. More reliability testing is desirable, particularly as the rating system depends on the judgment of the interviewer. Because the scale is broad in scope, it naturally sacrifices detail in most areas when compared with alternative scales. Nonetheless, where an expert rater is available to make the ratings and where summary ratings of a patient's problems (rather than assets) are required, this scale should be considered for use. Because of its semi-structured design, the method may be better suited for formulating rather than testing hypotheses.

Address

P.J. Tyrer, MD, FRCP, FRC Psych, Consultant Psychiatrist, Mapperley Hospital, Porchester Road, Nottingham, England NG3 6AA

References

(1) Remington M, Tyrer P. The Social Functioning Schedule—a brief semi-structured interview. Soc Psychiatry 1979;14:151–157.
(2) Tyrer PJ. Social Functioning Schedule—short version. (Manuscript, nd).
(3) Casey PR, Tyrer PJ, Platt S. The relationship between social functioning and psychiatric symptomatology in primary care. Soc Psychiatry 1985;20:5–9.
(4) Griggs SMLB, Tyrer PJ. Personality disorder, social adjustment and treatment outcome in alcoholics. J Stud Alcohol 1981;42:802–805.

THE INTERVIEW SCHEDULE FOR SOCIAL INTERACTION
(Scott Henderson, 1980)

Purpose

This is a research instrument that assesses the availability and supportive quality of social relationships. The interview was designed as a survey method to measure social factors associated with the development of neurotic illness; it may also be used to evaluate the outcomes of care for psychiatric patients.

Conceptual Basis

Henderson's approach to measuring social relationships was guided by his research goal of identifying how social support protects against neurotic disorders in the presence of adversity. Following the conceptual work of Robert Weiss, Henderson identified six benefits that are offered by lasting social relationships: a sense of attachment and security, social integration, the opportunity to care for others, the provision of reassurance as to one's personal worth, a sense of reliable alliance, and the availability of help and guidance when needed (1). The first of these themes, attachment, was considered especially important, and Henderson here drew on the concepts of Bowlby. Attachment refers to "that attribute of relationships which is characterized by affection and which gives the recipient a subjective sense of closeness. It is also pleasant and highly valued, commonly above all else" (3, p725).

Social ties may be evaluated in terms of their objective availability, or in terms of the person's subjective assessment of their adequacy. The Interview Schedule for Social Interaction (ISSI) "seeks to establish the availability of most of the six provisions proposed by Weiss by ascertaining the availability of persons in specified roles. Questions about adequacy follow each of the availability items" (1, p34).

Description

The ISSI is a 45-minute interview that records details of a person's network of social attachments, covering both quantity and quality of social support in the last 12 months. The interviewer mentions briefly a particular type of social relationship, and asks the respondent if he has such a relationship; the interviewer then asks if the amount of this type of relationship is adequate. The questions cover acquaintances, friendship, attachment, nurturance, reassurance of worth and reliable alliances (2). In addition, the respondent is asked to name the main person who provides each of several different facets of attachment relationships. This information is summarized on an attachment table that records the degree of closeness of the respondent to each of the people he cites as emotionally close to him. Details of the identity of these individuals are recorded, as is an indication of their accessibility to the respondent. The table is also used to indicate the extent to which social provisions are concentrated on few or many people. The instrument is too long to reproduce here; it is available, along with guide notes, in the appendices to Henderson's book (1). As an illustration, Exhibit 5.10 shows one question from the ISSI.

Initial analyses indicated that the results obtained from the questionnaire did not fully reflect the complexity of the conceptual formulation, so a simplified scoring system was proposed. Four scores summarize the extent and adequacy of social support:

> availability of attachment (8 items)
> adequacy of attachment (12 items)
> availability of social integration (16 items)
> adequacy of social integration (17 items)

A detailed discussion of scoring procedures is given by Duncan-Jones (2). The procedure is sophisticated in that it reflects the idea that scores should not necessarily increase or decrease monotonically: both too much and too little support may constitute less than ideal replies. An alternative, simpler scoring sys-

Exhibit 5.10 Example of an Item from the Interview Schedule for Social Interaction

---

33. At present, do you have someone you can share your most private feelings with (confide in) or not?

No one (Go to Q. 33D)	0
Yes	1

A. Who is this mainly? (Fill in only one on Attachment Table)

B. Do you wish you could share more with _____or is it about right?

About right	1
Depends on the situation	2
More	3
Not applicable	9

C. Would you like to have someone else like this as well, would you prefer not to use a confidant, or is it just about right for you the way it is?

Prefers no confidant	1
About right	2
Depends on the situation	3
Like someone else as well	4
Not applicable	9

(Go to Q. 34)

(If no one)

D. Would you like to have someone like this or would you prefer to keep your feelings to yourself?

Keep things to self	1
Like someone	2
Not applicable	9

Reprinted from *Neurosis and the social environment* by S. Henderson with D.G. Byrne and P. Duncan-Jones, Academic Press, Sydney, 1981, 214. With permission.

tem, and the questions that are included in forming the four scores shown above, are given in Appendix III of Henderson's book.

Reliability

The alpha internal consistency of four scores ranged from 0.67 to 0.79 (N = 756), and 18 day test-retest correlations ranged from 0.71 to 0.76 (N = 51) (1, p47). For 221 respondents, stability correlations were calculated using a structural modeling approach that corrects for the imperfect internal consistency of the scores. The stability results at 4, 8 and 12 months ranged from 0.66 to 0.88 (1, 3).

Validity

Preliminary comparisons were made between the structure of the scale and the conceptual definition of its content. A detailed presentation is given by Duncan-Jones (4). Henderson summarized the results by noting that:

> Dimensions of availability and adequacy of "reliable alliance" and "reassurance of worth" could be distinguished, but could not be measured as reliably, nor could these two dimensions be very well separated from friendship.

The attempt to measure Weiss's concept of "opportunity for nurturing" was not successful.

A more general dimension of "social integration" could be formed by combining acquaintance, friendship, reassurance of worth and reliable alliance. (1, p38).

The ISSI was shown to discriminate significantly between groups that would be expected to differ in social adjustment: recent arrivals in a city compared with residents, and separated or divorced people compared with those who were married (1).

Correlations between the four scores and trait neuroticism measured by the Eysenck Personality Inventory ranged from 0.18 to 0.31 for 225 respondents (1). Henderson described the pattern of associations as "coherent" (1). Correlations between the respondent's scores and an informant's score reflecting his perception of the respondent's social world ranged from 0.26 to 0.59 (N = 114) (3, p731). To estimate the effect of response sets, the scale was correlated with two lie scales, and a maximum of 10.6% of variance in the ISSI scores could be explained by socially desirable response styles (3). Other validity data include a comparison with the Health Locus of Control Scale: rho 0.40 with the availability of social integration score, showing greater social integration with greater internality (5).

In a study of predictive validity over four months, Henderson showed that 30% of the variance in the General Health Questionnaire was attributable to the ISSI in a population experiencing many life changes (6). Concurrent correlations between the GHQ-30 and the four ISSI scores ranged from −0.16 to −0.38 (6, Table 1).

Commentary

This recent instrument has already offered stimulating insights into the relationships between support, life change, coping and morbidity. Thus, for example, Henderson was able to show that the quality, rather than the quantity of support provided the best predictor of resistance to psychological disorder. The ISSI is one of the few scales that measures social support rather than social roles. Like Linn's SDRS and Brandt's Personal Resource Questionnaire (7), the ISSI assesses both availability and adequacy of relationships. Evidence for reliability and validity are quite good, and hopefully will continue to accumulate. It is noticeable that, as was the case with Weissman's scale, empirical analyses of the structure of the scale do not match the conceptual framework that it was designed to reflect. This seems to be a rather prevalent problem in this field, as with quality of life measurements. In comparison with the validity and reliability results of the other scales that we review, the ISSI is sufficiently successful that we recommend its use in studies where a 45-minute interview is practical. Where a shorter rating of social support is required, we recommend McFarlane's scale reviewed in this chapter, or one of the scales developed by Sarason, Brandt or Norbeck, described in the conclusion to the chapter.

Address

Scott Henderson, MD, Director, National Health and Medical Research Council, Social Psychiatry Research Unit, The Australian National University, Canberra, Australia 2600

References

(1) Henderson S, Byrne DG, Duncan-Jones P. Neurosis and the social environment. Sydney, Australia: Academic Press, 1981.
(2) Duncan-Jones P. The structure of social relationships: analysis of a survey instrument, part 1. Soc Psychiatry 1981;16:55–61.
(3) Henderson S, Duncan-Jones P, Byrne DG, Scott R. Measuring social relationships: the Interview Schedule for Social Interaction. Psychol Med 1980;10:723–734.
(4) Duncan-Jones P. The structure of social relationships: analysis of a survey instrument, part 2. Soc Psychiatry 1981;16:143–149.
(5) Thomas PD, Hooper EM. Healthy elderly: social bonds and locus of control. Res Nurs Health 1983;6:11–16.
(6) Henderson S. Social relationships, adversity and neurosis: an analysis of prospective observations. Br J Psychiatry 1981;138:391–398.
(7) Brandt PA, Weinert C. The PRQ—a social support measure. Nurs Res 1981;30:277–280.

THE STRUCTURED AND SCALED INTERVIEW TO ASSESS MALADJUSTMENT
(Barry J. Gurland, 1972)

Purpose

The Structured and Scaled Interview to Assess Maladjustment (SSIAM) provides a detailed clinical assessment of social role performance as an outcome indicator for psychotherapy. It has been used in both clinical and research applications (1).

Conceptual Basis

The relevance of measuring social maladjustment derives from the fact that much psychiatric treatment seeks to assist people in becoming more socially effective and in reducing distress, deviant behavior, and friction with others (2). The questions in the SSIAM "cover those aspects of social adjustment which are of interest to a clinician" (2). Gurland et al. distinguished between objective and subjective facets of maladjustment. Objectively, maladjustment is seen as ineffective performance of social roles; subjectively, it refers to a failure to obtain satisfaction from one's social activities (2). The SSIAM covers both facets of maladjustment. Assessments of maladjustment must also consider the patient's environment, because an unfavorable environment may in part explain distress or disturbed behavior. To cover this, the SSIAM includes a rating by the interviewer in each section asking how far the ratings are due to a currently unfavorable environment.

Description

The instrument contains 60 items, 45 of which are grouped into five "fields": work, social relations, family, marriage and sex. The remaining 15 items are used to record the interviewer's judgments about the level of stress in the patient's environment, about his prognosis, willingness to change and aspects of positive mental health, such as personality strengths.

Within each of the five fields the assessments follow a standard order: five deal with the patient's deviant behavior, one deals with friction between the patient and others, and three deal with the patient's distress (2). Questions refer to behavior over the past four months (1). Gurland describes the structure of the questions as follows:

> Each item has a caption indicating the disturbance covered, a question which the rater asks the patient, and a continuous scale with five anchoring definitions. The highest anchoring definition describes the maximum disturbance likely to be found in an outpatient psychoneurotic population. The lowest describes reasonable adjustment. The remaining three definitions represent successive levels of disturbance between the extremes. (2, pp261–262).

The questions are asked open-ended and the interviewer matches the reply to the answers printed on the interview schedule. If there is doubt about which rating best matches the reply, the interviewer reads the two most applicable categories (in a preset order), effectively implementing a forced-choice response (1). The scale positions of the defining phrases were determined by four psychotherapists in a scaling task (2). The response categories are unique to each item, thereby reducing the likelihood that an interviewer will use a particular response category across several questions. The questionnaire is too long to reproduce here, but an indication of the scope of the instrument is given in Exhibit 5.11. The interview takes about 30 minutes. Definitions of terms are given on the rating form as part of the item: an illustration is given in Exhibit 5.12. An instruction manual is included in the 30-page interview booklet (1).

Raw scores from 0 to 10 for each scale may be summed across each of the five fields, or each field may be scored in terms of deviant behavior, friction between the patient and others, and the patient's distress. Alternatively, factor scores may be used (see "Validity").

Reliability

Fifteen patients were each interviewed by one of three psychiatrists; all three then rated the patient, either during the interview or from a tape recording of it. Inter-rater reliability was tested by comparing the scores of the three raters.

Exhibit 5.11 Scope of the SSIAM Showing Arrangement of Items Within Each Section

Fields of Maladjustment	Type of Item	Caption of Items
Work	Behavior	Unstable, inefficient, unsuccessful, over-working, over-submissive
	Friction	Friction
	Distress	Disinterested, distressed, feeling inadequate
	Inferential	Rater's assessment of environmental stress
Social	Behavior	Isolated, constrained, unadaptable, apathetic in leisure, unconforming
	Friction	Friction
	Distress	Distressed by company, lonely, bored by leisure
	Inferential	Rater's assessment of environmental stress
Family	Behavior	Reticent, over-compliant, rebellious, family-bound, withdrawn
	Friction	Friction
	Distress	Guilt-ridden, resentful, fearful
	Inferential	Rater's assessment of environmental stress
Marriage	Behavior	Constrained, submissive, domineering, neglectful, over-dependent
	Friction	Friction
	Distress	Distressed, feeling deprived, feeling inadequate
	Inferential	Rater's assessment of environmental stress
Sex	Behavior	Undesirous, inadequate, inactive, cold, promiscuous
	Friction	Rejected by partner
	Distress	Tension, feeling deprived, unwanted urges
	Inferential	Rater's assessment of environmental stress
Overall	Global	Extent of patient's distress, exaggerating, minimizing
	Prognostic	Duration, contrast with previous state, willingness to change, pressure form others to change
	Positive mental health	Strengths and assets, resourcefullness, constructive effort

Reproduced from Gurland BJ, Yorkston NJ, Stone AR, Frank JD, Fleiss JL. The Structured and Scaled Interview to Assess Maladjustment (SSIAM): I. Description, rationale, and development. Arch Gen Psychiatry 1972;27:263. Copyright 1972, American Medical Association. With permission.

Exhibit 5.12 An Example of Two Items Drawn from the SSIAM: Social and Leisure Life Section

friction	*distress*
S6 FRICTION	***S7 DISTRESSED BY COMPANY**
Q: How smoothly and well do you get along with your friends and close acquaintances?	Q: Are you ill at ease, tense, shy or upset when with friends?
1) Rate overt behavior between the patient and others. The patient's subjective responses are rated under #S7.	1) Only rate distress occurring in friendly and informal company.
	2) Mild initial shyness or mild anticipatory anxiety should be rated as "reasonable"
	3) Include distress from any other source which interferes with the enjoyment of company.

Higher first	Lower first
Frequently has furious clashes or is studiously avoided by others.	Company is mainly a source of agonizing distress.
Often irritates others or is treated with reserve by them.	Company is mainly a source of marked distress.
Sometimes relationships with others somewhat uneasy and tense.	Company is sometimes a source of distress but often enjoyable.
Not provocative but can not handle delicate social situations.	Company is unnecessarily distressing only in special circumstances but usually enjoyable.
Reasonably diplomatic.	Company is enjoyed with reasonable ease.

__Not known	__Not known
__Not applicable	__Not applicable
scope	*scope*
The frequency and intensity of his aggressive actions towards others, and the seriousness of the reaction he provokes in others.	The frequency and intensity of distress when in company, and enjoyment of company.

Reproduced from Gurland BJ, Yorkston NJ, Stone AR, Frank JD. Structured and Scaled Interview to Assess Maladjustment (SSIAM). New York: Springer, 1974:10. With permission.

Intraclass correlations among raters were calculated for six factor scores; the lowest coefficient was 0.78, the highest 0.97 (3, p265). Analyses of variance showed no significant differences among the interviewers, but differences among raters were obtained for the scores on social isolation and friction in relationships with people other than family members (3).

Validity

Using a sample of 164 adults "considered suitable for outpatient psychother- apy" (70% of whom were students), 33 of the 45 subjective items were factor analyzed. Nine items on marriage and three on sex were omitted from the 45 questions because nearly two thirds of the sample had never been married. Twelve items were found not to load on factors and were discarded; the remaining 21 items loaded on six factors: social isolation, work inadequacy, friction with family, dependence on family, sexual dissatisfaction and friction outside the family (3). For 89 patients, a relative or close friend of the patient was interviewed to provide independent ratings of the six topics identified in the factor analysis. There was significant agreement between the SSIAM and the informants' ratings for all factors except sexual dissatisfaction (3).

Serban has reported on the performance of the SSIAM with 100 schizophre- nic patients (4,5). The correlations between the SSIAM scores and the total score derived from a psychiatrist's evaluation using the Psychiatric Assessment Interview ranged from 0.21 and 0.41 (4, Table 1). The SSIAM correlated 0.45 with the Social Stress and Functioning Inventory for Psychotic Disorders (4, p950). Serban showed that the SSIAM discriminated significantly between dif- ferent types of schizophrenic patients (5). The SSIAM has also been shown capable of identifying significant changes before and after psychotherapy (6).

Commentary

The descriptions of the SSIAM given by Gurland et al. are extremely clear. Great care has evidently been taken in the design of the questionnaire and the interviewer instructions are exemplary. The conceptual basis for this scale, contrasting objective and subjective indices of adjustment, corresponds well to other available approaches, and the approach used in the SSIAM has influ- enced the design of subsequent measurements such as the OARS Multidimen- sional Functional Assessment Questionnaire and Weissman's Social Adjust- ment Scale. The SSIAM is one of the more widely used of the social health indices, having been applied in studies of depression (7) and as an outcome indicator for psychotherapy (6).

The expectation that three manifestations of maladjustment (behavior, fric- tion and distress) would appear across all five fields of maladjustment received little empirical support from the factor analytic study, so that careful consid- eration must be given to how the instrument is scored. We would also like to see considerably more evidence for the validity of the instrument, including correlations with other social health measurement scales. With these reserva- tions, we recommend the SSIAM where time permits a thorough assessment of a broad range of types and levels of disorder.

Address

Barry J. Gurland, MRCP (London), FRC Psych, Columbia University Center for Geriatrics, 100 Haven Avenue, Tower 3-29F, New York, New York, USA 10032

References

(1) Gurland BJ, Yorkston NJ, Stone AR, Frank JD. Structured and Scaled Interview to Assess Maladjustment (SSIAM). New York: Springer, 1974.

(2) Gurland BJ, Yorkston NJ, Stone AR, Frank JD, Fleiss JL. The Structured and Scaled Interview to Assess Maladjustment (SSIAM): I. Description, rationale, and development. Arch Gen Psychiatry 1972;27:259–264.

(3) Gurland BJ, Yorkston NJ, Goldberg K, Fleiss JL, Sloane RB, Cristol AH. The Structured and Scaled Interview to Assess Maladjustment (SSIAM): II. Factor analysis, reliability, and validity. Arch Gen Psychiatry 1972;27:264–267.

(4) Serban G. Mental status, functioning, and stress in chronic schizophrenic patients in community care. Am J Psychiatry 1979;136:948–952.

(5) Serban G, Gidynski CB. Relationship between cognitive defect, affect response and community adjustment in chronic schizophrenics. Br J Psychiatry 1979;134:602–608.

(6) Cross DG, Sheehan PW, Khan JA. Short- and long-term follow-up of clients receiving insight-oriented therapy and behavior therapy. J Consult Clin Psychol 1982;50:103–112.

(7) Paykel ES, Weissman M, Prusoff BA, Tonks CM. Dimensions of social adjustment in depressed women. J Nerv Ment Dis 1971;152:158–172.

THE SOCIAL ADJUSTMENT SCALE
(Myrna M. Weissman, 1971)

Purpose

The Social Adjustment Scale (SAS) was designed as an outcome measurement to evaluate drug treatment and psychotherapy for depressed patients. It has since been used in studying a broader range of patients and healthy respondents.

Conceptual Basis

The development of this self-report scale reflected a growing interest in measuring successful adjustment to community living, as distinct from abnormal symptoms. This approach is particularly relevant to patients receiving psychotherapy who do not, for the most part, present with clinical symptoms (1). The conceptual approach and item content were derived from Gurland's SSIAM and from prior empirical studies by Paykel and Weissman. The scale assesses interpersonal relationships in various roles, covering feelings, satisfaction, friction and performance. The structure reflects two separate dimensions: six role areas (such as work, family) and five aspects of adjustment that are applied, depending on the appropriateness, to each role area (2).

Description

There are two versions of the SAS, an interview schedule that is available from Dr. Weissman and the self-report version, the SAS-SR, shown in Exhibit 5.13. The latter was developed from the interview, and its advantages are that it is inexpensive to administer and free from interviewer bias (1).

Both the interview and self-report versions contain 42 questions covering role performance in six areas of functioning: work (as employee, housewife or student) (questions 1–18), social leisure activities (questions 19–29), relationships with extended family (questions 30–37), and marital roles as spouse (questions 38–46), parent (questions 47–50) and member of the family unit (questions 51–54). The method provides alternative questions on work relations for students, housewives and the employed, so the scale includes a total of 54 questions of which respondents answer 42. In each area of functioning, questions relate to the past two weeks and cover the patient's performance (e.g., level of social contacts), the amount of friction he experiences with others, finer aspects of interpersonal relationships (e.g., level of independence), and inner feelings (e.g., shyness, boredom) and satisfaction. Five- or six-point response scales are used, with higher scores representing increasing impairment. Two scoring methods are used: a mean score for each section (e.g., work, leisure), or an overall score obtained by summing the item scores and dividing by the number of items checked. The self-report version takes 15 to 20 minutes to complete, while the interview version takes about 45 to 60 minutes and includes an additional six global judgments (1). The SAS-SR is usually completed in the presence of a research assistant, who can explain the format, answer questions and check on the completeness of replies.

Reliability

For 15 depressed patients the agreement between the patient's replies on the self-report instrument and a rating made by the spouse or other informant was 0.74; the correlation between patient and interviewer assessments was 0.70 (1, Table 5). Patients rated themselves as more impaired than the interviewer rated them. Scores on the self-report and interview versions of the SAS correlated 0.72 for 76 depressed patients; agreement for the various sections ranged from 0.40 to 0.76 (1, Table 3). Item-total correlations for the various role areas ranged between 0.09 and 0.83 for the interviewer-administered SAS (2, Table 2). An alpha internal consistency coefficient of 0.74 and a mean test-retest coefficient of 0.80 were reported (3, p324). Agreement between raters was assessed for the interview version for 31 patients. The raters agreed completely on 68% of all items, with a further 27% of ratings falling within one point of each other (4). Pearson correlations between the raters across all items averaged 0.83 (4, Table 3).

Exhibit 5.13 The Social Adjustment Scale—Self-Report

SOCIAL ADJUSTMENT SELF REPORT QUESTIONNAIRE

We are interested in finding out how you have been doing in the last *two weeks*. We would like you to answer some questions about york work, spare time and your family life. There are no right or wrong answers to these questions. Check the answers that best describes how you have been in the last *two weeks*.

WORK OUTSIDE THE HOME

Please check the situation that best describes you.

I am   1 ☐   a worker for pay   4 ☐   retired   (14)

       2 ☐   a housewife   5 ☐   unemployed

       3 ☐   a student

Do you usually work for pay more than 15 hours per week?

    1 ☐   YES   2 ☐   NO   (15)

Did you work any hours for pay in the last two weeks?

    1 ☐   YES   2 ☐   NO   (16)

Check the answer that best describes how you have been in the last two weeks.

1. How many days did you miss from work in the last two weeks?

    1 ☐   No days missed.   (17)

    2 ☐   One day.

    3 ☐   I missed about half the time.

    4 ☐   Missed more than half the time but did make at least one day.

    5 ☐   I did not work any days.

    8 ☐   On vacation all of the last two weeks.

If you have not worked any days in the last two weeks, go on to Question 7.

2. Have you been able to do your work in the last 2 weeks?

    1 ☐   I did my work very well.   (18)

    2 ☐   I did my work well but had some minor problems.

    3 ☐   I needed help with work and did not do well about half the time.

    4 ☐   I did my work poorly most of the time.

    5 ☐   I did my work poorly all the time.

3. Have you been ashamed of how you do your work in the last 2 weeks?

    1 ☐   I never felt ashamed.   (19)

    2 ☐   Once or twice I felt a little ashamed.

    3 ☐   About half the time I felt ashamed.

    4 ☐   I felt ashamed most of the time.

    5 ☐   I felt ashamed all the time.

4. Have you had any arguments with people at work in the last 2 weeks?

    1 ☐   I had no arguments and got along very well.   (20)

    2 ☐   I usually got along well but had minor arguments.

    3 ☐   I had more than one argument.

    4 ☐   I had many arguments.

    5 ☐   I was constantly in arguments.

5. Have you felt upset, worried, or uncomfortable while doing your work during the last 2 weeks?

    1 ☐   I never felt upset.   (21)

    2 ☐   Once or twice I felt upset.

    3 ☐   Half the time I felt upset.

    4 ☐   I felt upset most of the time.

    5 ☐   I felt upset all of the time.

6. Have you found your work interesting these last two weeks?

    1 ☐   My work was almost always interesting.   (22)

    2 ☐   Once or twice my work was not interesting.

    3 ☐   Half the time my work was uninteresting.

    4 ☐   Most of the time my work was uninteresting.

    5 ☐   My work was always uninteresting.

WORK AT HOME – HOUSEWIVES ANSWER QUESTIONS 7-12. OTHERWISE, GO ON TO QUESTION 13.

7. How many days did you do some housework during the last 2 weeks?

    1 ☐   Every day.   (23)

    2 ☐   I did the housework almost every day.

    3 ☐   I did the housework about half the time.

    4 ☐   I usually did not do the housework.

    5 ☐   I was completely unable to do housework.

    8 ☐   I was away from home all of the last two weeks.

8. During the last two weeks, have you kept up with your housework? This includes cooking, cleaning, laundry, grocery shopping, and errands.

    1 ☐   I did my work very well.   (24)

    2 ☐   I did my work well but had some minor problems.

    3 ☐   I needed help with my work and did not do it well about half the time.

    4 ☐   I did my work poorly most of the time.

    5 ☐   I did my work poorly all of the time.

9. Have you been ashamed of how you did your housework during the last 2 weeks?

    1 ☐   I never felt ashamed.   (25)

    2 ☐   Once or twice I felt a little ashamed.

    3 ☐   About half the time I felt ashamed.

    4 ☐   I felt ashamed most of the time.

    5 ☐   I felt ashamed all the time.

Validity

The SAS scores did not correlate significantly with age, social class, sex or history of previous depression (N = 76), suggesting that scores are unaffected by sociodemographic status (1). A factor analysis applied to the interview version produced six factors: work performance, interpersonal friction, inhibited communication, submissive dependency, family attachment and anxiety (2). These

---

SOCIAL ADJUSTMENT SELF REPORT QUESTIONNAIRE (Page 2 of 6)

10. Have you had any arguments with salespeople, tradesmen or neighbors in the last 2 weeks?

1 ☐ I had no arguments and got along very well. (26)
2 ☐ I usually got along well, but had minor arguments.
3 ☐ I had more than one argument
4 ☐ I had many arguments.
5 ☐ I was constantly in arguments.

11. Have you felt upset while doing your housework during the last 2 weeks?

1 ☐ I never felt upset. (27)
2 ☐ Once or twice I felt upset.
3 ☐ Half the time I felt upset.
4 ☐ I felt upset most of the time.
5 ☐ I felt upset all of the time.

12. Have you found your housework interesting these last 2 weeks?

1 ☐ My work was almost always interesting. (28)
2 ☐ Once or twice my work was not interesting.
3 ☐ Half the time my work was uninteresting.
4 ☐ Most of the time my work was uninteresting.
5 ☐ My work was always uninteresting.

FOR STUDENTS

Answer Questions 13-18 if you go to school half time or more. Otherwise, go on to Question 19.

What best describes your school program? (Choose one)

1 ☐ Full Time (29)
2 ☐ 3/4 Time
3 ☐ Half Time

Check the answer that best describes how you have been the last 2 weeks.

13. How many days of classes did you miss in the last 2 weeks?

1 ☐ No days missed. (30)
2 ☐ A few days missed.
3 ☐ I missed about half the time.
4 ☐ Missed more than half time but did make at least one day.
5 ☐ I did not go to classes at all.
8 ☐ I was on vacation all of the last two weeks.

14. Have you been able to keep up with your class work in the last 2 weeks?

1 ☐ I did my work very well. (31)
2 ☐ I did my work well but had minor problems.
3 ☐ I needed help with my work and did not do well about half the time.
4 ☐ I did my work poorly most of the time.
5 ☐ I did my work poorly all the time.

15. During the last 2 weeks, have you been ashamed of how you do your school work? (32)

1 ☐ I never felt ashamed.
2 ☐ Once or twice I felt ashamed.
3 ☐ About half the time I felt ashamed.
4 ☐ I felt ashamed most of the time.
5 ☐ I felt ashamed all of the time.

16. Have you had any arguments with people at school in the last 2 weeks?

1 ☐ I had no arguments and got along very well. (33)
2 ☐ I usually got along well but had minor arguments.
3 ☐ I had more than one argument.
4 ☐ I had many arguments.
5 ☐ I was constantly in arguments.
8 ☐ Not applicable; I did not attend school.

17. Have you felt upset at school during the last 2 weeks?

1 ☐ I never felt upset. (34)
2 ☐ Once or twice I felt upset.
3 ☐ Half the time I felt upset.
4 ☐ I felt upset most of the time.
5 ☐ I felt upset all of the time.
8 ☐ Not applicable; I did not attend school.

18. Have you found your school work interesting these last 2 weeks?

1 ☐ My work was almost always interesting. (35)
2 ☐ Once or twice my work was not interesting.
3 ☐ Half the time my work was uninteresting.
4 ☐ Most of the time my work was uninteresting.
5 ☐ My work was always uninteresting.

---

factors cut across the two-dimensional conceptual framework on which the method was constructed.

For 76 depressed patients, the self-report method was administered before and after four weeks of treatment. Significant improvements were recorded in all of the six areas covered in the questionnaire (1). Applied to samples of com-

Exhibit 5.13 *(continued)*

SOCIAL ADJUSTMENT SELF REPORT QUESTIONNAIRE (Page 3 of 6)

SPARE TIME – EVERYONE ANSWER QUESTIONS 19-27.

Check the answer that best describes how you have been in the last 2 weeks.

19. How many friends have you seen or spoken to on the telephone in the last 2 weeks?

   1 ☐ Nine or more friends.   (36)
   2 ☐ Five to eight friends.
   3 ☐ Two to four friends.
   4 ☐ One friend
   5 ☐ No friends.

20. Have you been able to talk about your feelings and problems with at least one friend during the last 2 weeks?

   1 ☐ I can always talk about my innermost feelings.   (37)
   2 ☐ I usually can talk about my feelings.
   3 ☐ About half the time I felt able to talk about my feelings.
   4 ☐ I usually was not able to talk about my feelings.
   5 ☐ I was never able to talk about my feelings.
   8 ☐ Not applicable; I have no friends.

21. How may times in the last two weeks have you gone out socially with other people? For example, visited friends, gone to movies, bowling, church, restaurants, invited friends to your home?

   1 ☐ More than 3 times.   (38)
   2 ☐ Three times.
   3 ☐ Twice.
   4 ☐ Once.
   5 ☐ None.

22. How much time have you spent on hobbies or spare time interests during the last 2 weeks? For example, bowling, sewing, gardening, sports, reading?

   1 ☐ I spent most of my spare time on hobbies almost (39) every day.
   2 ☐ I spent some spare time on hobbies some of the days.
   3 ☐ I spent a little spare time on hobbies.
   4 ☐ I usually did not spend any time on hobbies but did watch TV.
   5 ☐ I did not spend any spare time on hobbies or watching TV.

23. Have you had open arguments with your friends in the last 2 weeks?

   1 ☐ I had no arguments and got along very well.   (40)
   2 ☐ I usually got along well but had minor arguments.
   3 ☐ I had more than one argument.
   4 ☐ I had many arguments.
   5 ☐ I was constantly in arguments.
   8 ☐ Not applicable; I have no friends.

24. If your feelings were hurt or offended by a friend during the last two weeks, how badly did you take it?

   1 ☐ It did not affect me or it did not happen.   (41)
   2 ☐ I got over it in a few hours.
   3 ☐ I got over it in a few days.
   4 ☐ I got over it in a week.
   5 ☐ It will take me months to recover.
   8 ☐ Not applicable; I have no friends.

25. Have you felt shy or uncomfortable with people in the last 2 weeks?

   1 ☐ I always felt comfortable.   (42)
   2 ☐ Sometimes I felt uncomfortable but could relax after a while.
   3 ☐ About half the time I felt uncomfortable.
   4 ☐ I usually felt uncomfortable.
   5 ☐ I always felt uncomfortable.
   8 ☐ Not applicable; I was never with people.

26. Have you felt lonely and wished for more friends during the last 2 weeks?

   1 ☐ I have not felt lonely.   (43)
   2 ☐ I have felt lonely a few times.
   3 ☐ About half the time I felt lonely.
   4 ☐ I usually felt lonely.
   5 ☐ I always felt lonely and wished for more friends.

27. Have you felt bored in your spare time during the last 2 weeks?

   1 ☐ I never felt bored.   (44)
   2 ☐ I usually did not feel bored.
   3 ☐ About half the time I felt bored.
   4 ☐ Most of the time I felt bored.
   5 ☐ I was constantly bored.

Are you a Single, Separated, or Divorced Person not living with a person of opposite sex; please answer below:

   1 ☐ YES, Answer questions 28 & 29.   (45)
   2 ☐ NO, go to question 30.

28. How many times have you been with a date these last 2 weeks?

   1 ☐ More than 3 times.   (46)
   2 ☐ Three times.
   3 ☐ Twice.
   4 ☐ Once.
   5 ☐ Never.

munity residents, depressives, alcoholics and schizophrencis, the SAS demonstrated consistent, although not strong, contrasts in responses (3). In an earlier study, significant differences had been shown between depressed patients and nonpatients for 40 out of the 48 items (5).

Weissman et al. presented correlations with independent ratings for various

---

SOCIAL ADJUSTMENT SELF REPORT QUESTIONNAIRE (Page 4 of 6)

29. **Have you been interested in dating during the last 2 weeks. If you have not dated, would you have liked to?**

   1 ☐ I was always interested in dating. (47)
   2 ☐ Most of the time I was interested.
   3 ☐ About half of the time I was interested.
   4 ☐ Most of the time I was not interested.
   5 ☐ I was completely uninterested.

FAMILY

Answer Questions 30-37 about your parents, brothers, sisters, in laws, and children not living at home. Have you been in contact with any of them in the last two weeks?

   1 ☐ YES, Answer questions 30-37.
   2 ☐ NO, Go to question 36

30. **Have you had open arguments with your relatives in the last 2 weeks?**

   1 ☐ We always got along very well. (48)
   2 ☐ We usually got along very well but had some minor arguments.
   3 ☐ I had more than one argument with at least one relative.
   4 ☐ I had many arguments.
   5 ☐ I was constantly in arguments.

31. **Have you been able to talk about your feelings and problems with at least one of your relatives in the last 2 weeks?**

   1 ☐ I can always talk about my feelings with at least one relative. (49)
   2 ☐ I usually can talk about my feelings.
   3 ☐ About half the time I felt able to talk about my feelings.
   4 ☐ I usually was not able to talk about my feelings.
   5 ☐ I was never able to talk about my feelings.

32. **Have you avoided contacts with your relatives these last two weeks?**

   1 ☐ I have contacted relatives regularly. (50)
   2 ☐ I have contacted a relative at least once.
   3 ☐ I have waited for my relatives to contact me.
   4 ☐ I avoided my relatives, but they contacted me.
   5 ☐ I have no contacts with any relatives.

33. **Did you depend on your relatives for help, advice, money or friendship during the last 2 weeks?**

   1 ☐ I never need to depend on them. (51)
   2 ☐ I usually did not need to depend on them.
   3 ☐ About half the time I needed to depend on them.
   4 ☐ Most of the time I depend on them.
   5 ☐ I depend completely on them.

34. **Have you wanted to do the opposite of what your relatives wanted in order to make them angry during the last 2 weeks?**

   1 ☐ I never wanted to oppose them. (52)
   2 ☐ Once or twice I wanted to oppose them.
   3 ☐ About half the time I wanted to oppose them.
   4 ☐ Most of the time I wanted to oppose them.
   5 ☐ I always opposed them.

35. **Have you been worried about things happening to your relatives without good reason in the last 2 weeks?**

   1 ☐ I have not worried without reason (53)
   2 ☐ Once or twice I worried.
   3 ☐ About half the time I worried.
   4 ☐ Most of the time I worried.
   5 ☐ I have worried the entire time.
   8 ☐ Not applicable; my relatives are no longer living.

EVERYONE answer Questions 36 and 37, even if your relatives are not living.

36. **During the last two weeks, have you been thinking that you have let any of your relatives down or have been unfair to them at any time?**

   1 ☐ I did not feel that I let them down at all. (54)
   2 ☐ I usually did not feel that I let them down.
   3 ☐ About half the time I felt that I let them down.
   4 ☐ Most of the time I have felt that I let them down.
   5 ☐ I always felt that I let them down.

37. **During the last two weeks, have you been thinking that any of your relatives have let you down or have been unfair to you at any time?**

   1 ☐ I never felt that they let me down. (55)
   2 ☐ I felt that they usually did not let me down.
   3 ☐ About half the time I felt they let me down.
   4 ☐ I usually have felt that they let me down.
   5 ☐ I am very bitter that they let me down.

Are you living with your spouse or have been living with a person of the opposite sex in a permanent relationship?

   1 ☐ YES, Please answer questions 38-46. (56)
   2 ☐ NO, Go to question 47.

38. **Have you had open arguments with your partner in the last 2 weeks?**

   1 ☐ We had no arguments and we got along well. (57)
   2 ☐ We usually got along well but had minor arguments.
   3 ☐ We had more than one argument.
   4 ☐ We had many arguments.
   5 ☐ We were constantly in arguments.

---

subsamples. Table 5.2 shows the resulting correlations with four independent assessments: the Hamilton Depression Rating Scale and the Raskin Depression Scale, both applied by a clinician, and two self-administered scales: the Center for Epidemiologic Studies Depression Scale and the Symptom Checklist-90. A correlation of 0.42 was obtained with the Brief Psychiatric Rating

Exhibit 5.13 *(continued)*

SOCIAL ADJUSTMENT SELF REPORT QUESTIONNAIRE (Page 5 of 6)

39. Have you been able to talk about your feelings and problems with your partner during the last 2 weeks?

1 ☐ I could always talk freely about my feelings.　(58)
2 ☐ I usually could talk about my feelings.
3 ☐ About half the time I felt able to talk about my feelings.
4 ☐ I usually was not able to talk about my feelings.
5 ☐ I was never able to talk about my feelings.

40. Have you been demanding to have your own way at home during the last 2 weeks?

1 ☐ I have not insisted on always having my own way. (59)
2 ☐ I usually have not insisted on having my own way.
3 ☐ About half the time I insisted on having my own way.
4 ☐ I usually insisted on having my own way.
5 ☐ I always insisted on having my own way.

41. Have you been bossed around by your partner these last 2 weeks?

1 ☐ Almost never.　(60)
2 ☐ Once in a while.
3 ☐ About half the time.
4 ☐ Most of the time.
5 ☐ Always.

42. How much have you felt dependent on your partner these last 2 weeks?

1 ☐ I was independent.　(61)
2 ☐ I was usually independent.
3 ☐ I was somewhat dependent.
4 ☐ I was usually dependent.
5 ☐ I depended on my partner for everything.

43. How have you felt about your partner during the last 2 weeks?

1 ☐ I always felt affection.　(62)
2 ☐ I usually felt affection.
3 ☐ About half the time I felt dislike and half the time affection.
4 ☐ I usually felt dislike.
5 ☐ I always felt dislike.

44. How many times have you and your partner had intercourse?

1 ☐ More than twice a week.　(63)
2 ☐ Once or twice a week.
3 ☐ Once every two weeks.
4 ☐ Less than once every two weeks but at least once in the last month.
5 ☐ Not at all in a month or longer.

45. Have you had any problems during intercourse, such as pain these last two weeks?

1 ☐ None.　(64)
2 ☐ Once or twice.
3 ☐ About half the time.
4 ☐ Most of the time.
5 ☐ Always.
8 ☐ Not applicable; no intercourse in the last two weeks.

46. How have you felt about intercourse during the last 2 weeks?

1 ☐ I always enjoyed it.　(65)
2 ☐ I usually enjoyed it.
3 ☐ About half the time I did and half the time I did not enjoy it.
4 ☐ I usually did not enjoy it.
5 ☐ I never enjoyed it.

QUESTIONS 47-54 On Next Page.

Scale, and of 0.53 with a clinical rating of irritability (7, Table 2). Further details of the validation results are given in a review by Weissman et al. (4).

Reference Standards

Weissman et al. reported mean scores from a sample of 482 community respondents and 191 depressives (3).

SOCIAL ADJUSTMENT SELF REPORT QUESTIONNAIRE (Page 6 of 6)

CHILDREN

Have you had unmarried children, stepchildren, or foster children living at home during the last two weeks?

  1 ☐ YES, Answer questions 47-50.   (66)
  2 ☐ NO, Go to question 51.

47. **Have you been interested in what your children are doing – school, play or hobbies during the last 2 weeks?**

  1 ☐ I was always interested and actively involved.   (67)
  2 ☐ I usually was interested and involved.
  3 ☐ About half the time interested and half the time not interested.
  4 ☐ I usually was disinterested.
  5 ☐ I wasl always disinterested.

48. **Have you been able to talk and listen to your children during the last 2 weeks? Include only children over the age of 2.**

  1 ☐ I always was able to communicate with them.   (68)
  2 ☐ I usually was able to communicate with them.
  3 ☐ About half the time I could communicate.
  4 ☐ I usually was not able to communicate.
  5 ☐ I was completely unable to communicate.
  8 ☐ Not applicable; no children over the age of 2.

49. **How have you been getting along with the children during the last 2 weeks?**

  1 ☐ I had no arguments and got along very well.   (69)
  2 ☐ I usually got along well but had minor arguments.
  3 ☐ I had more than one argument.
  4 ☐ I had many arguments.
  5 ☐ I was constantly in arguments.

50. **How have you felt toward your children these last 2 weeks?**

  1 ☐ I always felt affection.   (70)
  2 ☐ I mostly felt affection.
  3 ☐ About half the time I felt affection.
  4 ☐ Most of the time I did not feel affection.
  5 ☐ I never felt affection toward them.

FAMILY UNIT

Have you ever been married, ever lived with a person of the opposite sex, or ever had children? Please check

  1 ☐ YES, Please answer questions 51-53.   (71)
  2 ☐ NO, Go to question 54.

51. **Have you worried about your partner or any of your children without any reason during the last 2 weeks, even if you are not living together now?**

  1 ☐ I never worried.   (72)
  2 ☐ Once or twice I worried.
  3 ☐ About half the time I worried.
  4 ☐ Most of the time I worried.
  5 ☐ I always worried.
  8 ☐ Not applicable; partner and children not living.

52. **During the last 2 weeks have you been thinking that you have let down your partner or any of your children at any time?**

  1 ☐ I did not feel I let them down at all.   (73)
  2 ☐ I usually did not feel that I let them down.
  3 ☐ About half the time I felt I let them down.
  4 ☐ Most of the time I have felt that I let them down.
  5 ☐ I let them down completely.

53. **During the last 2 weeks, have you been thinking that your partner or any of your children have let you down at any time?**

  1 ☐ I never felt that they let me down.   (74)
  2 ☐ I felt they usually did not let me down.
  3 ☐ About half the time I felt they let me down.
  4 ☐ I usually felt they let me down.
  5 ☐ I feel bitter that they have let me down.

FINANCIAL – *EVERYONE PLEASE ANSWER QUESTION 54.*

54. **Have you had enough money to take care of your own and your family's financial needs during the last 2 weeks?**

  1 ☐ I had enought money for needs.   (75)
  2 ☐ I usually had enough money with minor problems.
  3 ☐ About half the time I did not have enough money but did not have to borrow money.
  4 ☐ I usually did not have enough money and had to borrow from others.
  5 ☐ I had great financial difficulty.

Reproduced from Social Adjustment Scale obtained from Dr. Myrna M. Weissman. With permission.

Alternative Forms

An enlarged version (SAS-II), a semi-structured interview containing 56 items in eight role areas, has been developed for schizophrenic patients. The scale takes about one hour to complete, and information may be obtained either from the patient or from a significant other. Agreement between self-report and ratings by significant others was studied for 56 schizophrenics, giving intraclass

Table 5.2 Correlation of the SAS and Independent Rating Scales

	Correlation with				
Sample	Hamilton	Raskin	CES-D	SCL-90	(N)
Community sample	. . .	0.44	0.57	0.59	(482)
Acute depressives	0.36	0.18	0.49	0.66	(191)
Alcoholics	0.67	0.65	0.74	0.76	(54)
Schizophrenics	0.72	0.75	0.85	0.84	(47)

Adapted from Weissman MM, Prusoff BA, Thompson WD, Harding PS, Myers JK. Social adjustment by self-report in a community sample and in psychiatric outpatients. J Nerv Ment Dis 1978;166:324,Table 5.

correlations from 0.27 to 0.81 (8). The multiple correlation of the SAS with the section scores from the Brief Psychiatric Rating Scale was 0.58 for 98 schizophrenic patients (9). Data on the inter-rater reliability of this version are given by Glazer et al. (8).

Commentary

The Social Adjustment Scale was based on a defined conceptual approach to the topic, and drew items from another well-established scale, the SSIAM. The SAS has been extensively used in psychiatric research. Weissman provided a lengthy discussion of the dimensions of social health, and of the components that may be susceptible to modification through different forms of therapy for depressed patients. The scale is one of the few designed to measure the outcomes of psychotherapy, where the intention may be less to alleviate clinical symptoms than to improve interpersonal skills and relationships. From the results of the validation studies, it appears that the SAS closely reflects depression. Information on administering, scoring and interpreting the SAS are available from Dr. Weissman, along with a 12-page bibliography of studies that have used the instrument.

Weissman has reviewed some of the limitations of the scale, including the difficulty of scoring patients who are too sick to undertake some of the roles (such as work). As originally proposed, sections that are not applicable to an individual are omitted, but this means that a patient who subsequently assumes a role (such as starting to work, perhaps at a low level) may receive a low score, thereby appearing to have deteriorated (4). A more adequate scoring approach is required for such instances. Factor analyses suggested a grouping that cut across the two-dimensional conceptual schema on which the instrument was constructed. It is therefore not clear that providing scores for each role area as Weissman did subsequently (1, 4) is the optimal way to score the SAS; further examination of this issue would seem to be indicated if the SAS is to reach its potential as an outcome measurement.

Address

Myrna M. Weissman, PhD, Professor of Psychiatry and Epidemiology, Yale University School of Medicine, 350 Congress Avenue, New Haven, Connecticut, USA 06519

References

(1) Weissman MM, Bothwell S. Assessment of social adjustment by patient self-report. Arch Gen Psychiatry 1976;33:1111–1115.

(2) Paykel ES, Weissman M, Prusoff BA, Tonks CM. Dimensions of social adjustment in depressed women. J Nerv Ment Dis 1971;152:158–172.

(3) Weissman MM, Prusoff BA, Thompson WD, Harding PS, Myers JK. Social adjustment by self-report in a community sample and in psychiatric outpatients. J Nerv Ment Dis 1978;166:317–326.

(4) Weissman MM, Paykel ES, Prusoff BA. Social Adjustment Scale handbook: rationale, reliability, validity, scoring, and training guide. (Manuscript, nd).

(5) Weissman MM, Paykel ES, Siegel R, Klerman GL. The social role performance of depressed women: comparisons with a normal group. Am J Orthopsychiatry 1971;41:390–405.

(6) Paykel ES, Weissman MM. Social adjustment and depression. Arch Gen Psychiatry 1973;28:659–663.

(7) Weissman MM, Klerman GL, Paykel ES. Clinical evaluation of hostility in depression. Am J Psychiatry 1971;128:261–266.

(8) Glazer WM, Aaronson HS, Prusoff BA, Williams DH. Assessment of social adjustment in chronic ambulatory schizophrenics. J Nerv Ment Dis 1980;168:493–497.

(9) Glazer W, Prusoff B, John K, Williams D. Depression and social adjustment among chronic schizophrenic outpatients. J Nerv Ment Dis 1981;169:712–717.

CONCLUSION

In addition to the scales reviewed above, we considered a large number of others for inclusion in this chapter. Several of these are described in review articles by Linn (1), Donald et al. (2), and Weissman et al. (3, 4). Most of the scales that we reviewed but did not include showed strengths that commended them for certain applications, but most also suffered from weaknesses that made us unwilling to present them in full reviews. As with the ADL scales in Chapter 3, the most common reasons for not describing a scale were the simple lack of evidence for its validity or reliability, or else the fact that the method was old and little used. Some of these scales are mentioned briefly in the following paragraphs.

An extensive and useful conceptual discussion of social disability was given by Ruesch in presenting his Rating of Social Disability (5, 6). The scale itself summarizes physical and emotional impairment and describes the resulting impact on social role functioning; it is completed by a psychiatrist, social worker or psychologist. Ruesch's scale has seldom been reported in the literature and there is no published evidence for its validity.

The Community Adaptation Schedule was developed to evaluate the success of aftercare programs for mental patients discharged to the community (7, 8). It is a 202-item interview that covers work, family relationships, social interaction, social activities, and activities of daily living. It employs an interesting manner of collecting information in that each question is asked in three modes. The first records factual information on circumstances or describes behavior, the second covers affective responses to these and the third assesses the patient's cognitive responses: for example, the plans the patient has made or his understanding of how other people feel about him. The scale fell into disuse after a spate of validation studies in the early 1970s, most of which showed only modest agreement with other scales (results that did not deter the authors from inferring good construct validity for the method) (9, 10). The interpretation of the scale remains unclear and more evidence is required on its association with other social scales—such as those in the present chapter—before we can recommend its use. Further references to validation studies can be found in the article by Harris and Brown (10).

The Social Disability Questionnaire by Branch deserves mention as one of the few scales designed for use in general population surveys. It is a self-report instrument that estimates need for help in performing daily tasks among elderly people in the general population (11). An innovative feature is its provision of a high risk score that anticipates the possible development of future problems. Termed a social disability questionnaire, the scale resembles the IADL scales in Chapter 3, but it also considers social support and social interaction. The scale lacks evidence on reliability and validity, and has seen only limited use.

The Community Adjustment Profile System was designed for use in the long term monitoring of patients' adjustment. Using 60 questions, it covers ten aspects of adjustment and was designed for computer scoring. Test-retest reliability was quoted at 0.83 and internal consistency of the scales ranged from 0.70 to 0.92 (12, p533).

An early scale occasionally mentioned in introductory discussions, but seldom used in published studies, is the 1968 Personality and Social Network Adjustment Scale by Clark (13). This was designed to evaluate social adjustment among severe psychiatric patients receiving treatment in a therapeutic community. There is relatively good evidence for the validity and reliability of this scale and an abbreviated version is shown in Clark's report; it is worth consideration where a brief and simple rating is required. Another scale often cited as one of the seminal efforts in the field was developed by Renne (14). We have not described this as it has virtually no published validation data and has seldom been actually used.

Finally, a promising social support scale has been developed by Norbeck (15). The Norbeck Social Support Questionnaire is based on an explicit conceptual discussion of support, and showed test-retest reliability coefficients between 0.85 and 0.92 as well as high internal consistency (15, p267). Another instrument, the Personal Resource Questionnaire developed by Brandt and Weinert, is in two sections. The first provides descriptive information on the person's resources and satisfaction with these, and the second section includes questions that reflect Weiss's dimensions of social support (16). Alpha internal consistency for the second part is 0.89 and validity coefficients ranged from 0.30 to 0.44. Validity coefficients for the first part were somewhat lower, ranging from 0.21 to 0.23 (16, p279). We recommend that anyone planning to measure social support obtain recent evidence on the further testing of these scales.

Two types of scale have been reviewed in this chapter: social adjustment scales and measurements of social support. Among the former, the Social Adjustment Scale of Weissman is the most carefully developed and shows the highest levels of validity and reliability. Henderson's social interaction scale also shows careful attention to conceptual and empirical development, and data collected using it have made contributions to the literature on social aspects of disease. Among the social support scales, none is clearly superior, mainly because they are all comparatively new and few have been tested in more than a small number of studies. Of those we review, Sarason's scale appears to be the most promising, but we advise readers to check for more recent reports on the validity of the scales.

References

(1) Linn MW. Assessing community adjustment in the elderly. In: Raskin A, Jervik LF, eds. Assessment of psychiatric symptoms and cognitive loss in the elderly. Washington, DC: Hemisphere Press, 1979:187–204.

(2) Donald CA, Ware JE Jr, Brook RH, Davies-Avery A. Conceptualization and measurement of health for adults in the Health Insurance Study. Vol. IV, Social Health. Santa Monica, California: Rand Corporation, 1978.

(3) Weissman MM. The assessment of social adjustment: a review of techniques. Arch Gen Psychiatry 1975;32:357–365.

(4) Weissman MM, Sholomskas D, John K. The assessment of social adjustment: an update. Arch Gen Psychiatry 1981;38:1250–1258.

(5) Reusch J, Brodsky CM. The concept of social disability. Arch Gen Psychiatry 1968;19:394–403.

(6) Ruesch J, Jospe S, Peterson HW Jr, Imbeau S. Measurement of social disability. Compr Psychiatry 1972;13:507–518.

(7) Roen SR, Ottenstein D, Cooper S, Burnes A. Community adaptation as an evaluative concept in community mental health. Arch Gen Psychiatry 1966;15:36–44.

(8) Burnes AJ, Roen SR. Social roles and adaptation to the community. Community Ment Health J 1967;3:153–158.

(9) Cook PE, Looney MA, Pine L. The Community Adaptation Schedule and the Adjective Check List: a validational study with psychiatric inpatients and outpatients. Community Ment Health J 1973;9:11–17.

(10) Harris DE, Brown TR. Relationship of the Community Adaptation Schedule and the Personal Orientation Inventory: two measures of positive mental health. Community Ment Health J 1974;10:111–118.

(11) Branch LG, Jette AM. The Framingham Disability Study: 1. social disability among the aging. Am J Public Health 1981;71:1202–1210.

(12) Evenson RC, Sletten IW, Hedlund JL, Faintich DM. CAPS: an automated evaluation system. Am J Psychiatry 1974;131:531–534.

(13) Clark AW. The Personality and Social Network Adjustment Scale: its use in the evaluation of treatment in a therapeutic community. Hum Rel 1968;21:85–96.

(14) Renne KS. Measurement of social health in a general population survey. Soc Sci Res 1974;3:25–44.

(15) Norbeck JS, Lindsey AM, Carrieri VL. The development of an instrument to measure social support. Nurs Res 1981;30:264–269.

(16) Brandt PA, Weinert C. The PRQ—a social support measure. Nurs Res 1981;30:277–280.

6

Quality of Life and Life Satisfaction

Quality of life has been defined and studied from the perspectives of a variety of disciplines. Environmentalists have placed emphasis upon attributes and conditions of the physical and biological environment, economists on such measures as Gross National Product, psychologists on human needs and their fulfillment . . ." (1, p103).

Most recently, it has become common to allude to quality of life in health care research. Medical interest in the quality of life was stimulated largely by our skill and success in prolonging life, and from the growing realization that this may be a mixed blessing: patients want to live, not merely to survive. The quality of survival of people who in past years could not have been saved is at times questionable, so that debates over artificial life support, euthanasia and the definition of death itself have gained considerable prominence (2, 3). The theme, of course, is not new; the dilemma was well expressed by Jonathan Swift when he remarked that every man desires to live long, but no man wishes to be old. What is new is the development of formal ways to measure quality of life and their application in evaluative studies. As with measuring happiness, we have become intrepid to the point that the idea of measuring so abstract and complex a theme as quality of life no longer seems presumptuous.

Although concern over quality of life in the health field is comparatively new, in the social sciences there has been a long-standing interest in measuring quality of life in the general population. Conceptual work in the social sciences has clarified the definition of quality of life, distinguishing it from related themes such as life satisfaction, morale, happiness, or anomie (4). These concepts differ somewhat in their level of subjectivity. Quality of life relates both to the adequacy of material circumstances and to people's feelings about these circumstances. Life satisfaction generally refers to a personal assessment of one's condition, compared to an external reference standard, or to one's aspirations. Morale, a more subjective concept, refers to a person's mental orientation: enthusiasm, confidence, sadness or depression. Happiness is generally taken to refer to shorter-term, transient feelings of well-being in response to day-to-day events. These distinctions cannot, however, be taken as rigid, for changing social circumstances tend to bring changes in the definition of these concepts. For example, there has been a clear evolution in definitions of quality of life, from viewing it in material terms of income, possessions and outward symbols of career success towards emphasizing spiritual rewards such as satisfaction, personal development and participation in the community. A person's wealth or environment is not as important as his feelings about his circumstances, including his feelings about how his actual circumstances compare with his ideal (5). Empirical studies have shown that the association between objective and subjective indicators of life quality is often not strong; the mismatch may arise where levels of perceived need rise proportionately to improvements in material conditions. This theme leads to the fascinating political issue of whether to plan social programs on the basis of factual indicators, or on the basis of people's subjective responses (see, for example, reference 5).

The shift towards using subjective indicators of life quality, dating from the 1960s, brought the concept more in line with the orientation of health care researchers. Instead of counting the number of cars or television sets a family owns, quality of life measurements came to bear a strong resemblance to familiar indices of emotional well-being and life satisfaction used with the chronically sick and aged.* Likewise, quality of life came to form a focus of attention for studies in a wide range of other disciplines, each reviewing different factors that influence self-assessed quality of life. Many studies have reviewed the dimensions of quality of life that are considered important by the public, and the way in which subjective well-being can be explained by social circumstances, health, wealth or education (6–13). These studies emphasize the multidimensional nature of quality of life (14, 15). Health is generally cited as one of the most important determinants of overall life quality, which underscores the relevance of using quality of life as an ultimate outcome of health care. It may also be noted, in passing, that in most surveys of quality of life the measurement of the health component uses a single item global rating which, in the light of the more complex health measurement techniques described in this book, must be considered of limited value.

MEASURING QUALITY OF LIFE

While conceptual distinctions may be drawn between themes such as life satisfaction, happiness, morale and anomie, progress in developing measurements that can distinguish among these concepts has lagged far behind. Indeed, many of the early quality of life indices borrowed items from life satisfaction scales. Naturally, therefore, the correlation between the two types of scale was high (16) and for this reason the present chapter groups measurements of life satisfaction and quality of life together. Although in a few years the field may have developed sufficiently to merit separate treatment of measurements of these topics, at present we view quality of life as a convenient, if somewhat

---

*Life satisfaction scales must be distinguished from patient satisfaction measurements, which refer to the patient's evaluation of, and feelings about, the quality of care.

nebulous, term referring to overall subjective feelings of well-being that are also closely related to morale, happiness and satisfaction. Acceptance of the idea that we should consider the quality of life as well as the simple fact of survival has not shown us how to define it. One difficulty arises because the concept is intuitively familiar and therefore appears undeserving of close definition: everyone believes he knows when he is better or worse off. Although this represents the central theme, definitions of "well off" seem more closely to reflect the personal values or academic orientation of the researcher than an objective attempt to define the nature of the concept. As a result, a wide variety of measurements began to be called "quality of life" indicators, including scales that bear a striking resemblance to the functional disability indices described in Chapter 3. This development arose in part as a backlash against reliance on subjective quality of life measurements, which was seen as a disadvantage if it led to ignoring practical problems in daily functioning (13). A synthesis of these approaches has led to the design of newer quality of life indices that include a blend of functional capacity and questions on emotional well-being, as seen especially in scales designed for assessing the elderly. However, there has been little theoretical work that justifies the assumption that normal functioning is necessary for a high quality of life, and evidence of high levels of satisfaction among physically disabled persons may cast doubt on this view implicit in many measurements of life quality (5).

As will be seen from the scales described in this chapter, many measurements of quality of life and life satisfaction are psychometrically weak; considerable reliance has been placed on single item instruments. Although some of these are imaginative in their design (17) single items cannot capture the complexity of a theme that is generally argued to be multidimensional. Furthermore, with one or two exceptions, very scanty evidence has been collected to indicate the reliability and validity of these measurements.

Attempts to achieve rigor in defining quality of life are also complicated by its polemic overtones: the theme has become a rallying call for social planners, politicians and activists, and quality of life measurement is certainly controversial: a radical critique of the field might claim that attention to subjective quality of life represents a conservative and reactionary attempt to divert attention away from weaknesses in objective social circumstances. The radical could further argue that medical interest in quality of life represents a desire of the medical profession to influence facets of life that should remain the responsibility of the individual.

SCOPE OF THE CHAPTER

Reflecting the varied historical roots of the available measurement methods, the four scales reviewed in this chapter are diverse in their content. We begin with Spitzer's brief Quality of Life Index intended for terminally ill cancer patients. Like an index developed by Schipper (18), this scale exemplifies the quality of life measurements that include items on physical functioning. The second method we review is a set of single item scales that have been tested by

Table 6.1 Comparison of the Quality of Life Satisfaction Indices*

Measurement	Scale	Number of items	Application	Administered by (time)	Studies using method	Reliability		Validity	
						Testing thoroughness	Results	Testing thoroughness	Results
Quality of Life Index (Spitzer)	ordinal	5	clinical	self (2 min)	few	++	++	++	++
Four Single Item Indicators of Well-Being (Andrews)	interval	1†	survey	self (<1 min)	several	+	+	+	++
Life Satisfaction Index A (Neugarten & Havighurst)	ordinal	20	survey	self	many	+ (for LSIZ only)	++	+++	++
Philadelphia Geriatric Center Morale Scale (Lawton)	ordinal	22	clinical, survey	self	few	++	+++	++	++

*For an explanation of the categories used, see Chapter 1, pages 8–9.
†Andrews describes several, single item rating scales.

Andrews (17). Although we question the adequacy of single item scales, the prevalence of their use in measuring quality of life and their innovative design have led us to include some examples. More adequate scales in terms of measurement theory have been described in the gerontological literature, where considerable attention has been paid to developing and interpreting quality of life indices. Examples include the Life Satisfaction Index and the Philadelphia Geriatric Center Morale Scale reviewed in this chapter. These longer scales are based on a formal conceptual definition of the themes they address; both are intended for elderly people and both emphasize psychological feelings of well-being. Table 6.1 compares the scope and quality of these four measurement scales.

Because of the overlap between the themes of quality of life and psychological well-being, the reader will find scales in other chapters with similar content to those described here. Chapter 4 on psychological measurement touched on positive well-being and happiness, both closely linked to subjective quality of life, and so the Bradburn scale or Dupuy's General Well-Being Schedule may be of use to those who wish to cover the psychological aspects of life quality. Conversely, if the reader's approach to quality of life emphasizes physical functioning, several of the general health measurements in Chapter 8 include aspects of quality of life: the Multilevel Assessment Instrument and the Sickness Impact Profile are examples.

References

(1) Bubolz MM, Eicher JB, Evers SJ, Sontag MS. A human ecological approach to quality of life: conceptual framework and results of a preliminary study. Soc Indicat Res 1980;7:103–136.

(2) Jones MB. Health status indexes: the trade-off between quantity and quality of life. Socio Econ Plan Sci 1977;11:301–305.

(3) Kottke FJ. Philosophic considerations of quality of life for the disabled. Arch Phys Med Rehabil 1982;63:60–62.

(4) Horley J. Life satisfaction, happiness, and morale: two problems with the use of subjective well-being indicators. Gerontologist 1984;24:124–127.

(5) Najman JM, Levine S. Evaluating the impact of medical care and technologies on the quality of life: a review and critique. Soc Sci Med 1981;15F:107–115.

(6) Flanagan JC. Measurement of quality of life: current state of the art. Arch Phys Med Rehabil 1982;63:56–59.

(7) Berg RL, Hallauer DS, Berk SN. Neglected aspects of the quality of life. Health Serv Res 1976;11:391–395.

(8) Harwood P de L. Quality of life: ascriptive and testimonial conceptualizations. Soc Indicat Res 1976;3:471–496.

(9) Liu B-C. Quality of life: concept, measure and results. Am J Econ Sociol 1975;34:1–13.

(10) Ziller RC. Self-other orientations and quality of life. Soc Indicat Res 1974;1:301–327.

(11) Burt RS, Wiley JA, Minor MJ, Murray JR. Structure of well-being: form, content, and stability over time. Sociol Meth Res 1978;6:365–407.

(12) Gratton LC. Analysis of Maslow's need hierarchy with three social class groups. Soc Indicat Res 1980;7:463–476.

(13) Alexander JL, Willems EP. Quality of life: some measurement requirements. Arch Phys Med Rehabil 1981;62:261–265.

(14) Knapp MRJ. Predicting the dimensions of life satisfaction. J Gerontol 1976;31:595–604.

(15) Cutler NE. Age variations in the dimensionality of life satisfaction. J Gerontol 1979;34:573–578.

(16) Klemmack DL, Carlson JR, Edwards JN. Measures of well-being: an empirical and critical assessment. J Health Soc Behav 1974;15:267–270.

(17) Andrews FM, Withey SB. Social indicators of well-being: Americans' perceptions of life quality. New York: Plenum, 1976.

(18) Schipper H, Clinch J, McMurray A, Levitt M. Measuring the quality of life of cancer patients: the Functional Living Index—Cancer: development and validation. J Clin Oncol 1984;2:472–483.

THE QUALITY OF LIFE INDEX
(W.O. Spitzer, 1980)

Purpose

The Quality of Life Index (QL-Index) measures the general well-being of patients with cancer and other chronic diseases. It was intended to evaluate the effects of treatment and supportive programs such as palliative care.

Conceptual Basis

Quality of life was conceptualized as a variable with several dimensions, so that good quality of life would include a positive mood state, supportive relationships, and the absence of physical or psychological distress (1). Spitzer argued that a measurement of quality of life should consider physical, social and emotional function, attitudes to illness, the adequacy of family interactions and the cost of illness to the individual (2).

Description

Possible themes for inclusion in the QL-Index were selected empirically from an opinion survey of chronic disease patients, their relatives, health professionals and well people, concerning the factors that enhance or detract from the quality of life. Fourteen themes were identified, including absence of symptoms, mental alertness and financial independence. Questions measuring these themes were incorporated in draft versions of the QL-Index. Pilot testing on 339 patients led to the selection of five themes for the eventual index: activity level (including occupation), activities of daily living, feelings of healthiness, quality of social support and psychological outlook (2). The scale, which takes about two minutes to complete, is designed to be administered by a physician or other health professional and is shown in Exhibit 6.1. A self-administered

Exhibit 6.1 The Quality of Life Index: Scoring Form

Score each heading 2, 1 or 0 according to your most recent assessment of the patient.

Activity

During the last week, the patient

- has been working or studying full-time or nearly so, in usual occupation; or managing own household; or participating in unpaid or voluntary activities, whether retired or not — 2

- has been working or studying in usual occupation or managing own household or participating in unpaid or voluntary activities; but requiring major assistance or a significant reduction in hours worked or a sheltered situation or was on sick leave — 1 ☐

- has not been working or studying in any capacity and not managing own household — 0

Daily living

During the last week, the patient

- has been self-reliant in eating, washing, toileting and dressing; using public transport or driving own car — 2

- has been requiring assistance (another person or special equipment) for daily activities and transport but performing light tasks — 1 ☐

- has not been managing personal care nor light tasks and/or not leaving own home or institution at all — 0

Health

During the last week, the patient

- has been appearing to feel well or reporting feeling "great" most of the time — 2

- has been lacking energy or not feeling entirely "up to par" more than just occasionally — 1 ☐

- has been feeling very ill or "lousy," seeming weak and washed out most of the time or was unconscious — 0

Support

During the last week

- the patient has been having good relationships with others and receiving strong support from at least one family member and/or friend   2
- support received or perceived has been limited from family and friends and/or by the patient's condition   1   ☐
- support from family and friends occurred infrequently or only when absolutely necessary or patient was unconscious   0

Outlook

During the past week the patient

- has usually been appearing calm and positive in outlook, accepting and in control of personal circumstances, including surroundings   2
- has sometimes been troubled because not fully in control of personal circumstances or has been having periods of obvious anxiety or depression   1   ☐
- has been seriously confused or very frightened or consistently anxious and depressed or unconscious   0

QL-Index total   ☐☐

How confident are you that your scoring of the preceding dimensions is accurate? Please ring [circle] the appropriate category.

Absolutely confident	Very confident	Quite confident	Not very confident	Very doubtful	Not at all confident
1	2	3	4	5	6

Reproduced from Spitzer WO, Dobson AJ, Hall J, Chesterman E, Levi J, Shepherd R, Battista RN, Catchlove BR. Measuring the quality of life of cancer patients: a concise QL-Index for use by physicians. J Chronic Dis 1981;34:591,Figure 2, Pergamon Press Ltd.

version has been developed and correlates well with the rating scale approach. Scores of 0, 1 or 2 for each category reflect increasing well-being, and may be summed to give a total score ranging from 0 to 10. Differential weights for the categories are not used. Representative scores from well and ill respondents are given by Spitzer (2).

Reliability

Internal consistency was assessed on 91 patients in an Australian study, giving an alpha of 0.77 (2, p594). Alpha was also calculated for a sample of 261 patients in Canada, giving a value of 0.78, and 0.85 for a subset of cancer patients (1). Spearman rho correlations among the five items ranged from 0.21 to 0.71 (2, Table 1).

Inter-rater reliability was studied by comparing pairs of ratings made by different physicians; Spearman correlations for various samples ranged from 0.74 to 0.84 (2). Physicians' ratings were also compared with self-ratings made by 161 Australian patients (rho = 0.61); this was repeated for 51 Canadian patients (rho = 0.69) (2, p595). Pearson correlations between ratings made by patients and relatives was 0.63 for 261 Canadian patients; the correlation between patients' and physicians' ratings was lower, at 0.45 (1).

Validity

The content validity of the instrument was checked by asking 68 people, including patients, well people, physicians and research methodologists to judge the scope and design of the instrument (2). A majority of respondents judged the format and content of the scale to be satisfactory.

Ten items from the initial item pool that were not used in the QL-Index were formed into a more extensive quality of life scale. This instrument was administered with the QL-Index to 476 patients and well people in Australia. The correlations between the QL-Index and the comprehensive scale were highest for samples of cancer patients (rho = 0.61 to 0.71), intermediate for other chronically sick patients, and low (rho = 0.29 to 0.49) for well people (2, Table 2). Replication of these analyses in a Canadian study yielded correlations between 0.66 and 0.84 for cancer patients (1, Table 4). Spitzer also developed a visual analogue scale (the QL Uniscale) for rating overall life quality, and correlations with the QL-Index were higher for cancer patients (0.49 to 0.61) than for well people (0.17 to 0.39).

Spitzer et al. reported mean scores for healthy people and various patient groups, showing that the index discriminates between healthy people and various categories of patients (2).

Commentary

The emphasis in this scale is on practicality: it is brief and easy to administer and yet broad in scope. It has proved acceptable to clinicians and so may come to replace the use of older and less well validated scales such as Karnofsky's index. It has been used in Australia, Canada, Germany, and the United States. French and German versions also exist (1).

One expects a brief scale that is also broad in scope to sacrifice some psychometric properties, and so the internal consistency alphas of 0.77 and above are reassuringly high. As Suissa et al. noted, patients give themselves higher scores than do their physicians, so in a research application the scale must be consistently completed by one type of respondent only. The validity correlations appear to be adequate for patients, especially for the very sick, but the scale is not suitable for healthy respondents for whom Spitzer recommends using one of the longer scales such as the Sickness Impact Profile (2). As the emphasis in Spitzer's scale is on physical functioning, it will be desirable to compare the QL-Index with ADL and IADL scales and also to other quality of life scales with a more psychological orientation. Suissa et al. identified systematic differences in scores across age, sex and disease categories, suggesting that these confounding variables need to be controlled in research studies using the instrument (1).

Address

W.O. Spitzer, MD, Chairman, Department of Epidemiology and Biostatistics, McGill University, 1020 Pine Avenue West, Montreal, Quebec, Canada H3A 1A2

References

(1) Suissa S, Shenker SC, Spitzer WO. Measuring the quality of life of cancer and chronically ill patients: cross-validation studies of the Quality of Life Index. (Manuscript, 1984).
(2) Spitzer WO, Dobson AJ, Hall J, Chesterman E, Levi J, Shepherd R, Battista RN, Catchlove BR. Measuring the quality of life of cancer patients: a concise QL-Index for use by physicians. J Chronic Dis 1981;34:585–597.

FOUR SINGLE ITEM INDICATORS OF WELL-BEING
(F.M. Andrews, 1976)

Purpose

These scales may be used to assess satisfaction with life in general, or with more specific topics such as health, economic status or housing. They have most commonly been used in population surveys but can also be used in clinical settings.

Conceptual Basis

Andrews stressed the subjective, evaluative component of ratings of quality of life: "The quality of life is not just a matter of the conditions of one's physical, interpersonal and social setting but also of how these are judged and evaluated by oneself and others" (1, p12).

Description

Self-ratings of life satisfaction and quality of life are frequently made on single item response scales that vary in design and format; their use is exemplified in the studies by Campbell (2). Although no single author developed these methods, it is convenient to review them in a description of the work of Frank M. Andrews, who formally compared the validity of several single item scales.

Of the scales tested by Andrews, we have selected the four shown to be most valid in his analyses. They may refer to life as a whole: "How happy are you these days?" or to reactions to particular life concerns such as health, income or housing. In either case, the scales are used to assess the affective component of quality of life rather than the physical and social conditions in which a person lives. According to the question phrasing, the scales may refer to the present or to the past, or may be used to express the respondent's hopes for the future.

To measure change with these scales Andrews uses difference scores. If this approach is complicated by an attenuation of the range of improvement where the initial score is already high, scores can be expressed as a proportion of the possible change (F. Andrews, personal communication, 1984).

The four scales are:

1. The Delighted-Terrible Scale. This is a seven-point scale ranging from delighted to terrible (see Exhibit 6.2). Respondents are told "we want to find out how you feel about various parts of your life, and life in this country as you see it. Please indicate the feelings you have now—taking

Exhibit 6.2 Delighted-Terrible Scale

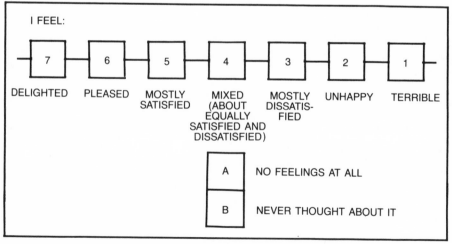

Reproduced from Andrews FM, Withey SB. Social indicators of well-being: Americans' perceptions of life quality. New York: Plenum, 1976:371. With permission.

Exhibit 6.3 Faces Scale

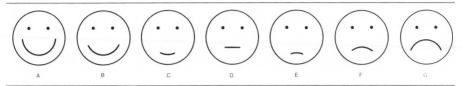

Reproduced from Andrews and Withey, p376. With permission.

into account what has happened in the last year and what you expect in the near future . . . How do you feel about _____?" (3, p5).

2. The Faces Scale. This is a seven-point scale consisting of stylized faces (see Exhibit 6.3). Each face consists of a circle with eyes that do not change and a mouth that varies from a smile of almost a half-circle to a similar half-circle upside down, representing gloom. Respondents were told "Here are some faces expressing various feelings . . . Which face comes closest to expressing how you feel about your _____ ?" (3, p5).

3. Ladder Scale. This scale (shown in Exhibit 6.4) is drawn as a ladder with nine rungs, derived from the ladder scale of Hadley Cantril (4). It has been used frequently and the instructions show slight variations (5– 7). The phrasing of Andrews and Withey is typical: the top rung is labeled "Best I could expect to have" and the bottom rung "Worst I could expect to have." Respondents are told "Here is a picture of a ladder. At the bottom of this ladder is the worst situation you might reasonably expect to have. At the top is the best you might expect to have. The other rungs are in between . . . Where on the ladder is your _____? On which rung would you put it?" The scale is often termed "self-anchoring" because ratings are made relative to each person's conception of his own maximum and minimum life satisfaction.

Exhibit 6.4 Ladder Scale

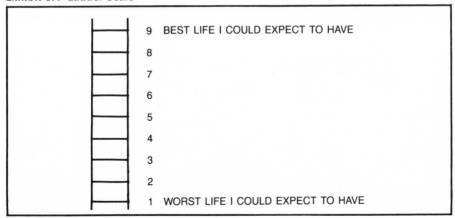

Reproduced from Andrews and Withey, p370. With permission.

Exhibit 6.5 Circles Scale

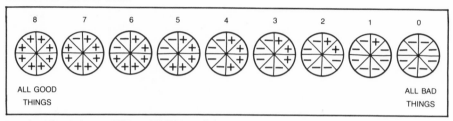

Reproduced from Andrews and Withey, p370. With permission.

4. The Circles Scale. Each of nine circles in this scale is divided into eight slices, each containing a plus or a minus sign. Circles are ordered so that they contain progressively more pluses and fewer minuses. The instruction reads "Here are some circles that we can imagine represent the lives of different people. Circle 0 has all minuses in it, to represent a person who has all bad things in his or her life. Circle 8 has all pluses in it, to represent a person who has all good things in his or her life. Other circles are in between. Which circle comes closest to matching how you feel about _____?" (3). The Circles Scale is shown in Exhibit 6.5.

Reliability

Reliability estimates from various surveys using the scales were combined by Andrews, who estimated an average test-retest reliability for each scale (applied twice in the same interview) of about 0.70. He noted that 92% of respondents provided an answer on retest that was identical or immediately adjacent to their previous answer (1). Two-year test-retest reliability in a community sample was 0.40 for the Ladder Scale and 0.41 for an 11-point satisfaction rating scale. For respondents who reported no major changes in life circumstances, coefficients were 0.47 and 0.43, respectively (8). Agreement between self-ratings and judgments by acquaintances averaged 0.33 for 16 areas rated on the Delighted-Terrible Scale. Correlations between alternative forms of the question stem (both using the Delighted-Terrible Scale) averaged 0.71 over 16 areas (9, Figure 1). Lehman et al. reported internal consistency reliabilities for the Delighted-Terrible Scales between 0.74 and 0.87 on a sample of chronic mental patients (10, p1272).

Validity

Validity analyses were carried out on a sample of 222 adults in Ohio. The analyses took the form of a multimethod-multitrait investigation in which six aspects of well-being were each assessed by the four methods, using the LISREL method of partitioning variance (3). The results show median validity coefficients of 0.82 for the Delighted-Terrible Scale, 0.82 for the Faces Scale, 0.70 for the Ladder Scale, and of 0.80 for the Circles Scale. Full results are presented by Andrews and Crandall (3, Table 1). The validity coefficients remained consistent when different aspects of life quality were assessed by the same method (3). Several other single item scales tested by Andrews showed much lower validity.

The Ladder Scale has been frequently used, although rarely validated. Using the Ladder Scale, Palmore and Kivett showed considerable stability in life satisfaction in a longitudinal study of 378 community residents aged 46 to 70 (5). Self-rated health levels formed the strongest predictors of overall life satisfaction, accounting for two thirds of the explained variance (5, 6). Atkinson showed significant associations between the Ladder Scale results and life events (8).

Lehman et al. showed the Delighted-Terrible Scale capable of showing consistent contrasts between mental patients living in the community and population reference values derived from Andrews's data (10). They also presented correlations between the subjective ratings and objective life circumstances, with coefficients falling in the range 0.07 to 0.57 (10, Table 3).

Commentary

These methods are equivalent to the numerical and visual analogue pain rating scales discussed in Chapter 7. The latter could presumably be used to measure quality of life, although they have not been frequently used in this way. The scales are simple to apply, and there are advantages to the nonverbal format. A scale such as the Faces Scale may provide a more direct representation of the feelings involved in quality of life than would a verbal translation of the response in a conventional question. The nonverbal scales may be used with children and others who would have difficulty completing a questionnaire. We presume that they provide measurements on an interval scale.

Because of their simplicity, these scales are likely to be widely used in survey research. However, it is strongly desirable that more evidence be collected on their reliability and validity. The Ladder Scale was originally used by Cantril without formal validation. Brown et al. used the Ladder Scale to examine life satisfaction among 84 people with various chronic conditions and their work represents an example of this type of study in the medical field (7). Andrews's validation studies represent a start, but employ complex analyses that may not be familiar to those working the health field. There is some data on the agreement between single item scales and Neugarten's Life Satisfaction Index (see Table 6.2 in the review that follows). Correlations ranged from 0.40 to 0.47: only about one quarter of the variance is shared by the two approaches, suggesting that although both may have some strengths, they do not agree closely as indicators of life satisfaction.

Address

F.M. Andrews, Survey Research Center, Institute for Social Research, University of Michigan, Ann Arbor, Michigan, USA 48106

References

(1) Andrews FM, Withey SB. Social indicators of well-being: Americans' perceptions of life quality. New York: Plenum, 1976.

(2) Campbell A, Converse PE, Rodgers WL. The quality of American life: perceptions, evaluations, and satisfactions. New York: Russell Sage, 1976.

(3) Andrews FM, Crandall R. The validity of measures of self-reported well-being. Soc Indicat Res 1976;3:1–19.

(4) Cantril H. The pattern of human concerns. New Brunswick, New Jersey: Rutgers University Press, 1965.

(5) Palmore E, Kivett V. Change in life satisfaction: a longitudinal study of persons aged 46–70. J Gerontol 1977;32:311–316.

(6) Palmore E, Luikart C. Health and social factors related to life satisfaction. J Health Soc Behav 1972;13:68–80.

(7) Brown JS, Rawlinson ME, Hilles NC. Life satisfaction and chronic disease: exploration of a theoretical model. Med Care 1981;19:1136–1146.

(8) Atkinson T. The stability and validity of quality of life measures. Soc Indicat Res 1982;10:113–132.

(9) Crandall R. Validation of self-report measures using ratings by others. Soc Meth Res 1976;4:380–400.

(10) Lehman AF, Ward NC, Linn LS. Chronic mental patients: the quality of life issue. Am J Psychiatry 1982;139:1271–1276.

THE LIFE SATISFACTION INDEX
(Bernice L. Neugarten and Robert J. Havighurst, 1961)

Purpose

The Life Satisfaction Index (LSI) covers general feelings of well-being among older people to identify "successful" aging (1).

Conceptual Basis

As used by Neugarten, Havighurst and Tobin, the concept of life satisfaction is closely related to morale, adjustment, and psychological well-being. Discussing these terms, they noted:

> The term "adjustment" is unsuitable because it carries the implication that conformity is the most desirable pattern of behavior. "Psychological well-being" is, if nothing else, an awkward phrase. "Morale," in many ways, captures best the qualities here being described, but there was the practical problem that there are already in use in gerontological research two different scales entitled Morale. The term Life Satisfaction was finally adopted on the grounds that, although it is not altogether adequate, it comes close to representing the five components." (1, p137).

Neugarten et al. criticized earlier, single-dimensional approaches to measuring morale or well-being; from a review of previous measurement instruments they identified five components of life satisfaction which the LSI was intended to measure. These include zest (as opposed to apathy), resolution and fortitude, congruence between desired and achieved goals, positive self-concept and mood tone (1). Positive well-being is indicated by the individual taking pleasure to his daily activities, finding life meaningful, reporting a feeling of success in achieving major goals, a positive self-image, and optimism (1).

Description

There exist several versions of the LSI. The original, the Life Satisfaction Index A (LSIA), comprises 20 items, of which 12 are positive and 8 are negative. An agree/disagree response format is used. A second and little used version, the LSIB, contains 12 questions using three-point answer scales (1). A third version, the LSIZ, was proposed by Wood et al. as a refinement of the LSIA and contains 13 of the 20 items (2, 3). Finally, Adams recommended deleting items 11 and 14 from the LSIA, forming an 18-item version which he also called the LSIA. This was later used by Harris in two large national surveys, although he confusingly named it the LSIZ (4). Exhibit 6.6 shows the original 20-item LSIA.

The LSIA was developed empirically by administering a draft version of the questionnaire to two groups of people known to differ in their level of life satisfaction. This difference had been established on the basis of the Life Satisfaction Rating Scale, also developed by Neugarten et al. The Rating Scale is scored by an expert and also reflects the five components of life satisfaction hypothesized by the authors (1). Questions in the draft scale that differentiated successfully between high and low scorers on the Rating Scale were selected for the LSIA, which is self-administered.

There are two ways to score the LSI. In the original method, a two-point agree/disagree score rated items 0 for a response indicating dissatisfaction and 1 for satisfaction. Problems with coding "undecided" responses then prompted the use of a three-point scale, rating a satisfied response as 2, an uncertain response as 1, and a dissatisfied response as 0 (3). This approach was used by Harris in his national surveys and is shown in Exhibit 6.6.

Reliability

Adams calculated item-total correlations for his 18-item LSIA, but only reported results for a few of the items (2). Wood et al. calculated the alpha internal consistency for her 13-item LSIZ at 0.79 (3, p467). Stock and Okun closely replicated this with 325 older persons, obtaining an alpha of 0.80 (5, p626). In a study of 1,288 older men, Dobson et al. used the 13-item LSIZ and reported alphas of 0.70 for two-point responses, and 0.76 for five-point answer scales (6, p571). Internal consistency appears to improve for the subset of ten items identified by Adams as loading on a factor analysis: Edwards and Klemmack obtained an alpha of 0.90 (7, p498).

Validity

The introduction to this chapter outlined two conceptual approaches to defining life satisfaction or quality of life: in terms of objective indicators such as wealth or via subjective feelings. The LSI is a subjective indicator and it is of interest to study whether or not it also reflects objective circumstances. Neu-

Exhibit 6.6 The Life Satisfaction Index A

Here are some statements about life in general that people feel differently about. Would you read each statement in the list, and if you agree with it, put a check mark in the space under "AGREE." If you do not agree with a statement, put a check mark in the space under "DISAGREE." If you are not sure one way or the other, put a check mark in the space under "?" *Please be sure to answer every question on the list.*

	Agree	Disagree	?
1. As I grow older, things seem better than I thought they would be.	_2_	_0_	_1_
2. I have gotten more of the breaks in life than most of the people I know.	_2_	_0_	_1_
3. This is the dreariest time of my life.	_0_	_2_	_1_
4. I am just as happy as when I was younger.	_2_	_0_	_1_
5. My life could be happier than it is now.	_0_	_2_	_1_
6. These are the best years of my life.	_2_	_0_	_1_
7. Most of the things I do are boring or monotonous.	_0_	_2_	_1_
8. I expect some interesting and pleasant things to happen to me in the future.	_2_	_0_	_1_
9. The things I do are as interesting to me as they ever were.	_2_	_0_	_1_
10. I feel old and somewhat tired.	_0_	_2_	_1_
11. I feel my age, but it does not bother me.	_2_	_0_	_1_
12. As I look back on my life, I am fairly well satisfied.	_2_	_0_	_1_
13. I would not change my past life even if I could.	_2_	_0_	_1_
14. Compared to other people my age, I've made a lot of foolish decisions in my life.	_0_	_2_	_1_
15. Compared to other people my age, I make a good appearance.	_2_	_0_	_1_
16. I have made plans for things I'll be doing a month or a year from now.	_2_	_0_	_1_
17. When I think back over my life, I didn't get most of the important things I wanted.	_0_	_2_	_1_
18. Compared to other people, I get down in the dumps too often.	_0_	_2_	_1_
19. I've gotten pretty much what I expected out of life.	_2_	_0_	_1_
20. In spite of what people say, the lot of the average man is getting worse, not better.	_0_	_2_	_1_

Reproduced from Neugarten BL, Havighurst RJ, Tobin SS. The measurement of life satisfaction. J Gerontol 1961;16:141. With permission. Scoring system based on Wood V, Wylie ML, Sheafor B. An analysis of a short self–report measure of life satisfaction: correlation with rater judgments. J Gerontol 1969;24:467.

garten and Havighurst showed that replies to the LSIA did not correlate with sex, socioeconomic status, age or geographical location, concluding that the scale is not merely an indicator of objective environmental circumstances (1,8). Other studies have not replicated this finding: Cutler obtained significant correlations with socioeconomic status (9). Harris found positive correlations with income, employment and education (4). Edwards studied correlates of the LSIA in a multiple regression analysis, and showed that socioeconomic status, perceived health status and social participation together explained 24% of the variance in LSIA scores (7). By contrast, Markides and Martin found that a self-rating health score, income and education explained 50% of the variance on the LSIA scores for males and 40% for females (10).

Neugarten et al. reported a correlation of 0.55 between the LSIA and the fuller Life Satisfaction Rating Scale for 92 respondents aged 50 to 90 years, and of 0.39 with a psychologist's clinical assessment of 51 respondents (1, p142). The comparison of the LSIA and the Rating Scale was replicated by Wood et al., with virtually identical results: a correlation of 0.56 (3, p467).

Lohmann compared the LSIA with other indicators of life satisfaction administered to 259 elderly people (11). The scales included the LSIA, the LSIB, the Wood's LSIZ, the Philadelphia Geriatric Center Morale Scale, the Kutner Morale Scale and a single global life satisfaction rating: "How satisfied are you with your life?" The results of the analyses are shown in Table 6.2. The Kutner Morale Scale shares four items with the LSIB, which may account for the high intercorrelation between the two scales. Stock and Okun reported correlations of 0.33 with the positive affect score on the Bradburn scale and of -0.39 with the negative affect score (5, Table 1).

Because the LSI is based on a specified conceptual definition of life satisfaction, several studies have examined its factor structure empirically. Adams identified three interpretable factors from a sample of 508 community respondents. The results showed an important general factor (34% of the variance) reflecting mood tone. The second factor corresponded to the original concept of zest for life, the third reflected congruence between desired and achieved goals. The interpretation of a fourth factor was unclear, and two items did not fall on any factor (2). More extensive exploratory and confirmatory factor analyses were carried out by Hoyt and Creech (N = 2,651) (12). The best model they identified was a three-factor solution that resembled Adams's results: congruence, mood tone and optimism (12). Using multiple regression analyses, Knapp showed that different demographic and health variables predicted each factor score, thus confirming the multidimensional nature of the scale (13). Although the LSI does cover several dimensions, Adams, like Hoyt and Creech, stressed that the empirical findings did not closely replicate the original conceptual formulation given by Neugarten and Havighurst (12, p115).

Reference Standards

Neugarten et al. obtained a mean LSIA score of 12.4 (SD, 4.4) (1, p.142). Very similar results have been obtained by other users for the 20-item scale and two-point responses: 11.6, (3, p466), 12.5, (2, p470) and 12.1 (SD, 3.9) (8, p76). For

Table 6.2 Correlations of the LSIA with Other Scales

	LSIA	LSIB	LSIZ	Kutner	PGC	Global rating
LSIA	1.00					
LSIB	0.63	1.00				
LSIZ	0.94	0.64	1.00			
Kutner	0.65	0.88	0.67	1.00		
PGC	0.76	0.74	0.79	0.74	1.00	
Global rating	0.41	0.40	0.40	0.40	0.47	1.00

Adapted from Lohmann N. Correlations of life satisfaction, morale and adjustment measures. J Gerontol 1977;32:74,Table 1.

the 18-item scale, using three-point responses, Harris reported mean scores of 26.7 for those 18 to 64 years (N = 1,457) and 24.4 for those over 65 years (N = 2,797) (4, p159).

Commentary

The Life Satisfaction Index has been extensively used and has several strengths, including reliability, strong correlations with other scales, and the availability of reference standards. The consistency of the validity findings and, in particular, of the factor structure, are striking: many other scales reviewed in this book show much less consistency between replications of factorial studies.

Despite these strengths, there have been a number of critical reviews of the LSI from which several points emerge. The question of precisely what the scale does measure is open to debate. It is agreed that the scale does not fully reflect the subtleties implied in the five component conceptual model of life satisfaction proposed by Neugarten and Havighurst. Hoyt and Creech were critical: their results "raise serious questions about the structure and interpretation of the measures in the LSIA" (12). As noted in the introduction to this chapter, measurement techniques (illustrated here by the LSI) have not managed to reflect the subtleties of the conceptual distinctions that have been drawn between concepts such as quality of life, anomie, happiness, or morale (6, 14). Klemmack et al. noted:

> Although the distinction between life satisfaction and social isolation may have some justification on theoretic grounds, there is no reason to anticipate, on the basis of our data, that the subtleties between the two concepts are reflected on an empirical level. (14, p270).

The failure of the measurement methods to reflect the distinctions among these concepts is shown by Lohmann's findings of strong associations between the LSI and the morale scales, although both were only weakly associated with a global life satisfaction rating scale of the type used by Andrews. This is probably due to the multidimensional nature of scales like the LSI, which introduces another criticism of the scale. Neugarten and Havighurst proposed a single score, which appears to obscure the multidimensional nature of the scale. A more adequate scoring system should be developed. Finally, Connidis has criticized the wording of some of the items in the LSI, suggesting that the values implicit in the wording may lead some respondents to disagree with the item even though they were not dissatisfied (15).

Some commentators have attempted to modify Neugarten and Havighurst's conceptual formulation to bring it more into line with empirical evidence. Lieberman noted:

> Life satisfaction, rather than being merely a reflection of a person's current level of goal achievement, is more like a set or orientation to one's environment which is acquired fairly early and remains moderately stable throughout life. (8, p75).

Despite the conceptual uncertainties over the LSI and despite its age, we do not recommend discarding it in favor of other life satisfaction scales, most of which have been less thoroughly evaluated. Its psychometric properties rival those of the best among comparable indices; the task is to identify clearly what, in conceptual terms, the scale measures.

Address

Bernice L. Neugarten, PhD, School of Education, Northwestern University, Evanston, Illinois, USA 60201

References

(1) Neugarten BL, Havighurst RJ, Tobin SS. The measurement of life satisfaction. J Gerontol 1961;16:134–143.
(2) Adams DL. Analysis of a Life Satisfaction Index. J Gerontol 1969;24:470–474.
(3) Wood V, Wylie ML, Sheafor B. An analysis of a short self-report measure of life satisfaction: correlation with rater judgments. J Gerontol 1969;24:465–469.
(4) Harris L. The myth and reality of aging in America. Washington, DC: National Council on the Aging, 1975.
(5) Stock WA, Okun MA. The construct validity of life satisfaction among the elderly. J Gerontol 1982;37:625–627.
(6) Dobson C, Powers EA, Keith PM, Goudy WJ. Anomie, self-esteem, and life satisfaction: interrelationships among three scales of well-being. J Gerontol 1979;34:569–572.
(7) Edwards JN, Klemmack DL. Correlates of life satisfaction: a re-examination. J Gerontol 1973;28:479–502.
(8) Lieberman LR. Life satisfaction in the young and the old. Psychol Rep 1970;27:75–79.
(9) Cutler SJ. Voluntary association participation and life satisfaction: a cautionary research note. J Gerontol 1973;28:96–100.
(10) Markides KS, Martin HW. A causal model of life satisfaction among the elderly. J Gerontol 1979;34:86–93.
(11) Lohmann N. Correlations of life satisfaction, morale and adjustment measures. J Gerontol 1977;32:73–75.
(12) Hoyt DR, Creech JC. The Life Satisfaction Index: a methodological and theoretical critique. J Gerontol 1983;38:111–116.
(13) Knapp MRJ. Predicting the dimensions of life satisfaction. J Gerontol 1976;31:595–604.
(14) Klemmack DL, Carlson JR, Edwards JN. Measures of well-being: an empirical and critical assessment. J Health Soc Behav 1974;15:267–270.
(15) Connidis I. The construct validity of the Life Satisfaction Index A and Affect Balance Scales: a serendipitous analysis. Soc Indicat Res 1984;15:117–129.

THE PHILADELPHIA GERIATRIC CENTER MORALE SCALE
(M. Powell Lawton, 1972)

Purpose

The Philadelphia Geriatric Center Morale Scale is designed to measure dimensions of emotional adjustment in persons aged 70 to 90. It is applicable both to community residents and to people in institutions.

Conceptual Basis

Lawton viewed morale as "a generalized feeling of well-being with diverse specific indicators" (1). The indicators of morale include "freedom from distressing symptoms, satisfaction with self, feeling of syntony between self and environment, and ability to strive appropriately while still accepting the inevitable" (1). The interrelationship among these components may or may not be close: a pessimistic ideology "may or may not accompany an ability to accept the status quo." Morale is viewed as a feeling and is not necessarily related to behavior; the relationship resembles that between attitudes and behavior (1).

> The person of high morale has a feeling of having attained something in his life, of being useful now, and thinks of himself as an adequate person.... High morale also means a feeling that there is a place in the environment for oneself... a certain acceptance of what cannot be changed. (1, p148).

Description

The morale scale is one of a series of geriatric assessment scales developed by the Philadelphia Geriatric Center. Their Multilevel Assessment Instrument is described in Chapter 8. Others include the Mental Status Questionnaire, the Instrumental Role Maintenance Scale, and the Minimal Social Behavior Scale (2).

A preliminary version of the morale scale with 41 items was tested on 300 healthy people with an average age of 78 years. Twenty-two items that were significantly associated with an independent ranking of the respondents according to morale, and that also loaded on a factor analysis, were retained for the main version of the scale, shown in Exhibit 6.7. Lawton subsequently recommended a further abbreviation of the scale to 17 items, as indicated by asterisks in the exhibit (3). Most of the items have a dichotomous response format; the method can be self- or interviewer-administered. Liang and Bollen suggested that scores be calculated to form three subscales (agitation, dissatisfaction and attitudes towards one's own aging), or an overall score reflecting global life satisfaction (4).

Reliability

Lawton studied reliability for several groups of respondents following varying delays. Test-retest correlations ranged from 0.91 after five weeks to 0.75 after three months (1, p150).

For 300 respondents a split-half reliability of 0.79 was obtained with the 22-item scale (1). The Kuder-Richardson internal consistency was 0.81. For three of the subscales, Morris and Sherwood obtained internal consistency reliabilities between 0.57 and 0.61 (5, p80). Other alpha values have been far higher (see "Validity").

Exhibit 6.7 The Philadelphia Geriatric Center Morale Scale
Note: Asterisks indicate the 17 items retained for the shortened version. Responses indicating satisfaction are shown on the right.

Item	Positive response
* 1. Things keep getting worse as I get older	no
* 2. I have as much pep as I did last year	yes
* 3. How much do you feel lonely? (not much, a lot)	not much
* 4. Little things bother me more this year	no
* 5. I see enough of my friends and relatives	yes
* 6. As you get older you are less useful	no
7. If you could live where you wanted, where would you live?	here
* 8. I sometimes worry so much that I can't sleep	no
* 9. As I get older, things are (better, worse, same) than/as I thought they would be	better
*10. I sometimes feel that life isn't worth living	no
*11. I am as happy now as I was when I was younger	yes
12. Most days I have plenty to do	no
*13. I have a lot to be sad about	no
14. People had it better in the old days	no
*15. I am afraid of a lot of things	no
16. My health is (good, not so good)	good
*17. I get mad more than I used to	no
18. Life is hard for me most of the time	no
*19. How satisfied are you with your life today? (satisfied, not satisfied)	satisfied
*20. I take things hard	no
21. A person has to live for today and not worry about tomorrow	yes
*22. I get upset easily	no

Derived from Lawton MP. The dimensions of morale. In: Kent DP, Kastenbaum R, Sherwood S, eds. Research planning and action for the elderly: the power and potential of social science. New York: Behavioral Publications, 1972:152–153. Also from Lawton MP. The Philadelphia Geriatric Center Morale Scale: a revision. J Gerontol 1975;30:78,Table 1.

Validity

For 199 elderly subjects, the 22-item scale correlated 0.47 with an independent ranking of their morale. Because of the low reliability of the independent ranking, this result probably represents an underestimate of the validity of the scale. A correlation of 0.57 was obtained with the Life Satisfaction Index, applied by a psychologist (1, p151).

Much attention has been paid to the factor structure of the morale scale. From the replies of 300 subjects in Lawton's original study, six factors were extracted: "surgency" or a feeling of optimism and willingness to be involved; attitudes towards own aging; satisfaction with the status quo; anxiety; depression versus optimism; and loneliness and dissatisfaction (1). Test-retest reliability on the factor scores ranged from 0.75 to 0.80. Morris and Sherwood examined the factorial structure in two samples of elderly and moderately handicapped patients (5). They obtained similar results from the two samples, but their findings differed from those of Lawton: satisfaction with the status quo and surgency were not replicated. Three factors (attitudes towards aging, agitation and loneliness) were, however, present in all samples.

Morris and Sherwood factor analyzed an abbreviated version of the scale. Three factors were obtained with internal consistencies ranging from 0.62 to 0.76 (5, p81). Lawton replicated this analysis on 828 elderly community residents (3). Seventeen items formed three factors which were comparable to those obtained by Morris and Sherwood: agitation (six items), attitude towards one's own aging (five items), and lonely dissatisfaction (six items). They provided alpha internal consistency coefficients of 0.85, 0.81 and 0.85 respectively (3, p87). Lawton recommended that these 17 items (indicated by asterisks in Exhibit 6.7) be referred to as the "Revised PGC Morale Scale," a conclusion supported by Morris and Sherwood (3).

Liang and Bollen analyzed the factor structure of the scale for a sample of 3,996 elderly respondents living in the community. Using a structural equation modelling approach, they identified three first-order factors (agitation, dissatisfaction, and attitudes towards one's own aging) and one second-order factor (global life satisfaction), which linked the three first-order factors (4). For a sample of 4,000 people aged 65 and older, Schooler factored a pool of morale-related items that included 21 of the original 22 items of the morale scale. The results "closely reproduced the three factors" obtained by Lawton (3).

Commentary

The Philadelphia Geriatric Center Morale Scale appears to be a reliable and internally consistent scale that correlates strongly with the most comparable alternative, the Life Satisfaction Index. More data are, however, needed on the validity of the scale in terms of its prediction and correlation with other quality of life scales. Nevertheless, the consistency of results across several studies suggests that Lawton's scale offers a reliable measurement of a relatively stable concept.

As Lawton noted, the morale scale might benefit from the addition of more positive affect items (3). There is some divergence of opinion over the number of items to include: Morris and Sherwood and Liang and Bollen found that two questions (numbers 3 and 5 in Exhibit 6.7) were conceptually different from the rest of the scale and should be omitted, but Lawton recommends retaining them. Liang and Bollen reviewed the scale in some detail and provide a thoughtful discussion of the alternative ways of scoring and interpreting the instrument (4).

Address

M. Powell Lawton, PhD, Philadelphia Geriatric Center, 5301 Old York Road, Philadelphia, Pennsylvania, USA 19141

References

(1) Lawton MP. The dimensions of morale. In: Kent DP, Kastenbaum R, Sherwood S, eds. Research planning and action for the elderly: the power and potential of social science. New York: Behavioral Publications, 1972:144–165.

(2) Lawton MP. Assessing the competence of older people. In: Kent DP, Kastenbaum R, Sherwood S, eds. Research planning and action for the elderly: the power and potential of social science. New York: Behavioral Publications, 1972:122–143.

(3) Lawton MP. The Philadelphia Geriatric Center Morale Scale: a revision. J Gerontol 1975;30:85–89.

(4) Liang J, Bollen KA. The structure of the Philadelphia Geriatric Center Morale Scale: a reinterpretation. J Gerontol 1983;38:181–189.

(5) Morris JN, Sherwood S. A retesting and modification of the Philadelphia Geriatric Center Morale Scale. J Gerontol 1975;30:77–84.

CONCLUSION

Quality of life remains more a fashionable idea than a rigorously defined concept in the health sciences. Although considerable good quality work has been devoted to establishing measurements, there is little agreement over the appropriate content for such indices or over how empirical measurements of quality of life relate to conceptual definitions of related themes such as morale and psychological well-being. Many of the measurement scales specify some form of conceptual framework, but these are not linked to the broader body of theoretical discussions in the literature. The current status of these measurements is in some ways the reverse of the situation in measuring functional capacity where the conceptual basis for measurement is straightforward, but the actual measurement techniques are rudimentary. Many of the quality of life indices are reliable and thoroughly tested, but this has not prevented disputes over their interpretation. While the theorists have split hairs over distinguishing between morale, happiness, and satisfaction, empirical measurements of these themes intercorrelate very highly and seem unable to reflect the conceptual distinctions. In the meanwhile, these subtleties are being ignored by many researchers who are willing to call almost any subjective well-being scale a quality of life indicator. The diversity is remarkable: under this general rubric we find indicators of life circumstances, of functional capacity, of emotional well-being, of satisfaction, and of feelings in general.

Despite this disarray, it seems that future years will see increasing attention paid to quality of life assessments as outcome measurements. This is especially true for terminally ill patients, but may also apply to general health surveys. With the growing emphasis on promoting health, quality of life holds some promise as a way to signal the final product of health care. Because quality of life scales are as much social indicators as health measurements, it will be desirable to establish a close liaison between health researchers and those with parallel interests in the social sciences and in philosophy. What is less clear is whether empirical measurements will ever be sufficiently precise to distinguish among these concepts that are obviously closely related, especially in the minds of those who will be answering the questions. We must also clarify the level at which measurements are aimed: do they refer to satisfaction and happiness in general, or do they refer to specific concerns? Do these subjective rating scales reflect objective life circumstances? Lehman et al. concluded that in some areas they do, but that the association is far from consistent: " . . . the objective and subjective indicators measured rather different aspects of quality of life. This finding argues for the use of both types of measures in quality of life assessment." (1, p1275).

The scales that have been developed show promise and will probably continue to be tested and used. The major emphasis in the coming years should be less on developing new measurements than on agreeing upon a common set of definitions and then on analyzing which of the existing indices reflect those concepts. Only when a definite gap in the coverage of existing indices has been identified should we attempt to develop new quality of life measurements.

Reference

(1) Lehman AF, Ward NC, Linn LS. Chronic mental patients: the quality of life issue. Am J Psychiatry 1982;139:1271–1276.

7

Pain Measurements

Several arguments have been raised to support the claim that pain measurement is the most challenging and difficult area of subjective health measurement. It has been argued that pain is a private and internal sensation that cannot be directly observed or measured, but whose measurement depends wholly on the subjective response of the person experiencing it. By contrast, the measurement of physical disability is more direct: we both define and measure it in terms of observable behaviors such as walking a given distance or climbing stairs. It is also clear that pain is multidimensional; a single assessment of intensity will not adequately reflect the contrast between, say, a pin prick, a toothache and a burn. Finally, pain measurement is, par excellence, the area in which subjective reports represent a blend of the strength of the underlying pain and of the person's emotional response to it. The anxiety and fear that so often accompany pain are strongly influenced by cultural norms and values and seriously complicate its measurement.

These comments are true, and yet they do not quite capture the essence of the difficulty of measuring pain; indeed, they can also apply to other areas of measurement—depression, anxiety, patient satisfaction. Like pain, depression is also an inner state, private and only measurable indirectly. Like pain, it has several aspects, such as intensity and temporal variation, but measuring depression differs from measuring pain in that we consider depression as a response, whereas we normally talk of pain as a stimulus. This may be the nub of the problem in pain measurement; we try to infer pain (as a stimulus) from the sufferer's subjective response to it. However, the way the pain is reported is influenced by many factors, biological, social and psychological. Biologically, there may not be a linear relationship between pain and the extent of tissue damage; minor damage may give rise to intense pain and vice versa. Numerous individual and cultural factors, including sex, upbringing, personality and age have been shown to influence a person's response to pain (1, 2). Psychological factors also modify the reaction to pain, and these may vary independently of the strength of the pain stimulus so that they cannot be predicted from it.

Thus, more than is the case with other areas of subjective measurement, reports of pain reflect the combined influence of the pain stimulus, environmental circumstances and the characteristics of the individual experiencing it. This is explicitly recognized in Melzack's gate control theory of pain, which accepts the relevance of psychological factors in mediating the pain response (3). Treatment for pain reflects these multiple influences on the pain experience; pain therapy may tackle either the physical pain stimulus or the patient's reaction to it. Psychological or behavioral approaches to therapy may be used to modify the response to intractable pain where the stimulus itself cannot be alleviated. Clinical experience also shows that the required dose of analgesics will vary according to the individual's pain threshold, larger doses being needed for those with lower thresholds.

A wide variety of pain measurement methods have been proposed to respond to this congeries of problems in measuring pain. Historically, these have evolved from a straightforward approach in which pain is defined and measured in terms of the person's subjective response, to a series of more complex methods that attempt to disentangle the subjective element in the response from an estimate of the underlying pain. The former approach has been long established and forms the basis for the majority of the current measurement techniques. As an example, Mersky's definition of pain speaks of it in terms of a single-dimensional subjective response:

> Pain is an unpleasant experience which we primarily associate with tissue damage, or describe in terms of tissue damage, . . . the presence of which is signalled by some form of visible or audible behavior (see 4, p195).

Subjective measurements of pain usually concentrate on its intensity, although some scales also examine the type of pain sensation or its temporal fluctuation. More recent measurements attempt to distinguish the stimulus strength from the subjective response bias, although these techniques are not yet widely used. They are mainly based on sensory decision theory, which was described in Chapter 2. In its application to pain measurement, this involves the repeated presentation of two stimuli: noise (e.g., a low level of electrical current) or experimentally induced pain, in random order. The respondent classifies each as painful or not, and from the resulting pattern of true and false positive responses indices of discriminability and of response bias can be derived (5). The first shows how accurately the respondent can distinguish between various levels of a pain stimulus; this index of perceptual performance reflects the functioning of the neurosensory system. The second index shows the threshold at which the respondent applies the term "pain" in describing these stimuli; it is related to his attitudes towards pain. A high response threshold suggests stoicism, a low one indicates an individual who readily reports pain. This analytic technique has been used in experimental studies to determine whether analgesics work by influencing discriminability (i.e., by making the stimulus feel less noxious), or by shifting the response bias (making the respondent more or less willing to call the stimulus "painful"). Clark showed that a placebo worked as an analgesic principally by reducing the respondent's tendency to label the experimental stimulus as "painful," rather than by altering the person's ability to feel it: the placebo seems to alter the affective response, not the perception of the stimulus (5).

Although they offer exciting research possibilities, measurement methods based on sensory decision theory are seldom used in clinical applications, which employ far simpler, intensity scales. The present chapter describes a range of methods of both types, partly in the hope of encouraging a shift away from the current heavy reliance on simple intensity measurements.

SCOPE OF THE CHAPTER

The techniques for collecting data to measure pain fall into three main categories: (1) those that record verbal or written descriptions of pain, (2) ratings that assess pain via its effect on the observable behavior of the person experiencing it, and (3) various analogue techniques, commonly used in laboratory studies, in which the respondent compares his pain with an experimentally induced pain stimulus of known intensity. Unfortunately, few studies have yet compared these different approaches, and the comparisons that have been made suggest a rather low agreement: they appear to be measuring different aspects of pain (6). General reviews of pain measurement techniques are given by Frederiksen et al. (1), Chapman (7) and Over (8).

QUESTIONNAIRE TECHNIQUES

The majority of pain questionnaires concentrate on intensity, and use adjectives (mild, moderate, severe) or a numerical scale to represent the intensity continuum. A variant of this has been to use visual analogue scales that represent the intensity dimension by a plain line without verbal or numerical guides (see the review of Huskisson's measurement technique). Intensity ratings may be extended to add a time dimension by using diaries or pain charts that record variations in pain over the course of a day, and may show the medications taken. Cumulative scores representing the duration of pain at each intensity level may be derived from the chart (9).

Extending the questionnaire approach to cover more than the intensity and duration of pain, Melzack's McGill Pain Questionnaire gives a qualitative description of the pain, and of the patient's affective response to pain. Subsequent refinements of the McGill method, such as Tursky's Pain Perception Profile, have sought to improve on its scale characteristics. The SAD index illustrates an alternative approach to scoring separate dimensions of pain.

The above methods concentrate on the sufferer's own pain level. Other questionnaires have been developed to assess the respondent's emotional response to pain other than his own, as a way to indicate his affective response to pain, presumed to influence the reporting of pain severity. One method consists of a color film depicting increasingly severe levels of pain applied to a human hand. The viewer's emotional response to the scenes is graded (10).

BEHAVIORAL MEASUREMENTS OF PAIN

Because pain causes changes in behavior (often involuntarily), such changes can be used as indicators of pain levels. This is analogous to the behavioral rating scales used to measure functional disability (see, for example, the Kenny scale in Chapter 3). Fordyce has discussed the correspondence between verbal responses and overt pain behavior (11). Whether recording behavior offers a more "objective" approach to measuring pain is open to debate; behavior could reflect the subjective response to pain as much as do verbal reports, but it may also be argued that pain behavior such as grimacing or wincing is involuntary and less influenced by attitudes than is answering questions.

There are several types of behavioral measurement of pain. An approach commonly used in clinical studies is to record reductions in functional performance due to pain, with the pain being graded according to how seriously it limits physical function. Examples of such scales are given by Kessler (12) and are illustrated by Jette's index, described in Chapter 3. Alternatively, pain may be inferred from health care utilization, including taking medications. This is a common approach in research on headaches, although medication use reflects both the pain and the attitudes of the sufferer to drugs. Third, other behaviors (voluntary and involuntary) such as gasping, grimacing, panting or rubbing parts of the body may be observed and recorded. An experimental procedure may be used in which the patient makes a series of body movements and the response is observed (13). Observation should evidently be as unobtrusive as possible, although this may be hard to standardize and may prove costly. Craig and Prkachin list a number of behavioral measurements of this type (14).

ANALOGUE METHODS

The analogue approach requires the person to match his "normal" pain with various levels of experimentally induced pain, typically radiant heat or an electric shock. Once a match is found, the clinical pain is described in terms of the strength of the stimulus used to induce the experimental pain. There are several alternative strategies. The respondent may be asked to apply a physical effort (such as squeezing a pressure bulb) at an intensity that matches his pain level; Peck had patients match the intensity of their pain with the intensity of a sound produced by an audiometer (15). Smith et al. described the submaximal effort tourniquet method, in which the blood circulation in the arm is stopped by an inflated blood pressure cuff; the respondent is then asked to squeeze a hand exerciser slowly 20 times. This produces an increasingly intense pain, and the time between squeezing the exerciser and the point at which the patient judges the experimental pain to match his "normal" pain gives a numerical indication of his clinical pain. The length of endurance until the pain becomes unbearable indicates the maximum pain tolerance level (7, 16). Clinical pain may be expressed as a percentage of the pain tolerance level. Sternbach has discussed the limitations of the tourniquet test. These include

Table 7.1 Comparison of the Quality of Pain Indices*

Measurement	Scale	Number of items	Application	Administered by (time)	Studies using method	Reliability		Validity	
						Testing thoroughness	Results	Testing thoroughness	Results
Visual Analogue Pain Rating Scale (Huskisson)	ratio	1	clinical, survey	self (30 sec)	several	+	+++	+	++
Oswestry Low Back Pain Disability Questionnaire (Fairbank)	ordinal	60	clinical	self (<5 min)	few	++	++	+	0
SAD Index for Clinical Assessment of Pain (Black & Chapman)	ordinal	see text	clinical	expert	few	0	0	0	0
McGill Pain Questionnaire (Melzack)	PRI(S) = interval PRI(R) = ordinal	20	survey, clinical	self (15–20 min)	many	+	+	++	++
Pain and Distress Scale (Zung)	ordinal	20	clinical	self	few	+	++	++	++
Back Pain Classification Scale (Leavitt & Garron)	interval	13	clinical	self (5–10 min)	several	++	++	++	++
Illness Behavior Questionnaire (Pilowsky & Spence)	ordinal	52	clinical	self	many	++	++	++	++
Pain Perception Profile (Tursky)	ratio	37	research	expert	few	+	0	0	0

*For an explanation of the categories used, see Chapter 1, pages 8–9.

variability in strength between individuals and problems of representing pain on a linear time scale when arguably pain does not rise as a linear function of time in the test; there may also be a practice effect (17).

There has also been a more general discussion of the validity of the analogue methods as indicators of clinical pain (6). Many of the affective features of the pain response normally seen in clinical settings may be modified in laboratory experiments. Much of the fear and anxiety that accompanies normal pain are absent: the sufferer knows the experimental pain is of a fixed duration and under the control of the experimenter. Over (8) commented that while laboratory experiments studying pain responses may constitute good psychophysics, they may have little relevance to pain outside the laboratory.

We have chosen to review measurement scales that illustrate some of the themes we have introduced. The scales are presented in order of increasing complexity. We begin with visual analogue scales that measure pain intensity, and follow this with Fairbank's Oswestry questionnaire as an example of a brief measurement that rates the disabling effect of low back pain. We then present two questionnaires that offer multidimensional pain ratings: the first is a very simple method developed by Black and Chapman known as the SAD index; the second is the longer McGill Pain Questionnaire by Melzack. The next two scales in the chapter distinguish between pain that reflects psychological disturbance and that based on organic causes: Zung's Pain and Distress Scale and Leavitt's Back Pain Classification Scale. The final two methods we describe, the Illness Behavior Questionnaire developed by Pilowsky and the Pain Perception Profile by Tursky, both distinguish between the affective response to pain and its underlying physical intensity. As in other chapters, Table 7.1 summarizes the characteristics of the scales reviewed.

References

(1) Frederiksen LW, Lynd RS, Ross J. Methodology in the measurement of pain. Behav Ther 1978;9:486–488.

(2) Tursky B, Jamner LD, Friedman R. The Pain Perception Profile: a psychophysical approach to the assessment of pain report. Behav Ther 1982;13:376–394.

(3) Melzack R. The puzzle of pain. New York: Basic Books, 1973.

(4) Bond MR. New approaches to pain. Psychol Med 1980;10:195–199.

(5) Clark WC, Yang JC. Applications of sensory decision theory to problems in laboratory and clinical pain. In: Melzack R, ed. Pain measurement and assessment. New York: Raven Press, 1983:15–25.

(6) Postlethwaite R, Grieve N, Santacroce T, Renfree L, Wilson G, Peck C. An analysis of pain produced by the submaximum effort tourniquet test. In: Peck C, Wallace M, eds. Problems in pain. Sydney, Australia: Pergamon Press, 1980:128–135.

(7) Chapman CR. Measurement of pain: problems and issues. In: Bonica JJ, Albe-Fessard DG, eds. Advances in pain research and therapy. Vol. I. New York: Raven Press, 1976:345–353.

(8) Over R. Clinical and experimental pain. In: Peck C, Wallace M, eds. Problems in pain. Sydney, Australia: Pergamon Press, 1980:94–100.

(9) Elton D, Burrows GD, Stanley GV. Clinical measurement of pain. Med J Aust 1979;1:109–111.

(10) Elton D, Burrows GD, Stanley GV. Apperception of pain. In: Peck C, Wallace M, eds. Problems in pain. Sydney, Australia: Pergamon Press, 1980:117–120.

(11) Fordyce WE. The validity of pain behavior measurement. In: Melzack R, ed. Pain measurement and assessment. New York: Raven Press, 1983:145–153.

(12) Kessler HH. Disability—determination and evaluation. Philadelphia: Lea & Febiger, 1970.

(13) Waddell G, McCulloch J, Kummel E, Venner R. Nonorganic physical signs in low back pain. Spine 1980;5:117–125.

(14) Craig KD, Prkachin KM. Nonverbal measures of pain. In: Melzack R, ed. Pain measurement and assessment. New York: Raven Press, 1983:173–179.

(15) Peck RR. A precise technique for the measurement of pain. Headache 1967;7:189–194.

(16) Smith GM, Lowenstein E, Hubbard JH, Beecher MK. Experimental pain produced by the submaximal effort tourniquet technique. Further evidence of validity. J Pharmacol Exp Ther 1968;163:468–474.

(17) Sternbach RA. The tourniquet pain test. In: Melzack R, ed. Pain measurement and assessment. New York: Raven Press, 1983:27–31.

VISUAL ANALOGUE PAIN RATING SCALES
(E.C. Huskisson, 1974)

Purpose

Visual analogue pain rating scales provide a simple way to record subjective estimates of pain intensity.

Conceptual Basis

Visual analogue measurements are normally used only to rate the overall severity of pain, although the technique could be applied in measuring other dimensions, such as levels of anxiety or emotional responses associated with pain.

Description

Visual analogue scales have been widely used in measuring pain; we have chosen to report the work of Huskisson, who is one of the leading exponents of this approach. Huskisson applied visual analogue scales, which had long been used in psychological measurement, to the problem of rating pain (1). A visual analogue scale is a straight line that represents the continuum of the symptom to be rated. The scale, conventionally 10 cm long, may be printed either vertically or horizontally. Each end of the scale is marked with labels that indicate the range being considered: in measuring pain Huskisson used the phrases "Pain as bad as it could be" and "No pain" (2, 3). The patient is asked to place a mark on the line at a point representing the severity of his pain. The scale requires only about 30 seconds to complete.

Alternative formats have been used. For example, descriptive terms may be placed at intervals along the line, such as "severe," "moderate," or "mild." A comparison of 5, 10, 15 and 25 cm lines suggested that the 5 cm line provided less reliable results than other lengths (4). Scott and Huskisson carried out a series of experiments to test which format provided the most valid results; they concluded that scales without adjectives along their length were the most suitable. Scales with adjectives tended to produce a clustering of responses beside the adjectives (see 1, Figures 2, 3). If adjectives are to be used, they should be printed so that they spread along the entire length of the line, as illustrated in Exhibit 7.1.

There are several ways to score the scales. The distance of the respondent's mark from the lower end of the scale, measured in millimeters, forms the basic score. Alternatively, a 20-point grid may be superimposed over the line to give a categorical rating. Huskisson justified this approach by noting that it represents the maximal level of discrimination people can use in recording pain levels (1). The distribution of results is not normal, and nonparametric statis-

Exhibit 7.1 Alternative Formats for Rating Scales Tested by Huskisson

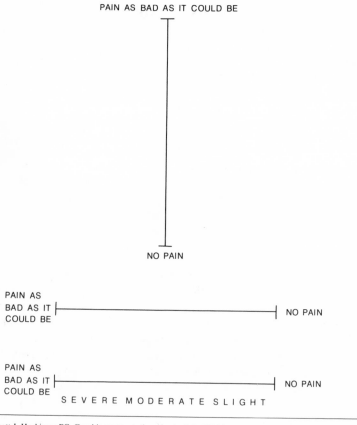

Adapted from Scott J, Huskisson EC. Graphic representation of pain. Pain 1976;2:176.

tical analyses are appropriate (2). Transformations may be applied to normalize the data (1, p1128); a critical review of scoring procedures was given by Maxwell (5). In estimating pain relief, Huskisson argued that it is not appropriate simply to compare scores before and after treatment, for the possible magnitude of this difference is determined by the initial score (1). Indeed, initial and subsequent pain ratings tend to be correlated; Huskisson reported coefficients of 0.62 and 0.63 (1, Figures 5, 6). Rather than comparing ratings before and after treatment, therefore, Huskisson recommended using a rating of pain relief. This can take the form of a descriptive scale (such as none, slight, moderate or complete relief) or a visual analogue scale ranging from no relief to complete relief of pain. Comparing the two methods, Huskisson showed that the simple descriptive scale gave better results when completed by patients without assistance (1).

Reliability

Scott and Huskisson studied the repeatability of visual analogue pain scales and also compared scales printed vertically and horizontally. One hundred rheumatology patients were given a vertical and a horizontal scale in random order. The correlation was 0.99 between the scores, although scores on the horizontal scale were slightly, but not significantly, lower than on the vertical scale (mean 10.85 versus 11.05) (6).

Validity

Huskisson reported a correlation of 0.75 between a visual analogue scale printed vertically and a four-point descriptive scale rating pain as slight, moderate, severe or agonizing (3). The association was probably attenuated by the restricted number of categories on the descriptive scale. Similar analyses on samples of 100 and 104 rheumatic patients gave correlations ranging from 0.71 to 0.78 between a four-point descriptive scale and visual analogue scales printed vertically or horizontally. Correlations between the vertical and horizontal scales ranged from 0.89 to 0.91 (7, Tables 1, 2). Elton et al. obtained correlations ranging from 0.60 to 0.63 between a visual analogue scale and Melzack's McGill Pain Questionnaire, although the latter was scored in an unconventional manner (8, Table 1).

Commentary

Huskisson summarized the advantages of visual analogue scales as follows:

> Visual analogue scales provide the patients with a robust, sensitive, reproducible method of expressing pain severity. Results correlate well with other methods of measuring pain. The method is applicable to all patients regardless of language and can be used by children aged 5 or more years. (2, p768).

Other commentators have been less enthusiastic. Downie et al. compared a visual analogue scale with a ten-point numerical rating scale as shown in

Exhibit 7.2, and argued that the latter "was to be preferred on the grounds of measurement error"—perhaps because the visual analogue scale offers a confusingly wide range of choice (7). Huskisson, indeed, noted that the visual analogue scale may cause difficulty for some respondents. Of 100 patients, seven were unable to understand the idea of the scale when it was first explained, even though all could use a descriptive scale (1). Scott and Huskisson recommended that patients complete the visual analogue scale under supervision before attempting it on their own. Other minor points have been raised, including the warning by Dixon and Bird that in using a vertical scale, distortion may result from perspective when the page lies flat on a table (9).

A debate has arisen over whether or not patients should be shown their initial pain ratings when reassessing pain on follow-up. Scott and Huskisson argued that, because increasing time between assessments leads to patients being less able to remember their initial rating, this reduces the validity of comparing ratings before and after treatment, and patients should be shown their previous scores when making subsequent judgments of pain severity (10). Dixon and Bird disagreed: although patients may find it easier to rate their current pain level when shown previous scores, such ratings may not agree with other indices of disease progress (9). They also showed that the accuracy with which a person could reproduce marks on a visual analogue scale varied according to the placement of the original mark: marks close to the ends or the centre of the line were more accurately reproduced than marks in other positions (9).

In conclusion, the agreement among the various ways of recording pain severity is close; the selection of a method may not be overly important. The choice between using a visual analogue scale and the categorical rating will depend upon the degree of sensitivity required: for research purposes, a four-point rating may be too crude, although it appears to be simpler for patients

Exhibit 7.2 Formats of the Numerical Rating (NRS) and Visual Analogue Scales (VAS) as Used by Downie et al.

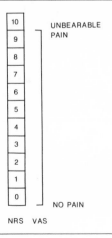

Reproduced from Downie WW, Leatham PA, Rhind VM, Wright V, Branco JA, Anderson JA. Studies with pain rating scales. Ann Rheum Dis 1978;37:378, Figure 1. With permission.

to complete. The data presented by Downie et al. suggest that a ten-point numerical scale may provide a compromise position between the four-point rating and the visual analogue methods.

Address

E.C. Huskisson, MD, FRCP, Department of Rheumatology, St. Bartholomew's Hospital, London, England EC1A 7BE

References

(1) Huskisson EC. Measurement of pain. Lancet 1974;2:1127–1131.
(2) Huskisson EC. Measurement of pain. J Rheumatol 1982;9:768–769.
(3) Scott J, Huskisson EC. Graphic representation of pain. Pain 1976;2:175–184.
(4) Revill SI, Robinson JO, Rosen M, Hogg MIJ. The reliability of a linear analogue for evaluating pain. Anaesthesia 1976;31:1191–1198.
(5) Maxwell C. Sensitivity and accuracy of the visual analogue scale: a psycho-physical classroom experiment. Br J Clin Pharmacol 1978;6:15–24.
(6) Scott J, Huskisson EC. Vertical or horizontal visual analogue scales. Ann Rheum Dis 1979;38:560.
(7) Downie WW, Leatham PA, Rhind VM, Wright V, Branco JA, Anderson JA. Studies with pain rating scales. Ann Rheum Dis 1978;37:378–381.
(8) Elton D, Burrows GD, Stanley GV. Clinical measurement of pain. Med J Aust 1979;1:109–111.
(9) Dixon JS, Bird HA. Reproducibility along a 10 cm vertical visual analogue scale. Ann Rheum Dis 1981;40:87–89.
(10) Scott J, Huskisson EC. Accuracy of subjective measurements made with or without previous scores: an important source of error in serial measurement of subjective states. Ann Rheum Dis 1979;38:558–559.

THE OSWESTRY LOW BACK PAIN DISABILITY QUESTIONNAIRE
(Jeremy Fairbank, 1980)

Purpose

The Oswestry questionnaire indicates the extent to which a person's functional level is restricted by pain. It was intended for clinical use and is completed by the patient.

Conceptual Basis

No information is available.

Description

The Oswestry Low Back Pain Disability Questionnaire is divided into ten sections, each containing six items. The first section rates the effect of analgesics in relieving pain. The remaining nine sections cover the disabling effect of increasingly severe levels of pain on typical daily activities: personal care, lifting, walking, sitting, standing, sleeping, sex life, social life and traveling. This questionnaire therefore concentrates on the effects, rather than the nature, of pain.

Exhibit 7.3 The Oswestry Low Back Pain Disability Questionnaire

How long have you had back pain?   .... Years .... Months .... Weeks

How long have you had leg pain?   .... Years .... Months .... Weeks

Please read:
This questionnaire has been designed to give the doctor information as to how your back pain has affected your ability to manage in everyday life. Please answer every section, and mark in each section only the *one box* which applies to you. We realise you may consider that two of the statements in any one section relate to you, but please just *mark the box which most closely describes your problem.*

Section 1 — Pain Intensity
- ☐ I can tolerate the pain I have without having to use pain killers.
- ☐ The pain is bad but I manage without taking pain killers.
- ☐ Pain killers give complete relief from pain.
- ☐ Pain killers give moderate relief from pain.
- ☐ Pain killers give very little relief from pain.
- ☐ Pain killers have no effect on the pain and I do not use them.

Section 2 — Personal Care (Washing, Dressing, etc)
- ☐ I can look after myself normally without causing extra pain.
- ☐ I can look after myself normally but it causes extra pain.
- ☐ It is painful to look after myself and I am slow and careful.
- ☐ I need some help but manage most of my personal care.
- ☐ I need help every day in most aspects of self care.
- ☐ I do not get dressed, wash with difficulty and stay in bed.

Section 3 — Lifting
- ☐ I can lift heavy weights without extra pain.
- ☐ I can lift heavy weights but it gives extra pain.
- ☐ Pain prevents me from lifting heavy weights off the floor, but I can manage if they are conveniently positioned, eg on a table.
- ☐ Pain prevents me from lifting heavy weights but I can manage light to medium weights if they are conveniently positioned.
- ☐ I can lift only very light weights.
- ☐ I cannot lift or carry anything at all.

Section 4 — Walking
- ☐ Pain does not prevent me walking any distance.
- ☐ Pain prevents me walking more than 1 mile.
- ☐ Pain prevents me walking more than ½ mile.
- ☐ Pain prevents me walking more than ¼ mile.
- ☐ I can only walk using a stick or crutches.
- ☐ I am in bed most of the time and have to crawl to the toilet.

Section 5 — Sitting
- ☐ I can sit in any chair as long as I like.
- ☐ I can only sit in my favourite chair as long as I like.
- ☐ Pain prevents me sitting more than 1 hour.
- ☐ Pain prevents me from sitting more than ½ hour.
- ☐ Pain prevents me from sitting more than 10 mins.
- ☐ Pain prevents me from sitting at all.

Section 6 — Standing
- ☐ I can stand as long as I want without extra pain.
- ☐ I can stand as long as I want but it gives me extra pain.
- ☐ Pain prevents me from standing for more than 1 hour.
- ☐ Pain prevents me from standing for more than 30 mins.
- ☐ Pain prevents me from standing for more than 10 mins.
- ☐ Pain prevents me from standing at all.

Section 7 — Sleeping
- ☐ Pain does not prevent me from sleeping well.
- ☐ I can sleep well only by using tablets.
- ☐ Even when I take tablets I have less than six hours sleep.
- ☐ Even when I take tablets I have less than four hours sleep.
- ☐ Even when I take tablets I have less than two hours sleep.
- ☐ Pain prevents me from sleeping at all.

Section 8 — Sex Life
- ☐ My sex life is normal and causes no extra pain.
- ☐ My sex life is normal but causes some extra pain.
- ☐ My sex life is nearly normal but is very painful.
- ☐ My sex life is severely restricted by pain.
- ☐ My sex life is nearly absent because of pain.
- ☐ Pain prevents any sex life at all.

Section 9 — Social Life
- ☐ My social life is normal and gives me no extra pain.
- ☐ My social life is normal but increases the degree of pain.
- ☐ Pain has no significant effect on my social life apart from limiting my more energetic interests, eg dancing, etc.
- ☐ Pain has restricted my social life and I do not go out as often.
- ☐ Pain has restricted my social life to my home.
- ☐ I have no social life because of pain.

Section 10 — Travelling
- ☐ I can travel anywhere without extra pain.
- ☐ I can travel anywhere but it gives me extra pain.
- ☐ Pain is bad but I manage journeys over two hours.
- ☐ Pain restricts me to journeys of less than one hour.
- ☐ Pain restricts me to short necessary journeys under 30 minutes.
- ☐ Pain prevents me from travelling except to the doctor or hospital.

Comments ....

....

- -

Scoring (not seen by patients)

For each section the total possible score is 5; if the first statement is marked the section score = 0, if the last statement is marked it = 5.

If all ten sections are completed the score is calculated as follows:

Example: $\frac{16}{50}$ (total scored) / (total possible score) x 100 = 32%

If one section is missed or not applicable the score is calculated:

Example: $\frac{16}{45}$ (total scored) / (total possible score) x 100 = 35.5%

Reproduced from Fairbank JCT, Couper J, Davies JB, O'Brien JP. The Oswestry Low Back Pain Disability Questionnaire. Physiotherapy 1980;66:272.

The patient marks the statement in each section that most accurately describes the effect of his pain; if two items are marked, the more severe is scored. For each section scores fall on a 0 to 5 scale, with higher values representing greater disability. The sum of the ten scores is expressed as a percentage of the maximum score. If the patient fails to complete a section, the percentage score is adjusted accordingly. Fairbank et al. interpreted the results as follows: scores from 0 to 20 represent minimal disability, 20 to 40 represent moderate disability, 40 to 60 represent severe disability, while scores of 60 and over indicate that the patient is severely disabled by pain in several areas of life (1).

When self-administered, the questionnaire takes less than five minutes to complete and one minute to score; if the questions are read to a patient, it requires about ten minutes. The questionnaire is shown in Exhibit 7.3.

Reliability

Twenty-two patients with low back pain completed the questionnaire twice, on consecutive days. A test-retest correlation of 0.99 was obtained (1, p273). Fairbank also reported "a good internal consistency," but offered no statistical summary of this (1).

Validity

The only available indication of validity was derived from a study of 25 patients suffering from a first attack of low back pain, expected to remit spontaneously. Over a three-week period, scores on the questionnaire showed a significant improvement (1).

Commentary

This questionnaire has been included as it represents a measurement of disability and handicap due to pain, rather than of pain as impairment. As such, it provides potentially valuable additional information to that offered by the measurements developed by Huskisson and Melzack. The preliminary nature of the validity and reliability tests, however, indicates that further analyses need to be carried out to assess the quality of this measurement.

Address

Jeremy C.T. Fairbank, MD, FRCS, Senior Orthopaedic Registrar, Orthopaedic Department, St. Bartholomew's Hospital, West Smithfield, London, England EC1A 7BE

Reference

(1) Fairbank JCT, Couper J, Davies JB, O'Brien JP. The Oswestry Low Back Pain Disability Questionnaire. Physiotherapy 1980;66:271–273.

THE SAD INDEX FOR CLINICAL ASSESSMENT OF PAIN
(Richard G. Black and C. Richard Chapman, 1976)

Purpose

The SAD Index provides a numerical score summarizing the severity of clinical pain and accompanying levels of anxiety and depression.

Conceptual Basis

The SAD Index is based on the recognition that expressions of pain reflect the level of the pain stimulus as modified by the patient's emotional reaction. These two elements must be distinguished for the provision of appropriate therapy. Otherwise, there is a danger that physical treatment could be applied to what was in reality a psychological complaint:

> unnecessary and even harmful surgery may be performed, often repeatedly, in a desperate attempt to eliminate a "pain" that may have no surgically correctable cause. Alternate, yet still inappropriate, management with strong analgesic medications prescribed in ever-escalating doses may lead the patient into a vicious circle of depression, confusion, and increased expression of pain. (1, p301).

The SAD Index provides a clinical tool for summarizing separately the somatic and psychological aspects of the pain response.

Description

The SAD Index assesses the patient's complaint of pain on three dimensions, "each a well-known clinical entity with an accepted, effective therapy. . . . each pain problem is defined in terms of Somatic input, Anxiety, and Depression" (1). Each of these dimensions of pain is rated by the therapist on a 0 to 10 scale of intensity, the three axes forming a three-dimensional system of coordinates. For research purposes, an overall pain (or "suffering") score can be represented by the vector sum of the dimensions represented on the three axes, using the formula

$$\text{Suffering} = 0.58\sqrt{S^2 + A^2 + D^2},$$

where S designates the somatic score, A, the level of anxiety and D, the level of depression (1). The coefficient 0.58 is a scaling factor that restricts the total score to a range of 0 to 10. For clinical applications, the scores may be presented separately as a profile. Black and Chapman cite as an illustration "the chronically depressed low-back cripple with minimum physical disability" with a pain profile of 1:4:8 (1).

The authors of the SAD Index did not specify exactly how data for each of the three ratings were to be collected. They suggested using one of the many established anxiety and depression scales, but noted that assigning scores on the somatic axis

> is a difficult problem involving quantification of clinical judgment as well as psychophysical assessment of the patient's subjective state. Variables that can be used

for this evaluation include: history and functional inquiry, activity diary, clinician's subjective impression, experience with comparable disease, pain description questionnaires, and pain matching tests . . . (1, p303).

Black and Chapman viewed the SAD Index primarily as a clinical tool, rather than as a research instrument. Because of this orientation, and because no standard set of questions was recommended, they did not report on the reliability or validity of the index.

Reliability

No information is available.

Validity

No information is available.

Commentary

Although the method is not fully developed, we have described the SAD Index because it represents an elegant approach to the problem of summarizing pain on several dimensions. It is intended to be practical to use in a clinical setting and, as such, the idea merits attention. Unfortunately, its authors have not proceeded further with the method, and developmental work is needed, including the selection of the most adequate indicators for each dimension so that a standard form of the index can be produced. It will then be necessary to collect reliability and validity data.

Address

C. Richard Chapman, PhD, Department of Anesthesiology RN-10, University of Washington, School of Medicine, Seattle, Washington, USA 98195

Reference

(1) Black RG, Chapman CR. SAD Index for clinical assessment of pain. In: Bonica JJ, Albe-Fessard D, eds. Advances in pain research and therapy. Vol. 1. New York: Raven Press, 1976:301–305.

THE McGILL PAIN QUESTIONNAIRE
(Ronald Melzack, 1975)

Purpose

The McGill Pain Questionnaire (MPQ) was designed to provide a quantitative profile of three aspects of pain (1). The method was originally used in evaluating pain therapies; its use as a diagnostic aid has also been described (2).

Conceptual Basis

Melzack's major contribution to pain measurement has been to emphasize that the pain experience comprises several distinct aspects. In 1973 he wrote:

> The problem of pain, since the beginning of this century, has been dominated by the concept that pain is purely a sensory experience. Yet it has a unique, distinctively unpleasant, affective quality that differentiates it from sensory experiences such as sight, hearing or touch. . . .
>
> The motivational-affective dimension of pain is brought clearly into focus by clinical studies on frontal lobotomy . . . Typically, these patients report after the operation that they still have pain but it does not bother them. . . . the suffering, the anguish are gone. . . . Similarly, patients exhibiting "pain asymbolia" . . . after lesions of portions of the parietal lobe or the frontal cortex are able to appreciate the spatial and temporal properties of noxious stimuli (for example, they recognize pin pricks as sharp) but fail to withdraw or complain about them. . . .
>
> These considerations suggest that there are three major psychological dimensions of pain: sensory-discriminative, motivational-affective, and cognitive-evaluative. (3, pp93–95).

Melzack argued that these three aspects of the pain experience are subserved by distinct systems in the brain (3) and he attempted to measure these dimensions with the MPQ. Melzack stressed that the questionnaire represented a first attempt at developing a measurement reflecting his theory of pain, and suggested that other investigators might ultimately refine it (1). Nonetheless, the method continues to be used in its original form.

Description

The complete MPQ comprises sections recording the patient's diagnosis, drug regimen, medical history concerning pain, present pain pattern, accompanying symptoms and modifying factors, effects of pain, and the list of words describing pain which is the part of the instrument most commonly used. The present discussion concerns only this latter section of the questionnaire.

Melzack and Torgerson selected 102 words describing pain from the literature and from existing questionnaires (4). They sorted these words into the three major classes proposed in Melzack's theory of pain: words concerned with the sensory qualities of pain (e.g., temporal, thermal), those covering affective qualities of pain (e.g., fear, tension), and "evaluative words that describe the subjective overall intensity of the total experience of pain" (4). Within the three major classes, Melzack and Torgerson grouped words that were qualitatively similar, as shown in Exhibit 7.4. The suitability of this *a priori* grouping was checked by 20 reviewers. At first there were 16 such subclasses, but four others were added to give a final questionnaire with 20 subclasses (1).

An equal-appearing interval scaling procedure was used to estimate the intensity of pain represented by the words in each subclass. Three groups of judges (140 students, 20 physicians, and 20 patients) rated each word on a seven-point scale (4). Where there was disagreement among the three groups of judges on the rank ordering of a word within a subclass, the word was

Exhibit 7.4 The McGill Pain Questionnaire

Patient's Name_____Date_____Time_____am/pm
Analgesic(s) _____ Dosage_____Time Given _____am/pm
             _____ Dosage_____Time Given_____am/pm

Analgesic Time Difference (hours):   +4 +1 +2 +3
PRI: S_____ A_____ E_____ M(S)_____ M(AE)_____ M(T)_____PRI(T)____
     (1-10)   (11-15) (16)   (17-19)   (20)   (17-20)   (1-20)

1 FLICKERING __	11 TIRING ___
QUIVERING __	EXHAUSTING __
PULSING __	12 SICKENING ___
THROBBING __	SUFFOCATING __
BEATING __	13 FEARFUL __
POUNDING __	FRIGHTFUL __
2 JUMPING __	TERRIFYING __
FLASHING __	14 PUNISHING __
SHOOTING __	GRUELLING __
3 PRICKING __	CRUEL __
BORING __	VICIOUS __
DRILLING __	KILLING __
STABBING __	15 WRETCHED __
LANCINATING __	BLINDING __
4 SHARP __	16 ANNOYING __
CUTTING __	TROUBLESOME __
LACERATING __	MISERABLE __
5 PINCHING __	INTENSE __
PRESSING __	UNBEARABLE __
GNAWING __	17 SPREADING __
CRAMPING __	RADIATING __
CRUSHING __	PENETRATING __
6 TUGGING __	PIERCING __
PULLING __	18 TIGHT __
WRENCHING __	NUMB __
7 HOT __	DRAWING __
BURNING __	SQUEEZING __
SCALDING __	TEARING __
SEARING __	19 COOL __
8 TINGLING __	COLD __
ITCHY __	FREEZING __
SMARTING __	20 NAGGING __
STINGING __	NAUSEATING __
9 DULL __	AGONIZING __
SORE __	DREADFUL __
HURTING __	TORTURING __
ACHING __	PPI
HEAVY __	0 No pain __
10 TENDER __	1 MILD __
TAUT __	2 DISCOMFORTING __
RASPING __	3 DISTRESSING __
SPLITTING __	4 HORRIBLE __
	5 EXCRUCIATING __

PPI_____ COMMENTS:

CONSTANT____
PERIODIC____
BRIEF____

ACCOMPANYING SYMPTOMS:	SLEEP:	FOOD INTAKE:
NAUSEA __	GOOD __	GOOD __
HEADACHE __	FITFUL __	SOME __
DIZZINESS __	CAN'T SLEEP __	LITTLE __
DROWSINESS __	COMMENTS:	NONE __
CONSTIPATION __		COMMENTS:
DIARRHEA __		
COMMENTS:	ACTIVITY:	COMMENTS:
	GOOD __	
	SOME __	
	LITTLE __	
	NONE __	

Reproduced from Melzack R. Psychologic aspects of pain. Pain 1980;8:145. With permission.

deleted from the questionnaire; scale values for the remaining words, were based on the ratings made by patients. These values are shown in Exhibit 7.5.

The words were originally read to the patient by an interviewer so that unfamiliar words could be explained. This took 15 to 20 minutes, reducing to 5 to 10 minutes for patients familiar with the method. Subsequent users have employed the checklist in a written format. The respondent is asked to select the one word in each subclass that most accurately describes his pain at that time (1). If none of the words applies, none is chosen. Other instructions have

Exhibit 7.5 Scale Weights for Scoring the McGill Pain Questionnaire

1			2			3		
	Flickering	1.89		Jumping	2.60		Pricking	1.94
	Quivering	2.50		Flashing	2.75		Boring	2.05
	Pulsing	2.56		Shooting	3.42		Drilling	2.75
	Throbbing	2.68					Stabbing	3.45
	Beating	2.70					Lancinating	3.50
	Pounding	2.85						
4			5			6		
	Sharp	2.95		Pinching	1.95		Tugging	2.16
	Cutting	3.20		Pressing	2.42		Pulling	2.35
	Lacerating	3.64		Gnawing	2.53		Wrenching	3.47
				Cramping	2.75			
				Crushing	3.58			
7			8			9		
	Hot	2.47		Tingling	1.60		Dull	1.60
	Burning	2.95		Itchy	1.70		Sore	1.90
	Scalding	3.50		Smarting	2.00		Hurting	2.45
	Searing	3.88		Stinging	2.25		Aching	2.50
							Heavy	2.95
10			11			12		
	Tender	1.35		Tiring	2.42		Sickening	2.75
	Taut	2.36		Exhausting	2.63		Suffocating	3.45
	Rasping	2.61						
	Splitting	3.10						
13			14			15		
	Fearful	3.30		Punishing	3.50		Wretched	3.16
	Frightful	3.53		Gruelling	3.73		Blinding	3.45
	Terrifying	3.95		Cruel	3.95			
				Vicious	4.26			
				Killing	4.50			
16			17			18		
	Annoying	1.89		Spreading	3.30		Tight	2.25
	Troublesome	2.42		Radiating	3.38		Numbing	2.10
	Miserable	2.85		Penetrating	3.72		Drawing	2.53
	Intense	3.75		Piercing	3.78		Squeezing	2.35
	Unbearable	4.42					Tearing	3.68
19			20					
	Cool			Nagging	2.25			
	Cold			Nauseating	2.74			
	Freezing			Agonizing	3.20			
				Dreadful	4.11			
				Torturing	4.53			

Adapted from Melzack R, Torgerson WS. On the language of pain. Anesthesiology 1971;34:54–55,Table 1.

been used: patients may be asked to describe their "average pain," their "most intense" pain (5), or how their pain "typically feels" (6).

Four scoring methods were proposed by Melzack:

1. The sum of the scale values for all the words chosen in a given category (sensory, etc.) or across all categories. This was called a Pain Rating Intensity Score using scale values: PRI(S). The scale weights are shown in Exhibit 7.5. (Note that no scale weights are available for category 19).

2. As above, but replacing the scale values by a code indicating the rank-placement of each word selected within its subclass: PRI(R).

3. The Number of Words Chosen: NWC.
4. The Present Pain Intensity score on a 0 to 5 scale from the pain description section of the questionnaire shown in Exhibit 7.4: PPI.

Reliability

Melzack reported a small test-retest study in which ten patients completed the questionnaire three times at intervals ranging from three to seven days, with an average consistency of response of 70.3% (1, p287).

Validity

Melzack reviewed the agreement among the four scoring methods (1). Correlations are presented in Table 7.2 and show that the PPI score is not closely reflected by the other scores.

Dubuisson and Melzack compared responses to the MPQ given by 95 patients suffering from one of eight distinct pain syndromes. Discriminant function analyses showed that 77% of patients could be correctly classified into diagnostic groups on the basis of their verbal description of pain (2, 7).

Correlations between MPQ scores and visual analogue scales for 40 patients ranged from 0.50 for the affective score to 0.65 for the PPI and for the total score (8, Table 2).

Several reviewers of the MPQ have addressed the question of whether Melzack's selection and grouping of words do indeed reflect the three dimensions he proposed. Studies in Canada (5), the United States (9), and in Britain (10), each using different types of pain patient, have reviewed the factor structure of the MPQ. A summary of such investigations is given by Prieto and Geisinger (11). The general aim of the studies was, in the words of Crockett et al., "to empirically determine the nature and minimum number of dimensions necessary to describe responses to the MPQ" (5). The three studies applied principal components analyses to the MPQ, using the scale values of the words chosen from each group as the scores for 20 variables in the analysis. Two of the studies extracted four factors (8, 9), and one found five (5); there is some correspondence between the factors obtained, although this is not great. Read-

Table 7.2 Pearson Correlations Among Four Scoring Procedures for the McGill Pain Questionnaire (N = 248)

	PRI(S)	PRI(R)	NWC	PPI
PRI(S)	. . .	0.95	0.97	0.42*
PRI(R)		. . .	0.89	0.42
NWC			. . .	0.32
PPI				. . .

*Melzack did not give a precise figure, but stated it was "virtually identical" to the 0.42 obtained between PPI and PRI(R).

Adapted from Melzack R. The McGill Pain Questionnaire: major properties and scoring methods. Pain 1975;1:285.

ing concluded that "Factorial investigations of the questionnaire provide support for the distinction between affective and sensory dimensions, but not for a distinctive evaluative component" (10).

Alternative Forms

A Finnish translation of the MPQ is described in Melzack's recent book on pain measurement (12), as is an extended version of the MPQ itself, which is presented in the book (13). The latter is called the McGill Comprehensive Pain Questionnaire, and covers details of the patient's illness, personality, milieu and coping resources.

Commentary

There can be no question that Melzack's McGill Pain Questionnaire is the leading instrument for describing the various dimensions of pain. It is based on a clear theory of pain and has been widely used in many different countries. Although Melzack originally presented the MPQ as a preliminary version of a measurement method, it has remained unmodified. Does it, in fact, succeed in reflecting Melzack's theory of pain?

Crockett et al. argued that the results of their factor analyses offered empirical validation of Melzack's *a priori* classification of pain descriptors, and concurred with Melzack's emphasis on the need to describe pain in terms of several dimensions rather than as a single intensity score. However, there remains concern over the structure of the MPQ, and there are several methodological problems in examining how closely it reflects Melzack's theory of pain. As well as the technical criticisms raised by Prieto et al., there are conceptual difficulties in using factor analysis to assess the validity of the questionnaire. Melzack and Torgerson recognized that words from different components (e.g., affective, evaluative) may correlate with one another, while different subclasses in each component will not necessarily intercorrelate (4). If this is the case, one would not necessarily expect words in, say, the sensory component to load on a single factor. Because the respondent selects only one word in each subclass, the correlations among words in each subclass will be zero, and so the grouping of words into subclasses cannot be tested empirically. Furthermore, because each word reflects both a type and an intensity of pain, a factor analysis may extract type of pain or intensity of pain factors, or both. This was illustrated by a study that departed from normal usage and presented the MPQ words in random order, asking subjects to check every word that described their pain (6). The seven factors that were interpretable cut across Melzack's groupings, and took words at similar levels of intensity from a wide range of subclasses.

Although it is hard to show that Melzack's questionnaire does reflect his conceptual definition of pain, the method is still the leading pain measurement scale, and we recommend its continued use until a superior method is available.

Address

Ronald Melzack, PhD, Professor, Department of Psychology, Stewart Biological Sciences Building, McGill University, 1205 Docteur Penfield Avenue, Montreal, Quebec, Canada H3A 1B1

References

(1) Melzack R. The McGill Pain Questionnaire: major properties and scoring methods. Pain 1975;1:277–299.
(2) Melzack R. Psychologic aspects of pain. Pain 1980;8:143–154.
(3) Melzack R. The puzzle of pain. New York: Basic Books, 1973.
(4) Melzack R, Torgerson WS. On the language of pain. Anesthesiology 1971;34:50–59.
(5) Crockett DJ, Prkachin KM, Craig KD. Factors of the language of pain in patient and volunteer groups. Pain 1977;4:175–182.
(6) Leavitt F, Garron DC, Whisler WW, Sheinkop MB. Affective and sensory dimensions of back pain. Pain 1978;4:273–281.
(7) Dubuisson D, Melzack R. Classification of clinical pain descriptions by multiple group discriminant analysis. Exp Neurol 1976;51:480–487.
(8) Taenzer P. Postoperative pain: relationships among measures of pain, mood, and narcotic requirements. In: Melzack R, ed. Pain measurement and assessment. New York: Raven Press, 1983:111–118.
(9) Prieto EJ, Hopson L, Bradley LA, Byrne M, Geisinger KF, Midax D, Marchisello PJ. The language of low back pain: factor structure of the McGill Pain Questionnaire. Pain 1980;8:11–19.
(10) Reading AE. The internal structure of the McGill Pain Questionnaire in dysmenorrhoea patients. Pain 1979;7:353–358.
(11) Prieto EJ, Geisinger KF. Factor-analytic studies of the McGill Pain Questionnaire. In: Melzack R, ed. Pain measurement and assessment. New York: Raven Press, 1983:63–70.
(12) Pöntinen PJ, Ketovuori H. Verbal measurement in non-English language: the Finnish Pain Questionnaire. In: Melzack R, ed. Pain measurement and assessment. New York: Raven Press, 1983:85–93.
(13) Monks R, Taenzer P. A comprehensive pain questionnaire. In: Melzack R, ed. Pain measurement and assessment. New York: Raven Press, 1983:233–237.

THE SELF-RATING PAIN AND DISTRESS SCALE
(William W.K. Zung, 1983)

Purpose

The self-rating Pain and Distress Scale was intended as a brief measurement of the mood and behavior changes that are associated with acute pain. It does not directly asssess the severity of the pain itself.

Conceptual Basis

No information is available.

Description

Zung's Pain and Distress Scale (PAD) describes the physical and emotional sequelae of pain. These include limitations in activities of daily living and psychological responses such as agitation, depression and decreased alertness. The PAD contains 20 items that were selected on clinical grounds and reflect problems (particularly psychological) that commonly accompany pain. Zung grouped the items on a conceptual basis: one item covers pain (item 18), six reflect mood changes (items 1, 2 and 16–19), while the remaining 13 items cover behavioral changes (see Exhibit 7.6).

The PAD scale is self-administered, and the questions use four-point response scales indicating the frequency with which that symptom is experienced; higher scores denote more frequent symptoms. The time period to which the items refer is not fixed; any appropriate period such as a week may be used. The scores for each question are summed and are expressed as a percentage of the maximum attainable score.

Reliability

Zung reported an alpha internal consistency of 0.89 based on data from 122 pain patients and 195 controls (1, p892).

Validity

A comparison of pain patients and controls showed that each of the 20 items discriminated significantly ($p < 0.01$) between them (1). A discriminant function analysis was used to identify 11 items that discriminated with a sensitivity of 84.4% and a specificity of 99.5% (1, p893). These 11 items represented both mood and behavior changes. A factor analysis identified six factors that cut across the conceptual assignment of items described above, in that most of the factors included both behavioral and mood change items.

Commentary

This new pain rating scale differs from others in this chapter in that it concentrates more on the distress associated with pain than on evaluating the pain itself. Many of the items reflect general anxiety and depressive responses, and are not phrased to refer specifically to pain as the source of the symptoms. Zung's method may be compared with two other scales we review: Pilowsky's Illness Behavior Questionnaire, which is designed to diagnose the psychological causes for an exaggerated pain response, and Leavitt's Back Pain Classification Scale, which also distinguishes pain of organic origin from that due to psychological causes. Zung's method, by contrast, covers psychological prob-

Exhibit 7.6 The Pain and Distress Scale

	None or a little of the time	Some of the time	Good part of the time	Most or all of the time
1. I feel miserable, low and down	☐	☐	☐	☐
2. I feel nervous, tense, and keyed up	☐	☐	☐	☐
3. I get tired for no reason	☐	☐	☐	☐
4. I can work for as long as I usually do	☐	☐	☐	☐
5. I am as efficient in my work as usual	☐	☐	☐	☐
6. I have trouble falling asleep	☐	☐	☐	☐
7. I have trouble sleeping through the night	☐	☐	☐	☐
8. I wake up earlier than I want to	☐	☐	☐	☐
9. I feel rested when I get out of bed	☐	☐	☐	☐
10. I am restless and can't keep still	☐	☐	☐	☐
11. I find it hard to do the things I usually do	☐	☐	☐	☐
12. I find it hard to think and remember things	☐	☐	☐	☐
13. My mind is foggy and I can't concentrate	☐	☐	☐	☐
14. I am as alert as I could be	☐	☐	☐	☐
15. I still enjoy the things I used to	☐	☐	☐	☐
16. I enjoy listening to the radio or watching TV	☐	☐	☐	☐
17. I enjoy visiting friends and relatives	☐	☐	☐	☐
18. I have aches and pains that bother me	☐	☐	☐	☐
19. I am more irritable than usual	☐	☐	☐	☐
20. Everything I do is an effort	☐	☐	☐	☐

Adapted from Zung WWK. A self-rating Pain and Distress Scale. Psychosomatics 1983;24:889,Table 2. Copyright W. Zung, 1982. All rights reserved. With permission.

lems *associated* with pain, commonly as responses to the pain rather than as causes.

Because it is new, there is very little information available on the reliability and validity of the PAD scale. It will, for example, be important to show how well the PAD scores correlate with those obtained from established pain measurement methods such as Melzack's MPQ. The validity testing used patients with acute, traumatic pain; the method has not been tested on chronic pain patients. Like the SAD index, Zung's method deliberately identifies separate aspects of pain, although the maneuver of combining these various dimensions into a single overall score would appear to some extent to vitiate his original purpose. It may be that future versions of the PAD scale will develop a more adequate scoring system that provides separate scores for different dimensions of the pain experience.

Address

William W.K. Zung, MD, Professor of Psychiatry, VA Medical Center, Durham, North Carolina, USA 27705

Reference

(1) Zung WWK. A self-rating Pain and Distress Scale. Psychosomatics 1983;24:887–894.

THE BACK PAIN CLASSIFICATION SCALE
(Frank Leavitt and David C. Garron, 1978)

Purpose

The Back Pain Classification Scale (BPCS) is a screening device that distinguishes low back pain due to psychological disturbance from that due to organic disease (1). It was principally intended as a clinical tool to identify patients with low back pain who would benefit from a more thorough psychological evaluation.

Conceptual Basis

Leavitt and Garron noted that there are many patients with low back pain for whom organic pathology cannot be demonstrated and for whom the pain may reflect psychological distress: "People in psychological distress are assumed to develop physical symptoms as a means of communicating and/or managing emotional or interpersonal difficulties." (1, p149). Diagnosis of such problems is hard: "Patients are habitually silent about psychological problems, and even the most astute of physicians are by their training poorly equipped to evaluate these highly complex processes with any degree of sophistication." (2, p79). Because of the difficulty in diagnosis, the existence of a psychological basis for pain is commonly inferred from the absence of organic pathology, rather than being positively demonstrated in its own right (1). As an alternative approach, several studies have used MMPI scales to detect an emotional basis for pain complaints; the MMPI Low Back Scale is capable of identifying consistent patterns of response apparently reflecting pain of a psychosomatic origin (1). However, the MMPI produces a high rate of misclassification and is long and not readily accepted by pain patients. Leavitt therefore developed the BPCS as an alternative means to distinguish between organic and psychological bases for low back pain.

Description

The BPCS was derived from the observation that patients whose pain reflected psychological disturbance used verbal pain descriptors differently than did patients whose pain had an organic basis (3). Patients with pain attributable to a psychological cause (termed "functional pain") described their pain as more variable, diffuse, and intense. They used a wider variety of words to describe their pain, typically endorsing more of the affective and skin pressure types of pain descriptor (2, 3).

The BPCS forms one component of the longer Low Back Pain Symptom Checklist shown in Exhibit 7.7. This comprises 103 adjectives taken from the McGill Pain Questionnaire and other sources. The 103 words include 71 that may be scored to provide seven pain scales and the 13 words that form the Back Pain Classification Scale (4). These are randomly distributed through the questionnaire, and all 103 items are normally asked even if only the 13 words comprising the BPCS are to be analyzed. The results reported below refer only to the Classification Scale that is shown in Exhibit 7.8. The other seven scales were identified via factor analyses and describe various aspects of the pain experience. The first factor describes emotional discomfort, while the second is a mixed emotional and sensory factor. The remaining five cover sensory aspects of pain (5). The Low Back Pain Symptom Checklist is self-administered and takes between five and ten minutes to complete.

The BPCS was developed empirically from a comparison of the responses of 62 patients whose back pain was explained organically and 32 patients whose pain was judged (via a battery of mental and psychological tests) to have a psychological origin (1). A discriminant analysis identified the 13 words that distinguished between the two types of patient (1, p152). The BPCS is scored using weights derived from the discriminant function analyses, shown in Exhibit 7.8. The weights for the items selected by the respondent are added, and a positive total implies pain of psychological origin, whereas a negative score reflects pain of organic origin. The higher the score (in either direction) the more likely is the diagnosis.

Exhibit 7.7 The Low Back Pain Symptom Checklist

WHAT DOES YOUR PAIN USUALLY FEEL LIKE?

DIRECTIONS: The words below describe different qualities of pain. Place an ⊠ in the boxes beside the words that best describe how your pain typically feels. You may check as many boxes as you wish that describe your typical pain **this last week.**

9	☐ squeezing	44	☐ splitting	8	☐ continuous
10	☐ aching	45	☐ torturing	9	☐ transient
11	☐ gruelling	46	☐ pricking	10	☐ pulling
12	☐ periodic	47	☐ troublesome	11	☐ tender
13	☐ nagging	48	☐ throbbing	12	☐ intermittent
14	☐ quivering	49	☐ numb	13	☐ suffocating
15	☐ radiating	50	☐ nauseating	14	☐ taut
16	☐ heavy	51	☐ drilling	15	☐ frightful
17	☐ boring	52	☐ jumping	16	☐ crushing
18	☐ miserable	53	☐ dreadful	17	☐ pinching
19	☐ cutting	54	☐ drawing	18	☐ flashing
20	☐ cruel	55	☐ rasping	19	☐ killing
21	☐ penetrating	56	☐ blinding	20	☐ fearful
22	☐ annoying	57	☐ spreading	21	☐ beating
23	☐ exhausting	58	☐ tearing	22	☐ cramping
24	☐ wrenching	59	☐ rhythmic	23	☐ lacerating
25	☐ pounding	60	☐ shooting	24	☐ wretched
26	☐ momentary	61	☐ hurting	25	☐ intense
27	☐ dull	62	☐ hot	26	☐ pins and needles
28	☐ pulsing	63	☐ punishing	27	☐ superficial
29	☐ stinging	64	☐ burning	28	☐ deep
30	☐ brief	65	☐ sharp	29	☐ localized
31	☐ cold	66	☐ tiring	30	☐ unlocalized
32	☐ flickering	67	☐ scalding	31	☐ spasms
33	☐ unbearable	68	☐ gnawing	32	☐ diffuse
34	☐ tugging	69	☐ stabbing	33	☐ surface
35	☐ agonizing	70	☐ tingling	34	☐ stiff
36	☐ piercing	71	☐ freezing	35	☐ skin pain
37	☐ smarting	72	☐ tight	36	☐ muscle pain
38	☐ steady	73	☐ itchy	37	☐ bone pain
39	☐ constant	74	☐ pressing	38	☐ joint pain
40	☐ lancinating	75	☐ sore	39	☐ moving pain
41	☐ terrifying	76	☐ sickening	40	☐ electrical
42	☐ vicious	77	☐ searing	41	☐ shock-like
43	☐ cool				

Reproduced from the Low Back Pain Symptom Checklist, obtained from Dr. Frank Leavitt. With permission.

Exhibit 7.8 The Back Pain Classification Scale,
Showing Discriminant Function Coefficients

Note: Words with positive coefficients reflect pain of
psychological origin, those with negative coefficients
indicate organic pain.

Pain variables	Unstandardized coefficients
Squeezing	0.67
Nagging	−0.67
Exhausting	0.50
Dull	−0.49
Sickening	0.69
Troublesome	0.47
Throbbing	−0.33
Tender	0.66
Intermittent	−0.51
Numb	0.66
Shooting	−0.30
Punishing	−1.64
Tiring	0.49

Reproduced from Leavitt F, Garron DC. The detection of psychological disturbance in patients with low back pain. J Psychosom Res 1979;23:152,Table 2. With
permission.

Reliability

A test-retest reliability of 0.86 after 24 hours was obtained from a hospitalized
sample (N = 114). A split-half reliability of 0.89 was obtained from 158
patients hospitalized with low back pain (2, p83).

Validity

To check the discriminant analysis used to select the adjectives included in the
BPCS, Leavitt and Garron carried out a cross-validation study on a different
sample of pain patients. The scale correctly classified 132 out of 159 cases: a
rate of 83% (1, p152).

Leavitt studied 91 patients with low back pain that could not be attributed
to organic disease. This group was divided into 59 patients with clinically manifest symptoms of psychological disorders and 32 patients without. The BPCS
achieved a 78% correct classification of these two types of pain patient, compared with 64.5% for the MMPI scales measuring hypochondriasis and hysteria, and 37.4% for the MMPI Low Back Scale (4, pp302–303).

In a further examination of the discriminal ability of the BPCS, a sample of
120 patients with low back pain was divided into two groups on the basis of
their BPCS scores: 79 patients whose pain apparently had an organic basis and
41 whose pain was classified as nonorganic (6). All patients were examined by
a clinical psychologist who also administered the MMPI. The group identified

by the BPCS as exhibiting pain of psychological origin gave higher scores on all ten clinical scales of the MMPI, eight of these differences being statistically significant ($p < 0.01$) (6, Table 2). The clearest differences were on the MMPI hypochondriasis and hysteria scales.

In a prospective study, 108 patients were divided into those for whom an organic basis could be identified clinically for their pain versus those for whom there was none (7). All were treated medically and were followed for 14 weeks after discharge. The BPCS scores at admission were used to classify the group without organic signs into two subgroups: those showing psychological symptoms and those showing none. Over a 14-week follow-up period the progress of the two latter groups differed, with the group exhibiting psychological symptoms showing less improvement (7). Patients with no organic basis for their pain reported as much pain on retesting 14 weeks after treatment as the organic group did prior to treatment (2). Sanders compared the classification made by the scale with one made on the basis of a medical record review. The BPCS correctly classified 80% of the low back pain patients, but only 60% of 50 headache patients (8).

Demographic variables including age, sex, education, religion and race do not predict scores on the BPCS, so that it can be used in comparing patients with different sociodemographic backgrounds (2). In a multiple regression study, Garron and Leavitt showed that the MMPI hypochondriasis scale explained 15.5% of the variance in the BPCS (9, p62). Adding a battery of other tests and MMPI scales to the regression analysis raised the variance explained to 34%.

Commentary

The Back Pain Classification Scale performs a diagnostic and screening task similar to that of Zung's Pain and Distress Scale and Pilowsky's Illness Behavior Questionnaire. The rationale for the BPCS was to provide a means for positively identifying patients whose pain was due to psychological distress. The scale appears to succeed in this, and it can also demonstrate that not all patients for whom no organic basis can be found for their pain do, in fact, suffer from psychological disorders. Thus, for example, Leavitt and Garron used the BPCS to classify patients into four categories according to the presence or absence of organic and psychological problems (3). The discriminal ability of the BPCS is high and appears to exceed that of the MMPI. Leavitt and Garron concluded that the BPCS provides a viable clinical alternative to the more cumbersome MMPI for distinguishing between pain of organic and of psychosomatic origin.

As with some of the psychological screening tests described in Chapter 4, the exact interpretation of the BPCS scores may not be clear (8). The 13 discriminating words came from several of the factors that underlie the complete pain scale (1). As Leavitt noted:

> Why this particular set of verbal pain descriptors works as discriminators and others do not is unclear from research to date. The shared variance of pain words with

MMPI items is only 21%, and does not seem to fit any particular pattern in terms of the sensory and affective divisions of pain experience. Much research is still needed to understand the apparently heterogeneous content of the scale as it reflects some pain experience and/or personal characteristics that are as of yet not apparent. . . . Although the BPCS indicates with a high degree of probability that a psychological disturbance exists, it does not identify the specific nature of the emotional problems. (2, pp83–84).

These comments echo the conclusions drawn by Dohrenwend et al. concerning the interpretation of psychological screening scales such as the Heath Opinion Survey or Langner's 22-item scale: they represent at best indicators of nonspecific distress and do not guide the user to any specific clinical interpretation of the nature of the psychological problem involved. Accordingly, this scale appears to be of value where a screening test is needed; as there is no clear explanation for how the method works it will be of less value where more detailed, diagnostic information is required.

Address

Frank Leavitt, PhD, Department of Psychology and Social Sciences, Rush-Presbyterian-St. Luke's Medical Center, 1753 West Congress Parkway, Chicago, Illinois, USA 60612

References

(1) Leavitt F, Garron DC. The detection of psychological disturbance in patients with low back pain. J Psychosom Res 1979;23:149–154.
(2) Leavitt F. Detecting psychological disturbance using verbal pain measurement: the Back Pain Classification Scale. In: Melzack R, ed. Pain measurement and assessment. New York: Raven Press, 1983:79–84.
(3) Leavitt F, Garron DC. Psychological disturbance and pain report differences in both organic and non-organic low back pain patients. Pain 1979;7:187–195.
(4) Leavitt F. Comparison of three measures for detecting psychological disturbance in patients with low back pain. Pain 1982;13:299–305.
(5) Leavitt F, Garron DC, Whisler WW, Sheinkop MB. Affective and sensory dimensions of back pain. Pain 1978;4:273–281.
(6) Leavitt F, Garron DC. Validity of a Back Pain Classification Scale for detecting psychological disturbance as measured by the MMPI. J Clin Psychol 1980;36:186–189.
(7) Leavitt F, Garron DC. Validity of a Back Pain Classification Scale among patients with low back pain not associated with demonstrable organic disease. J Psychosom Res 1979;23:301–306.
(8) Sanders SH. Cross-validation of the Back Pain Classification Scale with chronic, intractable pain patients. Pain 1985;22:271–277.
(9) Garron DC, Leavitt F. Psychological and social correlates of the Back Pain Classification Scale. J Pers Assess 1983;47:60–65.

THE ILLNESS BEHAVIOR QUESTIONNAIRE
(I. Pilowsky and N.D. Spence, 1975, Revised 1983)

Purpose

The Illness Behavior Questionnaire (IBQ) assesses maladaptive responses to illness. It covers hypochondriacal responses, denial and changes in affect, and was designed to indicate the extent to which such psychological states may explain apparently exaggerated responses to illness. Although it is applicable to any illness, it has been most widely used in studies of pain.

Conceptual Basis

A patient's psychological reaction to his condition exerts an important influence on the way he reports symptoms. The IBQ is designed to identify psychological syndromes that may account for a discrepancy between the objective level of pathology and the patient's response to it, termed abnormal illness behavior. The IBQ was developed from a hypochondriasis questionnaire developed for this purpose, the Whiteley Index of Hypochondriasis, which is incorporated within the IBQ (1–3). The IBQ is a more general assessment tool which covers other syndromes in addition to hypochondriasis and is based on Mechanic's concept of illness behavior. Illness behavior refers both to overt actions, such as consulting a physician, and to the patient's emotional and psychological reaction to illness (3), covering "the ways in which symptoms may be differentially perceived, evaluated and acted (or not acted) upon by different kinds of persons" (4, p62). Illness behavior refers to "the patient's psychological transactions with his/her physical symptoms" (5, p222), and can take normal or abnormal forms. Pilowsky proposed that a number of common psychiatric syndromes such as hypochondriasis, conversion reaction, neurasthenia and malingering may be viewed as forms of abnormal illness behavior. In each case, there is a discrepancy between the objective somatic pathology present and the patient's response to it:

> patients with intractable pain may be described as displaying "abnormal" or "maladaptive" illness behaviour in so far as their behaviour deviates from that regarded as appropriate to the degree of somatic pathology observed, and is not modified by suitable explanation and reassurance provided by a doctor. (4, p62).

Pilowsky argued that experiencing intractable pain may serve as a form of psychological atonement in response to guilt or it may permit denial or avoidance of conflicts. Pain may also occur in conjunction with chronic muscular activity, perhaps brought on for psychological reasons (4). The questions in the IBQ are concerned with the attitudinal and emotional components of illness behavior, rather than with overt behavior.

Description

The IBQ is a self-administered questionnaire that uses a yes/no response format. The version most commonly reported contains 52 questions, although the expanded, 62-item version shown in Exhibit 7.9 is the one the authors now recommend. A 30-item version has also been used (6). Ten of the questions were taken from the Whiteley Index of Hypochondriasis (2, 3). The IBQ is introduced to the patient as a survey containing "a number of questions about your illness and how it affects you" (6).

The 62 questions are grouped into seven dimensions identified empirically via factor analysis. Pilowsky describes these dimensions as follows (1, p3):

1. General Hypochondriasis. A general factor marked by phobic concern about one's state of health. Associated with a high level of arousal or anxiety and with some insight into inappropriateness of attitudes. A high score also suggests an element of interpersonal alienation, but one that is secondary to the patient's phobic concern.

2. Disease Conviction. Characterised by affirmation that physical disease exists, symptom preoccupation, and rejection of the doctor's reassurance.

3. Psychological vs Somatic Perception of Illness. A high score indicates that the patient feels somehow responsible for (and in fact deserves) his illness, and perceives himself to be in need of psychiatric rather than medical treatment. A low score indicates a rejection of such attitudes and a tendency to somatise concerns.

4. Affective Inhibition. A high score indicates difficulty in expressing personal feelings, especially negative ones, to others.

5. Affective Disturbance. Characterised by feelings of anxiety and/or sadness.

6. Denial. A high score indicates a tendency to deny life stresses, and to attribute all problems to the effects of illness.

7. Irritability. Assesses the presence of angry feelings, and interpersonal friction.

A total score for the questionnaire may be obtained by counting the responses that represent problems—these are indicated by asterisks in the exhibit. Alternatively, scores may be provided for the seven dimensions; the numbers in the last column in Exhibit 7.9 show the scale on which the question is scored. High scores "suggest maladaptive ways of perceiving, evaluating, or acting in relation to one's state of health" (4).

Reliability

Test-retest correlations for the seven scales of the 62-item version were reported for 42 cases. After a delay of one to 12 weeks, correlations ranged from 0.67 to 0.87, with only three coefficients below 0.84 (1, Appendix E). The ten hypochondriasis items previously tested showed a test-retest correlation of 0.81 (N = 71) (1, 3).

Comparisons of patient scores and ratings made by their spouses on the seven scales provided correlations ranging between 0.50 and 0.78 for 42 patients (1, p37).

Validity

Pilowsky reported evidence for the validity of the ten questions on hypochondriasis from the Whiteley Index (3). The scores of 118 patients were compared

Exhibit 7.9 The Illness Behavior Questionnaire, Showing the Response that Is Scored and the Factor Placement of 30 Items which Loaded on One of Seven Factors

Here are some questions about you and your illness. Circle either YES or NO to indicate your answer to each question.

			Scale
1. Do you worry a lot about your health?	YES	NO	—
2. Do you think there is something seriously wrong with your body?	YES*	NO	2
3. Does your illness interfere with your life a great deal?	YES*	NO	2
4. Are you easy to get on with when you are ill?	YES	NO*	7
5. Does your family have a history of illness?	YES	NO	—
6. Do you think you are more liable to illness than other people?	YES	NO	—
7. If the doctor told you that he could find nothing wrong with you, would you believe him?	YES	NO*	2
8. Is it easy for you to forget about yourself and think about all sorts of other things?	YES	NO	—
9. If you feel ill and someone tells you that you are looking better, do you become annoyed?	YES*	NO	1
10. Do you find that you are often aware of various things happening in your body?	YES*	NO	2
11. Do you ever think of your illness as a punishment for something you have done wrong in the past?	YES*	NO	3
12. Do you have trouble with your nerves?	YES*	NO	5
13. If you feel ill or worried, can you be easily cheered up by the doctor?	YES	NO	—
14. Do you think that other people realise what it's like to be sick?	YES	NO	—
15. Does it upset you to talk to the doctor about your illness?	YES	NO	—
16. Are you bothered by many pains and aches?	YES	NO*	3
17. Does your illness affect the way you get on with your family or friends a great deal?	YES*	NO	7
18. Do you find that you get anxious easily?	YES*	NO	5
19. Do you know anybody who has had the same illness as you?	YES	NO	—
20. Are you more sensitive to pain than other people?	YES*	NO	1
21. Are you afraid of illness?	YES*	NO	1
22. Can you express your personal feelings easily to other people?	YES	NO*	4
23. Do people feel sorry for you when you are ill?	YES	NO	—
24. Do you think that you worry about your health more than most people?	YES*	NO	1
25. Do you find that your illness affects your sexual relations?	YES	NO	—
26. Do you experience a lot of pain with your illness?	YES	NO	—
27. Except for your illness, do you have any problems in your life?	YES	NO*	6
28. Do you care whether or not people realise you are sick?	YES	NO	—
29. Do you find that you get jealous of other people's good health?	YES*	NO	1
30. Do you ever have silly thoughts about your health which you can't get out of your mind, no matter how hard you try?	YES*	NO	1
31. Do you have any financial problems?	YES	NO*	6
32. Are you upset by the way people take your illness?	YES*	NO	1
33. Is it hard for you to believe the doctor when he tells you there is nothing for you to worry about?	YES	NO	—
34. Do you often worry about the possibility that you have got a serious illness?	YES	NO	—
35. Are you sleeping well?	YES	NO*	2
36. When you are angry, do you tend to bottle up your feelings?	YES*	NO	4
37. Do you often think that you might suddenly fall ill?	YES*	NO	1

38. If a disease is brought to your attention (through the radio, television, newspapers or someone you know) do you worry about getting it yourself?	YES*	NO	1
39. Do you get the feeling that people are not taking your illness seriously enough?	YES	NO	—
40. Are you upset by the appearance of your face or body?	YES	NO	—
41. Do you find that you are bothered by many different symptoms?	YES*	NO	2
42. Do you frequently try to explain to others how you are feeling?	YES	NO	—
43. Do you have any family problems?	YES	NO*	6
44. Do you think there is something the matter with your mind?	YES*	NO	3
45. Are you eating well?	YES	NO	—
46. Is your bad health the biggest difficulty of your life?	YES	NO*	3
47. Do you find that you get sad easily?	YES*	NO	5
48. Do you worry or fuss over small details that seem unimportant to others?	YES	NO	—
49. Are you always a co-operative patient?	YES	NO	—
50. Do you often have the symptoms of a very serious disease?	YES	NO	—
51. Do you find that you get angry easily?	YES*	NO	7
52. Do you have any work problems?	YES	NO	—
53. Do you prefer to keep your feelings to yourself?	YES*	NO	4
54. Do you often find that you get depressed?	YES*	NO	5
55. Would all your worries be over if you were physically healthy?	YES*	NO	6
56. Are you more irritable towards other people?	YES*	NO	7
57. Do you think that your symptoms may be caused by worry?	YES*	NO	3
58. Is it easy for you to let people know when you are cross with them?	YES	NO*	4
59. Is it hard for you to relax?	YES*	NO	5
60. Do you have personal worries which are not caused by physical illness?	YES	NO*	6
61. Do you often find that you lose patience with other people?	YES*	NO	7
62. Is it hard for you to show people your personal feelings?	YES*	NO	4

*The asterisks indicate the response that is scored. Note that we have added these to the questionnaire presented by Pilowsky and Spence.

Derived from Pilowsky I, Spence ND. Manual for the Illness Behaviour Questionnaire (IBQ). 2nd ed. Adelaide, Australia: University of Adelaide, 1983, Appendix A. With permission.

with their spouse's perception of what the patient's response would have been. A correlation of 0.59, or 0.65 when corrected for attenuation, was obtained (3, p90). A factor analysis of the ten items provided three factors that reflected clinically relevant aspects of hypochondriasis: bodily preoccupation, disease phobia and conviction of the presence of disease with refusal to be reassured (3).

Much of Pilowsky and Spence's development work on the IBQ concerned factor analyses of the 52 items using a small sample of only 100 patients with chronic pain of various types (1, 4, 7). Seven factors were identified, which accounted for 63% of the variance (5). Forty items loaded on these factors, as shown in Exhibit 7.9. This analysis has been replicated on other groups of pain patients with comparable results. Most of the applications of the IBQ report scale scores based on these seven factors.

Speculand et al. used the 30-item IBQ to compare 24 patients suffering from

intractable facial pain with 24 age- and sex-matched dental patients. Two of
the seven factor scores showed significant differences: disease conviction and
psychological versus somatic perception of disease (6). Other studies have
shown that certain of the factor scores discriminate between different types of
pain patients (5, 8–11). Speculand et al. used a discriminant analysis to compare responses of dental patients with patients with chronic facial pain, and
from their results a sensitivity of 87.5% at a specificity of 62.5% can be calculated (6, Table 3).

Two reports discuss the validity of a 62-item version of the IBQ. Pilowsky
et al. applied the method to patients who underwent coronary artery bypass
surgery and used a discriminant function analysis to contrast 38 patients who
showed relief of angina with 12 whose angina was not improved (2). Six factor
scores provided an 82% correct classification. In a cross-cultural study
Pilowsky et al. developed a discriminant function equation from interviews
with 100 pain patients and 78 general practice patients in Seattle, Washington,
and then applied the equation to 100 patients attending a pain clinic and 155
general practice patients in Adelaide, Australia, to evaluate its discriminal ability. Pilowsky reported a sensitivity of 97% at a specificity of 73.6% (12, p206).

Correlations between the affective disturbance scale (factor 5) and the Zung
Depression Scale and the Levine-Pilowsky Depression Questionnaire were
0.54 and 0.56. This scale also correlated significantly with the Spielberger state
anxiety (0.59) and trait anxiety (0.76) scales (1, p10).

Reference Standards

The Manual of the IBQ reports reference standards from samples of 231 pain
clinic patients, 147 general practice patients, 540 psychiatric patients, and 217
general hospital patients (1, Appendix F).

Commentary

The Illness Behavior Questionnaire has been used in Australia, North America, Europe and India, mostly in descriptive studies comparing different types
of pain patients. The widespread use of the method suggests that it fills a gap
in the range of measurements currently available. A strength of the IBQ is its
foundation on a clear conceptual analysis of pain responses (13), and this
advantage makes it unfortunate that we do not yet have methodologically
strong evidence for the validity of the questionnaire.

The factor analytic studies have used unacceptably small samples, often analyzing 52 questions with as few as 100 cases. The numerous comparisons that
have been presented between various types of patients unfortunately cannot be
used to indicate the validity of the IBQ, as no empirical or theoretical evidence
is provided to indicate how the groups should be expected to score on the
questionnaire.

Pilowsky's questionnaire covers a field similar to that of Zung's Pain and

Distress Scale. They differ in that the IBQ is intended principally for explaining chronic, intractable pain which is not readily explicable in terms of the level of tissue damage observed, while Zung's method provides a simple description of the psychological sequelae of pain. Pilowsky's method is similar in intent to Leavitt's Back Pain Classification Scale, but differs in being applicable to a far broader range of ailments. Recently, Pilowsky has described the Illness Behavior Assessment Schedule, which is a standardized clinical interview tool covering the the same fields as the IBQ (14). The IBQ has considerable potential; the Manual provides good documentation and readers interested in using the method should consult recent literature to see whether additional validity data have been published.

Address

Professor I. Pilowsky, Department of Psychiatry, Royal Adelaide Hospital, Adelaide, South Australia 5001

References

(1) Pilowsky I, Spence ND. Manual for the Illness Behaviour Questionnaire (IBQ). 2nd ed. Adelaide, Australia: University of Adelaide, 1983.

(2) Pilowsky I, Spence ND, Waddy JL. Illness behaviour and coronary artery by-pass surgery. J Psychosom Res 1979;23:39–44.

(3) Pilowsky I. Dimensions of hypochondriasis. Br J Psychiatry 1967;113:89–93.

(4) Pilowsky I, Spence ND. Illness behaviour syndromes associated with intractable pain. Pain 1976;2:61–71.

(5) Demjen S, Bakal D. Illness behavior and chronic headache. Pain 1981;10:221–229.

(6) Speculand B, Goss AN, Spence ND, Pilowsky I. Intractable facial pain and illness behaviour. Pain 1981;11:213–219.

(7) Pilowsky I, Spence ND. Is illness behaviour related to chronicity in patients with intractable pain? Pain 1976;2:167–173.

(8) Chapman CR, Sola AE, Bonica JJ. Illness behavior and depression compared in pain center and private practice patients. Pain 1979;6:1–7.

(9) Pilowsky I, Spence ND. Pain and illness behaviour: a comparative study. J Psychosom Res 1976;20:131–134.

(10) Pilowsky I, Chapman CR, Bonica JJ. Pain, depression and illness behaviour in a pain clinic population. Pain 1977;4:183–192.

(11) Pilowsky I, Spence ND. Pain, anger and illness behaviour. J Psychosom Res 1976;20:411–416.

(12) Pilowsky I, Murrell TGC, Gordon A. The development of a screening method for abnormal illness behaviour. J Psychosom Res 1979;23:203–207.

(13) Pilowsky I. A general classification of abnormal illness behaviours. Br J Med Psychol 1978;51:131–137.

(14) Pilowsky I, Bassett D, Barrett R, Petrovic L, Minniti R. The Illness Behavior Assessment Schedule: reliability and validity. Int J Psychiatry Med 1983–84;13:11–28.

THE PAIN PERCEPTION PROFILE
(Bernard Tursky, 1976)

Purpose

The Pain Perception Profile (PPP) offers quantitative estimates of the intensity, unpleasantness and type of pain a person experiences. It was intended for clinical use by behavior therapists treating pain patients (1).

Conceptual Basis

Tursky's PPP was developed at about the same time as Melzack's McGill Pain Questionnaire and, like the MPQ, it tackles the problem of how best to devise numerical ratings for the words that people typically use to describe their pain. Unlike the category scaling used in the MPQ, however, Tursky used magnitude estimation procedures (see Chapter 2) to scale the characteristic pain response of each individual. Tursky argued that the MPQ is limited in its ability to provide quantitative pain information, and that the use of categorical scales constrains the patient's ability to adequately rate his pain (1). However, to provide more adequate numerical estimates of pain, considerably more information must be collected from the respondent.

Description

The patient is given a pain diary which includes pain descriptors based on those used in the McGill Pain Questionnaire. Before the diary is completed, a set of optional experimental procedures may be applied to provide precise estimates of the way in which each respondent uses the adjectives to describe pain. These procedures identify the respondent's pain sensation and tolerance thresholds, his ability to judge reliably between differing levels of pain stimulation and his characteristic use of the pain descriptors. The preliminary stages can be omitted; if used, the full profile comprises four measurement stages, described below.

The first part of the PPP establishes the respondent's pain sensation threshold. An experiment is performed in which gradually increasing levels of electrical stimulation are applied to the respondent, who is asked to indicate at what level he experiences sensation, discomfort, pain and his limit of tolerance. The stimulation is applied through an electrode on the forearm; the equipment is portable and does not have to be used in a laboratory setting. Its major purpose is to provide the clinician with a better understanding of the patient's pain response and possible bias in rating pain; the level of electrical stimulation required to produce each response may be compared to reference standards to identify abnormal pain responses. The difference between pain threshold and pain tolerance indicates the patient's pain sensitivity range, a predictor of his ability to endure pain (1). This may be useful in prescribing treatment, and may be used to study the effect of treatment, including psychological intervention.

The second part of the PPP uses magnitude estimation methods to examine the respondent's rating of the painfulness of a series of electrical stimuli, and identifies the mathematical power function (see Chapter 2), which describes the relationship between the intensity of the experimental stimulus and the person's judgment of pain. These judgments and the power exponent can be compared to standards to evaluate the patient's ability to make normal judgments of pain stimulation.

> A greater exponent may be indicative of hypersensitivity, a lesser exponent indicative of hyposensitivity, and a significantly non-linear relationship may indicate a possible neurologic malfunction or an attempt on the part of the patient to manipulate his self-report. Changes in the exponent or the intercept may reflect alterations in the patient's pain responsivity as a function of treatment intervention. (1, p383).

In the third part of the assessment, the patient uses a cross-modality matching procedure (page 18) to rate the intensity of pain represented by the descriptors that are part of the pain diary. The adjectives cover three dimensions of pain: 14 describe pain intensity, 11 cover the emotional reaction to pain (unpleasantness) and 13 describe the sensation of pain (see Exhibit 7.10). The words were selected primarily from the McGill Pain Questionnaire and were tested in preliminary scaling studies (1). Reference scale values are available for the words (1, Table 2).

The fourth and final phase in administering the PPP involves the use of the daily pain diary shown in Exhibit 7.10. Using the three categories of pain descriptors scaled previously, the patient records his pain at specified times of the day. The diary also records the source of the discomfort, its time of onset, duration, and the medication taken for each reported pain period. Instructions for using the diary are given by Tursky et al. (1, p390).

Reliability

Some data on the reliability of the four parts of the PPP were provided by Tursky et al. The test-retest reliability for 20 pain patients in making judgments of pain thresholds and discomfort levels were reported as showing close agreement, although Tursky did not summarize the data statistically (1).

Validity

No information is available.

Commentary

The Pain Perception Profile differs from most other measurements in this book in that it lacks published validity and reliability data, and yet we have included it as an example of a sophisticated rating technique that could illustrate the types of methodological development to be anticipated in future health measurement methods. Our description of the method does not provide sufficient

Exhibit 7.10 The Pain Perception Profile: Sample Page from a Pain Diary, Including Lists of Pain Descriptors

INTENSITY	UNPLEASANTNESS	FEELING
Moderate	Distressing	Stinging
Just Noticeable	Tolerable	Grinding
Mild	Awful	Squeezing
Excruciating	Unpleasant	Burning
Very Strong	Unbearable	Shooting
Very Intense	Uncomfortable	Numbing
Severe	Intolerable	Throbbing
Intense	Bearable	Stabbing
Very Weak	Agonizing	Itching
Strong	Miserable	Aching
Weak	Distracting	Cramping
Not Noticeable	Not Unpleasant	None
		Pressure

PRESCRIBED MEDICATION	HOW OFTEN	DOSE SIZE	HOW MANY

Date 7-28-77 Thursday

AVERAGE DISCOMFORT NUMBER 140

Type of Discomfort	TIME		DISCOMFORT RATING				MEDICATION		
	Dur.	Begin	Intensity Word	Unpleasant Word	Feeling Word	Numb.	Name	How Many	Dose
headache		5:30 AM	Strong	distracting	throbbing	80	all		
same headache		12:45 PM	Moderate	tolerable	throbbing	40	meds		
same headache		6:45 PM	Strong	distracting	throbbing	80	as prescribed		
RATING FOR THE DAY			strong	distracting	throbbing	80			

HOURS SLEPT LAST NIGHT 5 hrs (Intermittent) 12:30 PM to 5:30 AM

STRESSFUL EVENTS & COMMENTS Nausea, Diarrhea, dizziness (morning) Went to sleep with headache (strong) Sweated

Reproduced from Tursky B, Jamner LD, Friedman R. The Pain Perception Profile: a psychophysical approach to the assessment of pain report. Behav Ther 1982;13:389. With permission.

information for the reader to apply the PPP; fuller details on its administration are contained in Tursky's report.

Although this method is the most detailed and mathematically complex of the pain measurement methods reviewed, Tursky argues that it is sufficiently simple to be used in a clinician's office by personnel with basic training in its administration. However, it remains to be seen whether the method will achieve widespread use. It is also necessary that data on the validity be collected to indicate how far the results of the magnitude estimation procedures produce results that differ from the simpler estimates obtained from the McGill Pain Questionnaire.

Address

Bernard Tursky, Laboratory for Behavioral Research, Political Science Department, State University of New York, Stony Brook, New York, USA 11794

Reference

(1) Tursky B, Jamner LD, Friedman R. The Pain Perception Profile: a psychophysical approach to the assessment of pain report. Behav Ther 1982;13:376–394.

CONCLUSION

The history of the development of pain measurements is a fascinating one that well illustrates several of the themes in our book. In many ways it has been one of the most successful areas of health measurement. For instance, there have been clear links between conceptual work on the definition of pain and the development of measurement scales, so that the results obtained using these methods have led to refinements in the conceptual definitions of pain found in the literature. Some of the leading measurement methods have been used in large numbers of studies, and have been used in consistent ways that permit direct comparisons of the results obtained in different studies. Close attention has been paid to reliability and validity in the development of the measurement methods. Furthermore, the link between clinical interests in pain management and the measurement techniques has been closer in this field than in, say, functional disability. The pressure from clinical studies to evaluate ways to manage pain led to the development of methods that distinguish between the objective experience of pain and the subjective facets of the pain response, one of the only areas of measurement in which this has been attempted. This field has also benefited from some of the most recent statistical analytic procedures. Finally, the reader gains the impression that the many researchers working on the problem of pain measurement, who come from widely differing disciplines, benefit from the existence of a single journal *(Pain)* that has published a number of the leading articles on pain measurement. By contrast, other fields of measurement lack a clearly identifiable journal that deals comprehensively with measurement and conceptual issues.

There remain, of course, gaps in the repertoire of pain measurements. It will be desirable to see greater application of high quality pain measurement methods in clinical studies than is now the case: frequently clinical studies rely on four-point verbal pain scales. More cross-validation is desirable among the pain measurement methods, especially exploring the equivalence of verbal, behavioral and analogue methods. The few studies that have compared the various approaches do not suggest close equivalence; this may well indicate an area for further investigation that would be of interest to health measurement theory in general.

8

General Health Measurements

Chapter 3 reviewed measurements of physical functioning and the chapters that followed have covered the social and emotional aspects of health. Several indices combine these themes in one instrument and these are included in the present chapter. Some, such as the Sickness Impact Profile, are flexible in their design and enable the user to select only required components, effectively offering self-contained measurements of physical, social or emotional well-being. Others, such as the Multidimensional Functional Activities Questionnaire, are intended to be used in their entirety, although this principle is not always followed by subsequent users.

Most of the general health measurements are newer than the instruments that assess physical or emotional functioning alone, and this mirrors the historical trend towards making global assessments of well-being. They reflect a multivariate formulation of health, emphasizing not only the level of functioning in several components, but also the balance between them. These newer instruments tend to be designed with research applications in mind, and have in general been more thoroughly tested for reliability and validity than the scales reviewed in Chapter 3. They represent some of the most successful applications of test development procedures to health measurement and, as can be seen from Table 8.1, the resulting methods are often of high quality.

SCOPE OF THE CHAPTER

The methods we review range from those that have primarily a research orientation, such as Bush's Quality of Well-Being Scale with its complex and somewhat radical approach to health measurement, to far simpler methods such as the Arthritis Impact Measurement Scale or the Nottingham Health Profile that may be used both clinically and in research studies. We include three extensive scales that are designed to provide comprehensive appraisals of the well-being of elderly people living in the community: the CARE instruments, the Multidimensional Functional Activities Questionnaire developed by the OARS group and the Multilevel Assessment Instrument. In their full

Table 8.1 Comparison of the Quality of General Health Measurements*

Measurement	Scale	Number of items	Application	Administered by (time)	Studies using method	Reliability		Validity	
						Testing thoroughness	Results	Testing thoroughness	Results
Arthritis Impact Measurement Scale (AIMS) (Meenan)	ordinal (Guttman)	45	clinical	self (15 min)	few	++	++	++	++
Physical and Mental Impairment-of-Function Evaluation (PAMIE) (Gurel)	ordinal	77	clinical	expert (10–15 min)	few	+	++	+	+
Functional Assessment Inventory (Crewe & Athelstan)	ordinal	40	clinical	expert (5 min)	few	++	++	++	++
Nottingham Health Profile (Martini & Hunt)	interval	38	clinical, survey	self (<10 min)	several	++	++	++	++
Sickness Impact Profile (Bergner)	interval	136	survey	self (20–30 min)	many	+++	+++	++	++
Multilevel Assessment Instrument (Lawton)	ordinal	147	survey	interviewer (50 min)	few	++	++	++	++
Multidimensional Functional Assessment Questionnaire (OARS)	ordinal	120 (Part A)	clinical	interviewer (30 min)	several	++	++	++	++
CORE-CARE (Gurland)	ordinal	329	clinical	interviewer	several	++	++	+++ (full CARE, not CORE-CARE)	++
Quality of Well-Being Scale (Bush)	ratio	18	research	interviewer (15 min)	several	++	+++	+	++

*For an explanation of the categories used, see Chapter 1, pages 8–9.

versions these require lengthy interviews, but provide results that seem to show good validity and reliability. We describe two other clinical scales, the Physical and Mental Impairment-of-Function Evaluation, which is appropriate for patients living in institutions and covers the more severe levels of disability, and the Functional Assessment Inventory, which focuses on a patient's potential for vocational rehabilitation. Finally, the Sickness Impact Profile represents one of the most generally applicable of all instruments, and provides a broad-ranging coverage that can be used with relatively sick patients and in general population surveys. Table 8.1 compares the quality of the scales in the chapter, while Table 8.2 summarizes their content.

THE ARTHRITIS IMPACT MEASUREMENT SCALE
(Robert F. Meenan, 1980)

Purpose

The Arthritis Impact Measurement Scale (AIMS), a self-administered scale covering physical, social and emotional well-being, was intended as an indicator of the outcome of care for arthritic patients.

Conceptual Basis

Meenan et al. criticized the measurements traditionally used with arthritic patients for their focus on disease activity and functional abilities to the exclusion of other components identified in the WHO definition of health (1). The AIMS was intended to be comprehensive and practical, with an emphasis on proven reliability and validity (2).

Description

The instrument consists of 45 items grouped into nine scales that assess mobility, physical activity (walking, bending, lifting), dexterity, household activity (managing money, medications, housekeeping), social activities, activities of daily living, pain, depression and anxiety. There are an additional 19 questions, not considered here as an integral part of the AIMS, that cover general health, health perceptions and demographic details. The dexterity and pain scales were developed by the author, and other items were adapted from Katz's Index of ADL, the Rand and the Bush instruments (1). Items were selected for inclusion on the basis of Guttman analyses and internal consistency correlations (2). For each scale the items are listed in Guttman order so that a patient indicating disability on one question will tend also to indicate disability on the items falling below it in that section.

In scoring the AIMS, the Guttman characteristics are ignored and each item is scored separately, with higher scores indicating greater limitation. No item weights are used. Certain questions use a reversed phrasing, so that care must be taken in coding replies to these. To convert section scores to a standard range of 0 to 10, Meenan provided simple standardization formulae for each

Table 8.2 Comparison of the Content of General Health Measurements, Showing Numbers of Questions on each Topic

Measurement	Self-care	Mobility	Travel	Body movement	Home management	Medical condition	Senses
Arthritis Impact Measurement Scale (AIMS) (Meenan)	3	7	2	6	6	5	
Physical and Mental Impairment-of-Function Evaluation (Gurel)	15	2				8	2
Functional Assessment Inventory (Crewe & Athelstan)	2	1		5		1	2
Nottingham Health Profile (Martini & Hunt)	1	5		2		11	
Sickness Impact Profile (Bergner)	12	24	4	7	10	9	
Multilevel Assessment Instrument (Lawton)	5	2	4	1	6	45	2
Multidimensional Functional Assessment Questionnaire (OARS)	5	2	1	1	7	27	2
CORE-CARE (Gurland)		27		39		107	25
Quality of Well-Being Scale (Bush)	1	3	2	4		4	

Self-care includes: dressing, grooming, feeding, bathing, toileting, bladder and/or bowel control

Mobility includes: lower limb abilities, standing, walking, running, stair climbing, transferring

Travel includes: use of transport, driving

Body movement includes: upper limb abilities (e.g., reaching, lifting), bending, moving in bed or confined to bed, hand dexterity (e.g., cutting toenails, turning faucets), carrying, dialing a phone

Home management includes: housework, meal preparation, shopping, managing money

Medical condition includes: diagnosis, signs, symptoms, limb abnormalities, medication, pain, diet

Senses includes: sight, hearing

section (3). He recommended forming a total health score by adding the values for six scales: mobility, physical and household activities, dexterity, pain and depression. These details are provided in a three-page User's Guide, available from Dr. Meenan (3). The questions are shown in Exhibit 8.1 (the questionnaire was obtained from Dr. Meenan; note that this is a newer, slightly modified version of that shown in reference 2, p149). Most of the questions refer to problems during the past month. Phrasing of the responses is shown below the exhibit. The instrument is self-administered and takes about 15 minutes to complete.

Reliability

During the process of item selection, the Guttman scale characteristics of the questions were evaluated using a sample of 104 arthritic patients. Coefficients of scalability and reproducibility exceeded 0.60 and 0.90, respectively, for all but the household activity scale, which had a coefficient of reproducibility of 0.88 (2, Table 2). The alpha internal consistencies of the nine scales all exceeded 0.60, with six in excess of 0.80 (2).

| Mental capacity | | | | Work | Resources | Social support | Social interaction | Hobbies | Behavior problems | Communication | Other | Total questions |
Cognition	Anxiety	Depression	Other									
	6	6					4					45
14	5	7					11		12	1		77
6		2	8		4	2	2			1	4	40
	3	7	1				3				5	38
10	3	3	1	9			20	8		9	7	136
10	1	7	3		25	7	27	2				147
6	2	4	15	7	27	4	6	2	2			120
19		29		7	34	34					8	329
				4								18

Mental capacity includes: cognition, anxiety, depression, other mental assessments
Work includes: education, retirement, housework (as an occupational category)
Resources includes: social, economic, environmental
Hobbies includes: leisure activities, sports
Communication includes: speech, reading
Other includes: sleep

In a study of 625 arthritics, Guttman reproducibility coefficients for all scales exceeded 0.90. Alpha coefficients of internal consistency exceeded 0.70 for all scales except physical activity (0.63) and social activity (0.69) (4, Table 2). Test-retest correlations for the nine scales exceeded 0.80 after a two-week delay, the mean test-retest correlation being 0.87 for 100 patients (1, 4). The reliability results were replicated in several diagnostic groups (4).

Validity

Correlations between the scales and a number of criterion variables were examined. These included age (on the expectation of a reduction in function with age), the patient's perception of his general health and of recent disease activity, and a physician's report of functional activity, joint count and disease activity (2). Meenan et al. commented:

> The performance-oriented scales generally correlated closely with age, and all 9 scales were significantly correlated with the patient's estimates of general health and disease activity. Finally, when the psychological scales are excluded, agreement between the scale scores and the doctor's report was significant in 16 of 21 pairs (76%). (2, p150).

Exhibit 8.1 The Arthritis Impact Measurement Scale: Questionnaire Items

Mobility
- 4   Are you in bed or chair for most or all of the day because of your health?
- 3   Do you have to stay indoors most or all of the day because of your health?
- 2   When you travel around your community, does someone have to assist you because of your health?
- 1   Are you able to use public transportation?

Physical activity
- 5   Are you unable to walk unless you are assisted by another person or by a cane, crutches, artificial limbs, or braces?
- 4   Do you have any trouble either walking one block or climbing one flight of stairs because of your health?
- 3   Do you have any trouble either walking several blocks or climbing a few flights of stairs because of your health?
- 2   Do you have trouble bending, lifting, or stooping because of your health?
- 1   Does your health limit the kind of vigorous activities you can do such as running, lifting heavy objects, or participating in strenuous sports?

Dexterity
- 5   Can you easily write with a pen or pencil?
- 4   Can you easily turn a key in a lock?
- 3   Can you easily tie a pair of shoes?
- 2   Can you easily button articles of clothing?
- 1   Can you easily open a jar of food?

Household activity
- 7   If you had a telephone, would you be able to use it?
- 6   If you had to take medicine, could you take all your own medicine?
- 5   Do you handle your own money?
- 4   If you had a kitchen, could you prepare your own meals?
- 3   If you had laundry facilities (washer, dryer, etc.), could you do your own laundry?
- 2   If you had the necessary transportation, could you go shopping for groceries or clothes?
- 1   If you had household tools and appliances (vacuum, mops, etc.), could you do your own housework?

Social activity
- 4   About how often were you on the telephone with close friends or relatives during the past month?
- 3   During the past month, about how often did you get together socially with friends or relatives?
- 2   During the past month, about how often have you had friends or relatives to your home?
- 1   During the past month, how often have you visited with friends or relatives at their homes?

Activities of daily living
- 4   How much help do you need to use the toilet?
- 3   How well are you able to move around?
- 2   How much help do you need in getting dressed?
- 1   When you bathe, either a sponge bath, tub or shower, how much help do you need?

Pain
- 4   During the past month, how long has your morning stiffness usually lasted from the time you wake up?
- 3   During the past month, how often have you had pain in two or more joints at the same time?
- 2   During the past month, how often have you had severe pain from your arthritis?
- 1   During the past month, how would you describe the arthritis pain you usually have?

Depression
6   During the past month, how often did you feel that others would be better off if you were dead?
5   How often during the past month have you felt so down in the dumps that nothing could cheer you up?
4   How much of the time during the past month have you felt downhearted and blue?
3   How often during the past month did you feel that nothing turned out for you the way you wanted it to?
2   During the past month, how much of the time have you been in low or very low spirits?
1   During the past month, how much of the time have you enjoyed the things you do?

Anxiety
6   How often during the past month did you find yourself having difficulty trying to calm down?
5   How much have you been bothered by nervousness, or your "nerves" during the past month?
4   During the past month, how much of the time have you felt tense or "high strung"?
3   How much of the time during the past month were you able to relax without difficulty?
2   How much of the time during the past month have you felt calm and peaceful?
1   How much of the time during the past month did you feel relaxed and free of tension?

Response Phrasing for the AIMS Questions:

The *Mobility, Physical Activity* and *Dexterity* questions use yes/no responses.

The *Household Activity* questions use a three-point scale: without help, with some help and completely unable.

The *Social Activity* questions use a six-point scale of frequency: every day, several days a week, about once a week, 2 or 3 times in the past month, once in the past month and not at all in the past month.

The *Activities of Daily Living* questions use the following responses. Question 1: no help at all, help with reaching some parts of the body, help in bathing more than one part of the body. Question 2: no help at all, only need help tying shoes, need help getting dressed. Question 3: able to get in and out of bed or chairs without the help of another person, need help of another person, and don't get out of bed. Question 4: no help at all, some help in getting to or using the toilet, not able to get to the bathroom at all.

Pain is measured on three different six-point frequency scales. The question describing pain grades it as: very severe, severe, moderate, mild, very mild or none. The question concerning the frequency of the pain and that about pain in two or more joints use: always, very often, fairly often, sometimes, almost never and never. The response modes for the duration of morning stiffness are: over 4 hours, 2 to 4 hours, 1 to 2 hours, 30 minutes to an hour, less than 30 minutes and do not have morning stiffness.

The 12 *Depression and Anxiety* questions use three response scales. Questions on enjoying things, feeling tense, low spirits, feeling relaxed, feeling downhearted and blue, feeling calm, and relaxing without difficulty use: all of the time, most of the time, a good bit of the time, some of the time, a little of the time, and none of the time. The questions about difficulty trying to calm down, feeling nothing turns out, feeling others would be better off if you were dead and feeling down in the dumps use: always, very often, fairly often, sometimes, almost never and never. The scale for how much you have been bothered by nervousness is: extremely so, very much, quite a bit, some, just a little bit and not bothered at all.

Reproduced from the Arthritis Impact Measurement Scale obtained from Dr. Robert F. Meenan. With permission.

Similar analyses were carried out using the data from the study of 625 arthritics. For 444 of the patients, the nine scales were correlated with disease activity (r between 0.14 and 0.52) and with the American Rheumatism Association functional class (r between 0.24 and 0.52) (4). Coefficients were significant at $p < 0.001$; scales measuring physical functioning showed higher associations with the disease indicators than did the psychological and social scales.

A factor analysis of summary scores for each of the nine sections provided three factors. The first included five physical function scales, the second included two psychological scales and the third included the pain scale (4). Reflecting the existence of a three-component factorial structure, the results of using a multivariate approach to criterion validation showed stronger associations than did the single-variate analyses reported above. Using multiple regression analyses, the AIMS scores achieved multiple correlation coefficients of 0.61 with disease activity and 0.66 with the ARA functional class index (4, p1050). Multiple correlations with a 3-item measure of global health status and a visual analogue measure of arthritis impact were 0.84 and 0.75, respectively (4, p1050).

Evidence was also given that the AIMS can reflect change in the health status of patients following treatment. Changes in the score were correlated with changes in a rating of health following treatment for 120 patients, with correlations falling between 0.24 and 0.67 (1, 4).

Commentary

This recently developed scale is well documented, clearly described in the literature, and presents strong preliminary evidence for its reliability and validity. The emphasis on Guttman scaling as a means for selecting items is appropriate for the questions covering physical disability, and the scaling results obtained for the AIMS appear to be superior to those obtained for other instruments that have used Guttman scaling, such as the OECD questionnaire. The AIMS deserves serious consideration as an outcome indicator for use with arthritic patients.

Address

Robert F. Meenan, MD, MPH, Department of Medicine, Boston City Hospital, 818 Harrison Avenue, Boston, Massachusetts, USA 02118

References

(1) Meenan RF. The AIMS approach to health status measurement: conceptual background and measurement properties. J Rheumatol 1982;9:785–788.
(2) Meenan RF, Gertman PM, Mason JH. Measuring health status in arthritis: the Arthritis Impact Measurement Scales. Arthritis Rheum 1980;23:146–152.
(3) Boston University Multipurpose Arthritis Center. AIMS user's guide. Boston University, Boston. (Manuscript, nd).

(4) Meenan RF, Gertman PM, Mason JH, Dunaif R. The Arthritis Impact Measurement Scales: further investigations of a health status measure. Arthritis Rheum 1982;25:1048–1053.

THE PHYSICAL AND MENTAL IMPAIRMENT-OF-FUNCTION EVALUATION
(Lee Gurel, 1972, Revised 1973)

Purpose

The Physical and Mental Impairment-of-Function Evaluation (PAMIE) records physical, psychological and social disability in the institutionalized elderly. It was intended for use with psychiatric and nonpsychiatric chronically ill patients (1).

Conceptual Basis

No information is available.

Description

The 77-item PAMIE is a modification of two previous instruments, the Self-Care Inventory and the 43-item Patient Evaluation Scale (1). Factor analyses of the latter scale guided the content of the PAMIE, which covers 12 topics (1):

Ambulation
Self-care
Verbal hostility
Bedfastness
Sensory and motor functions
Mental confusion
Cooperation
Withdrawal/apathy
Deteriorated appearance
Anxiety/depression
Irritability
Paranoia and suspicion

Empirical testing of the instrument indicated that scores are best presented for ten factors, rather than the 12 hypothesized. The analyses did not confirm the existence of separate factors for irritability and cooperation, and verbal hostility was renamed belligerent/irritable.

The items are mainly concerned with observable behavior during the preceding week; all but the first three use a yes/no answer format. The instrument is completed in 10 to 15 minutes by a caregiver, generally a nurse familiar with the patient (1). Exhibit 8.2 shows the questionnaire (note this is a slightly revised version of that shown in reference 1, Table 1, and was obtained from Dr. Gurel). Scores may be provided for each of ten factors, as indicated by

Exhibit 8.2 The Physical and Mental Impairment-of-Function Evaluation

On the basis of your knowledge of the patient at the present time will you please rate the following items. Answer items 1, 2 and 3 on this page by circling the number beside the most correct statement. For all other items check either Yes or No. Please do not leave any item unanswered.

1. Which of the following *best* fits the patient? (Circle one)
   - 5 Has no problem in walking
   - 4 Slight difficulty in walking, but manages; may use cane
   - 3 Great difficulty in walking, but manages; may use crutches or stroller
   - 2 Uses wheelchair to get around by himself
   - 1 Uses wheelchair pushed by others
   - 0 Doesn't get around much; mostly or completely bedfast, or restricted to chair

   (Factor X)

2. As far as you know, has the patient had one or more strokes (CVA)? (Circle one)
   - 0 No stroke
   - 1 Mild stroke(s)
   - 2 Serious stroke(s)

   (Factor VIII)

3. Which of the following *best* fits the patient? (Circle one)
   - 4 In bed all or almost all day
   - 3 More of the waking day in bed than out of bed
   - 2 About half the waking day in bed, about half out of bed
   - 1 More of the waking day out of bed than in bed
   - 0 Out of bed all or almost all day

   (Factor V)

	Yes	No	(Check either Yes or No)
4.	___	___	Eats a regular diet
5.	V	___	Is given bed baths
6.	II	___	Gives sarcastic answers
7.	___	I	Takes a bath/shower without help or supervision
8.	VI	___	Leaves his clothes unbuttoned
9.	VI	___	Is messy in eating
10.	II	___	Is irritable and grouchy
11.	IX	___	Keeps to himself
12.	VII	___	Says he's not getting good care and treatment
13.	II	___	Resists when asked to do things
14.	IV	___	Seems unhappy
15.	III	___	Doesn't make much sense when he talks to you
16.	II	___	Acts as though he has a chip on his shoulder
17.	V	___	Is IV or tube fed once a week or more
18.	VIII	___	Has one or both hands/arms missing or paralyzed
19.	___	II	Is cooperative
20.	V	___	Is toileted in bed by catheter and/or enema
21.	___	___	Is deaf or practically deaf, even with hearing aid
22.	IX	___	Ignores what goes on around him
23.	___	V	Knows who he is and where he is
24.	II	___	Gives the staff a "hard time"
25.	VII	___	Blames other people for his difficulties
26.	VII	___	Says, without good reason, that he's being mistreated or getting a raw deal

	Yes	No	(Check either Yes or No)
27.	II	___	Gripes and complains a lot
28.	VII	___	Says other people dislike him, or even hate him
29.	___	___	Says he has special or superior abilities
30.	___	___	Has hit someone or been in a fight in the last six months
31.	___	I	Eats without being closely supervised or encouraged
32.	IV	___	Says he's blue and depressed
33.	IX	___	Isn't interested in much of anything
34.	III	___	Has taken his clothes off at the wrong time or place during the last six months
35.	___	___	Makes sexually suggestive remarks or gestures
36.	II	___	Objects or gives you an argument before doing what he's told
37.	VII	___	Is distrustful and suspicious
38.	___	VI	Looks especially neat and clean
39.	IV	___	Seems unusually restless
40.	II	___	Says he's going to hit people
41.	III	___	Receives almost constant safety supervision (for careless smoking, objects in mouth, self-injury, pulling catheter, etc.)
42.	VI	___	Looks sloppy
43.	III	___	Keeps wandering off the subject when you talk with him
44.	VI	___	Is noisy; talks very loudly
45.	___	I	Does things like brush teeth, comb hair, and clean nails without help or urging
46.	___	___	Has shown up drunk or brought a bottle on the ward
47.	IV	___	Cries for no obvious reason
48.	___	___	Says he would like to leave the hospital
49.	I	___	Wets or soils once a week or more
50.	III	___	Has trouble remembering things
51.	VIII	___	Has one or both feet/legs missing or paralyzed
52.	X	___	Walks flight of steps without help
53.	___	V	When needed, takes medication by mouth
54.	IV	___	Is easily upset when little things go wrong
55.	___	I	Uses the toilet without help or supervision
56.	___	V	Conforms to hospital routine and treatment program
57.	VIII	___	Has much difficulty in speaking
58.	III	___	Sometimes talks out loud to himself
59.	___	IX	Chats with other patients
60.	I	___	Is shaved by someone else
61.	II	___	Seems to resent it when asked to do things
62.	___	I	Dresses without any help or supervision
63.	II	___	Is often demanding
64.	IX	___	When left alone, sits and does nothing
65.	VII	___	Says others are jealous of him
66.	III	___	Is confused
67.	___	___	Is blind or practically blind, even with glasses
68.	___	I	Decides things for himself, like what to wear, items from canteen (or canteen cart), etc.

279

Exhibit 8.2 (continued)

	Yes	No	(Check either Yes or No)
69.	II	___	Swears; uses vulgar or obscene words
70.	III	___	When you try to get his attention, acts as though lost in a dream world
71.	IV	___	Looks worried and sad
72.	III	___	Most people would think him a mental patient
73.	___	I	Shaves without any help or supervision, other than being given supplies
74.	II	___	Yells at people when he's angry or upset
75.	I	___	Is dressed or has his clothes changed by someone
76.	X	___	Gets own tray and takes it to eating place
77.	III	___	Is watched closely so he doesn't wander

Reproduced from the Physical and Mental Impairment-of-Function Evaluation form obtained from Dr. Lee Gurel. With permission.

Roman numerals beside each item in the exhibit. Where no numeral is given, the question did not load on a factor in the analyses. The scoring system for the first three questions is shown in the exhibit, while for the remaining questions the position of the Roman numeral indicates the response that is scored. Factor scores may be added to give three more general scores representing physical infirmity (factors I, V, VIII, X), psychological deterioration (factors III, VI, IX) and psychological agitation (factors II, IV, VII) (1). Weighted and unweighted factor scores provided essentially identical results, so the unweighted scores are generally used.

Reliability

Alpha internal consistency coefficients for the factor scores ranged from 0.67 to 0.91 (1, Table 2).

Validity

The PAMIE scale was tested on 845 male veterans in nursing homes. Their mean age was 66 years; 47% were general medical and surgical patients, while the remainder had predominantly psychiatric problems, often accompanied by additional medical complaints (1). The factor structure of the PAMIE scale was examined, and nine factors were derived. However, Gurel et al. chose to separate questions on ambulation from the self-care factor, effectively forming a tenth factor (1). To assess the stability of the factor solution, the analysis was repeated on medical/surgical and psychiatric patients separately, with considerable agreement between them, as indicated by a Harman's coefficient of congruence of 0.86 (1, p85). Several of the factors were substantially correlated, and a second-order factor analysis provided three factors, which the authors named physical infirmity (including ambulation, sensory and motor functions, bedfastness), psychological deterioration (including mental confusion, withdrawal/apathy, deterioration in behavior and appearance) and psychological agitation (including paranoia and suspicion, irritability and belligerence, anxiety/depression) (1).

The sample was grouped into those scoring high or low on each of 19 measures reflecting diagnostic and severity ratings. All of the PAMIE scores succeeded in distinguishing between contrasting subgroups in at least three cases. Scores reflecting physical abilities (especially bedfastness, self-care, ambulation) provided significant discriminations between almost all of the criterion dichotomies (1).

Commentary

The PAMIE is a relatively old scale that has not been widely used, but it has the advantage of an identifiable internal structure, broad scope, and relevance for the institutionalized elderly—a group for whom all too often only ADL questions are used.

Address

Lee Gurel, PhD, Chief, Research in Mental Health and Behavioral Science, Veterans Administration Medical Center, 50 Irving Street, NW, Washington, DC, USA 20422

Reference

(1) Gurel L, Linn MW, Linn BS. Physical and Mental Impairment-of-Function Evaluation in the aged: the PAMIE scale. J Gerontol 1972;27:83–90.

THE FUNCTIONAL ASSESSMENT INVENTORY
(Nancy M. Crewe and Gary T. Athelstan, 1981, Revised 1984)

Purpose

The Functional Assessment Inventory (FAI) was developed for clinical use to describe a client's potential for vocational rehabilitation. It summarizes functional limitations and the personal and environmental resources that a client can use to help cope with problems (1). It was intended to be applicable to all types of disability.

Conceptual Basis

The FAI is the first component of a two-part Functional Assessment System. The second part is a goal attainment scaling instrument called the Rehabilitation Goals Identification Form that measures treatment outcomes (1).

The FAI identifies a person's strengths and limitations (whether modifiable or not) that predict ability to return to work, and which should be taken into account in developing a vocational rehabilitation plan. "Pinpointing the obstacles to rehabilitation can be helpful in determining what services are needed even if no attempt will be made to directly modify the limitations" (1, p304). Crewe and Turner noted that existing physical assessment methods such as the Barthel or PULSES scales are not broad enough to assess the potential for vocational rehabilitation: "The vocational counselor . . . requires general information about capacities in a wide variety of physical, emotional, intellectual and social areas that may be relevant to work" (2, p1).

Description

The Functional Assessment Inventory is a rating scale of 30 items describing functional limitations and a ten-item checklist of assets or unusual strengths. The strength items are rated as present or absent and are meant to accommodate the instances when a particular asset may compensate for a patient's limitations: considering a patient's strengths may improve the prediction of success in vocational rehabilitation. The functional limitations questions are rated on four-point scales representing current levels of impairment (with aids when used): none, mild, moderate and severe. The FAI identifies problems that may improve following rehabilitation. Space does not permit showing the complete inventory; the item topics are shown in Exhibit 8.3. Note that the exhibit refers to a revised version, which differs from that published by Crewe and Athelstan (1, p301), two items having been substituted and the order of the items changed. Printed copies of the FAI, an instruction sheet and an interviewer manual are available from the Materials Development Center of the Stout Vocational Rehabilitation Institute, University of Wisconsin—Stout, Menomonie, Wisconsin, USA 54751. Full definitions of each level are given in the questionnaire and the accompanying instruction sheet. As an example, item 25 reads as follows:

> 25. Skills (See instructions)
>
>   0. No significant impairment.
>   1. No available skills that are job-specific. However, possesses general skills (i.e., educational or interpersonal) that could be used in a number of jobs.
>   2. Has few general skills. Job-specific skills are largely unusable due to disability or other factors.
>   3. Has no job-specific skills and has very few general or personal skills transferable to a job situation.

The instruction sheet adds:

> This item refers to skills which the individual possesses after onset of disability.

The Functional Assessment Inventory is completed by a rehabilitation counselor, using information available from interviews, observations of the patient and from medical records to rate the patient. The ratings concern observable behavior; problems that can only be inferred (e.g., pain, low self-esteem) are excluded (2). The FAI takes five minutes to complete. A total, unweighted functional limitation score is provided by adding the raw scores for each item. Alternatively, scores may be provided for the seven sections indicated in Exhibit 8.3.

Exhibit 8.3 The Functional Assessment Inventory: Items

Cognition
    1. Learning ability
    2. Ability to read and write
    3. Memory
    4. Spatial and form perception

Vision
    5. Vision

Communication
    6. Hearing
    7. Speech
    8. Language functioning

Motor function
    9. Upper extremity function
    10. Hand function
    11. Motor speed

Physical condition
    12. Mobility
    13. Capacity for exertion
    14. Endurance
    15. Loss of time from work
    16. Stability of condition

Vocational qualifications
    17. Work history
    18. Acceptability to employers
    19. Personal attractiveness
    20. Skills
    21. Economic disincentives
    22. Access to job opportunities
    23. Need for specialized placement or accommodations

Adaptive behavior
    24. Work habits
    25. Social support system
    26. Accurate perception of capabilities & limitations
    27. Effective interaction with employers and co-workers
    28. Judgment
    29. Congruence of behavior with rehabilitation goals
    30. Initiative and problem-solving ability

    The strength items include exceptional assets in the following areas:
    31. Physical appearance
    32. Personality
    33. Intelligent or has verbal fluency
    34. Vocational skill in demand
    35. Suitable educational qualifications
    36. Supportive family
    37. Financial resources
    38. Vocational motivation
    39. Job available with employer
    40. Initiative and problem-solving ability

Adapted from the Functional Assessment Inventory obtained from Dr. Nancy M. Crewe. Copyright University of Minnesota. With permission.

The original version of the FAI (as shown in reference 1) was field tested in three studies, first on 351 physically or mentally disabled patients who were assessed by one of 30 vocational rehabilitation counselors (1). Later it was tested on 1,716 vocational rehabilitation patients, and subsequently on 1,488 patients representing six types of disability: visual, hearing, orthopedic, mental illness, mental retardation and addictions (2).

Reliability

Alpha internal consistency coefficients were calculated for five subscales of the questionnaire for 351 patients; the resulting values ranged from 0.70 to 0.85 (1). To assess inter-rater reliability, a series of 51 interviews was observed and rated by pairs of psychologists. Seventy-five percent of the ratings made by the pairs of observers were identical; only 3% of all ratings differed by more than one point on the four-point scales (1, 2).

Validity

The replies of the 351 patients were factor analyzed, providing eight factors that agree quite closely with the item placements shown in Exhibit 8.3 (1, Table 4). The factor structure held relatively constant when responses from subgroups of the 351 patients with different types of disability were analyzed separately, and analyses of other samples produced similar results (2).

Concurrent validity was assessed by comparing the total FAI limitation and assets scores with two judgments made by rehabilitation counselors concerning employability and severity of disability. (Note that these do not represent independent ratings from the FAI responses, as they were recorded by the same rater). For the 351 patients the correlations with the FAI limitation score were -0.61 for employability and 0.60 for severity of disability (1, p303). For the sample of 1,716 cases the equivalent correlations were -0.57 and 0.55 (3). As might be expected, the correlation between the FAI strength scores and the counselor rating of employability (0.53) was higher than that with disability (-0.21) (1, p303). In a multiple regression analysis, the total functional limitation score plus the total strength score gave a multiple correlation coefficient of 0.70 ($R^2 = 0.49$) with the employability rating. The R^2 value for predicting severity of disability was 0.41 (1, p304).

The third sample of 1,488 patients was divided into those who were admitted for rehabilitation services, those excluded as being too severely disabled, and those excluded as having no impairment. Analyses of variance showed that all FAI scores except for vision and communication distinguished significantly between these groups (2). Strong and logical contrasts were also obtained between different diagnostic groups (2).

Alternative Forms

A self-administered version called the Personal Capabilities Questionnaire is being developed. This version provides the counselor with information on how the client perceives his own limitations.

Commentary

This recently developed instrument includes clear documentation and instructions. The incorporation of both limitations and assets is a welcome and relatively unusual approach in assessing disability and would seem to have considerable potential benefit.

The Functional Assessment Inventory differs from many other instruments in that it can be completed from existing information, so that the patient does not necessarily have to be present. Guidelines on scoring the FAI are contained in the manual available from the address above. The topic of how best to combine the positive and the limitation questions is currently being addressed by Dr. Crewe.

The validity and reliability evidence assembled so far are very promising and use large samples of patients. Because the FAI is intended to assess the potential for vocational rehabilitation, the results of predictive validity testing will be of particular importance. Testing is under way, although the preliminary evidence for predictive validity is not strong. Crewe and Turner reported results from 255 of the 351 patients: the data suggest that only about one half of the FAI items correlated with rehabilitation outcome scores and the total FAI score did not significantly predict outcome (2). Nonetheless, we strongly recommend the FAI as a clinical rating of rehabilitation potential on the basis of the quality of its documentation and its validity and reliability results.

Address

Nancy M. Crewe, PhD, Department of Physical Medicine and Rehabilitation, 860 Mayo Memorial Building, Box 297, University of Minnesota Hospitals, 420 Delaware Street Southeast, Minneapolis, Minnesota, USA 55455

References

(1) Crewe NM, Athelstan GT. Functional assessment in vocational rehabilitation: a systematic approach to diagnosis and goal setting. Arch Phys Med Rehabil 1981;62:299–305.
(2) Crewe NM, Turner RR. A functional assessment system for vocational rehabilitation. In: Halpern A, Fuhrer M, eds. Functional assessment in rehabilitation. Baltimore: Paul H Brooks, 1984.
(3) Crewe NM, Athelstan GT, Meadows GK. Vocational diagnosis through assessment of functional limitations. Arch Phys Med Rehabil 1975;56:513–516.

THE NOTTINGHAM HEALTH PROFILE
(Carlos Martini and Sonja Hunt, 1977, Revised 1981)

Purpose

There exist two forms of this method: an early scale (that we will designate as version 1) named the Nottingham Health Index, and a later one (version 2) called the Nottingham Health Profile (NHP). Both are intended to give brief and simple indications of perceived physical, social and emotional health problems (1). Version 1 indicates a patient's ability to carry on a normal life, and may be used in primary medical care settings as a routine measurement to be completed by patients in the waiting room (2). The second version assesses demand for care in population health surveys and has also been used in clinical studies.

Conceptual Basis

The design and content of the Nottingham indices were influenced by the Sickness Impact Profile. One difference, however, is that the NHP asks about feelings and emotional states directly, rather than via changes in behavior. The emphasis is on the respondent's subjective assessment of his health status: this is seen as the major factor predicting use of medical services and satisfaction with outcomes (3). The questions reflect the WHO concept of disability and the scale may be viewed as an indicator of perceived distress.

Description

Both versions are similar in content; they were constructed from the same pool of items. The existence of the two versions reflects their differing original purpose and the fact that two teams worked on developing the instrument. The items used in the scales were collected empirically from a survey of 768 patients with various acute and chronic ailments, and from other health indices such as the Sickness Impact Profile. Each item refers to

> departures from "normal" functioning because, in the field of health especially, it is easier to obtain, record, and provide some measure of departures from the norm than it is to specify the norm itself. Respondents were asked to answer "Yes" or "No" according to whether or not they feel the item applies to them "in general."
> (4, p282).

Both versions are self-administered questionnaires that take under ten minutes to complete. The first version contains 33 items, selected on the basis of item analyses of interviews with rehabilitation patients (5) and surgical patients undergoing hip replacements (2). This version has not received further testing. Version 2, presented here, contains 38 items that can be grouped into six sections (6). These cover physical mobility (PM = 8 items), pain (P = 8), sleep (S = 5), social isolation (SI = 5), emotional reactions (ER = 9) and energy level (EL = 3). The items were scaled for severity using a paired comparisons technique involving 1,200 outpatient interviews (7), although a simpler, unweighted scoring system is normally used in which the number of affirmative responses in each section is counted. Section scores may be presented as a profile, or an overall score may be calculated. Exhibit 8.4 shows the items in the order in which they are presented and the section that they pertain to. All items use a yes/no answer format.

Exhibit 8.4 The Nottingham Health Profile (Version 2), Showing the Sections on which Each Item Is Scored

Note: EL = energy level, P = pain, ER = emotional reactions, S = sleep, SI = social isolation, PA = physical abilities

- Listed below are some problems people can have in their daily life.
- Please read each one carefully.
- If it is TRUE for you, put a tick ($\checkmark$) in the box under Yes.
- If it is NOT TRUE, put a tick ($\checkmark$) in the box under No.
- If you are not sure whether to answer yes or no to a problem, ask yourself whether it is true for you *in general*.

Note: it is important that you answer every question.

	Yes	No	Section
I'm tired all the time	☐	☐	EL
I have pain at night	☐	☐	P
Things are getting me down	☐	☐	ER
I have unbearable pain	☐	☐	P

	Yes	No	
I take tablets to help me sleep	☐	☐	S
I've forgetten what it's like to enjoy myself	☐	☐	ER
I'm feeling on edge	☐	☐	ER
I find it painful to change position	☐	☐	P
I feel lonely	☐	☐	SI

	Yes	No	
I can walk about only indoors	☐	☐	PA
I find it hard to bend	☐	☐	PA
Everything is an effort	☐	☐	EL
I'm waking up in the early hours of the morning	☐	☐	S

	Yes	No	
I'm unable to walk	☐	☐	PA
I'm finding it hard to make contact with people	☐	☐	SI
The days seem to drag	☐	☐	ER
I have trouble getting up and down stairs or steps	☐	☐	PA
I find it hard to reach for things	☐	☐	PA

	Yes	No	
I'm in pain when I walk	☐	☐	P
I lose my temper easily these days	☐	☐	ER
I feel there is nobody I am close to	☐	☐	SI
I lie awake for most of the night	☐	☐	S

	Yes	No	
I feel as if I'm losing control	☐	☐	ER
I'm in pain when I'm standing	☐	☐	P
I find it hard to dress myself	☐	☐	PA
I soon run out of energy	☐	☐	EL

	Yes	No	
I find it hard to stand for long	☐	☐	PA
(e.g. at the kitchen sink, waiting for a bus)			
I'm in constant pain	☐	☐	P
It takes me a long time to get to sleep	☐	☐	S
I feel I am a burden to people	☐	☐	SI

Exhibit 8.4 (*continued*)

Worry is keeping me awake at night	☐	☐	ER
I feel that life is not worth living	☐	☐	ER

	Yes	No	
I sleep badly at night	☐	☐	S
I'm finding it hard to get on with people	☐	☐	SI
I need help to walk about outside	☐	☐	PA
(e.g. a walking aid or someone to support me)			

	Yes	No	
I'm in pain when going up and down stairs or steps	☐	☐	P
I wake up feeling depressed	☐	☐	ER
I'm in pain when I'm sitting	☐	☐	P

Adapted from the Nottingham Health Profile obtained from Dr. S.M. Hunt. Copyright Hunt SM, McEwen J, McKenna SP. With permission.

Reliability

For the first version, Kuder Richardson 20 internal consistency coefficients for different sections ranged from 0.90 to 0.94 (8). The correlations of items with section scores were examined in two studies (2, 5). The four-week test-retest reliability of the second version was reported by Hunt et al. for 58 arthritics and 93 patients with peripheral vascular disease; coefficients for the six sections ranged from 0.75 to 0.88 (1, Table 2; 9).

Validity

Considerable attention was paid in the initial development of the method to establishing content validity. The items were drawn from interviews with patients about their actual experience. Formal tests of linguistic clarity were applied to analyze the wording of the items using the Fry graph and Flesch test methods.

Discriminal ability of the first version was tested on patients before and after hip replacement surgery. Evidence that the groups did differ was provided by independent assessments, including the McGill Pain Questionnaire and a physical assessment made by a physiotherapist (2). Differences in NHP scores for the two groups of patients were strong (10). A further study showed clear differences between hip replacement patients and their spouses who served as controls (11). The scale also showed clear contrasts between rehabilitation patients with physical and mental handicaps (5, Table 5).

The second version was used in interviews with four groups of elderly respondents ranging from those with diagnosed chronic illness and physical, social and emotional disabilities, to groups of physically fit people who had recently sought medical care (4). Kruskal Wallis tests showed significant differences on all six areas between the groups ($p < 0.001$). A summary of several studies that compare profile scores for nine different patient groups is given by Hunt et al. (1). The results showed clear and clinically plausible contrasts.

The correlation between the first version and the McGill Pain Questionnaire was 0.74, with a range from 0.50 for the social activities section to 0.78 for the pain section (10). The overall score correlated 0.65 with a physiotherapist's rating; correlations for each item range from 0.16 to 0.47 (2, Table 3). Equivalent data were collected in the rehabilitation study, correlations being drawn between the questionnaire and a set of ratings made by a physician (5). Kendall correlations for the walking questions ranged from 0.47 to 0.56, while those for dressing and self-care ranged between 0.40 and 0.48; coefficients for body movements ranged from 0.44 to 0.55 (5, Table 4).

Thirty-three of the items in the first version were factored for the 98 hip replacement patients; they fell on eight factors, reflecting pain, mobility, body movement, sleep, anxiety, getting out of the house, loneliness and depression (2).

Reference Standards

Reference scores for version 2 were given by Hunt et al. for healthy people and various categories of patients (1, Table 1).

Commentary

The second version has been used in a variety of medical and nonmedical settings: miners and firemen selected as being in good physical health (12), elderly people and patients frequently visiting their general practitioner (13), and in a study of social class differences in perceived health (1). The strengths of the method include its simplicity, its sensitivity and its broad coverage. The authors caution that, to avoid false positives, the items were designed to represent rather severe problems and therefore healthy populations or those with minor ailments will have low scores, making change scores difficult to compare. As Hunt notes, however, the scoring may prove cumbersome as it gives a profile of six scores. The method also covers only negative aspects of health and so cannot show change beyond an absence of relatively severe experiences; zero scores do not necessarily indicate a total absence of problems (1). The method continues to be used and tested, however, and holds considerable promise as a survey and as a clinical instrument. A postal survey version is currently being developed.

Address

Sonja Hunt, PhD, Senior Research Fellow, Research Unit in Health and Behavioural Change, University of Edinburgh, Edinburgh, Scotland EH1 2Q2

References

(1) Hunt SM, McEwen J, McKenna SP. Measuring health status: a new tool for clinicians and epidemiologists. J R Coll Gen Pract 1985;35:185–188.
(2) McDowell IW, Martini CJM, Waugh W. A method for self-assessment of disability before and after hip replacement operations. Br Med J 1978;2:857–859.

(3) Hunt SM, McKenna SP, McEwen J, Williams J, Papp E. The Nottingham Health Profile: subjective health status and medical consultations. Soc Sci Med 1981;15A:221–229.

(4) Hunt SM, McKenna SP, McEwen J, Backett EM, Williams J, Papp E. A quantitative approach to perceived health status: a validation study. J Epidemiol Community Health 1980;34:281–286.

(5) Martini CJ, McDowell I. Health status: patient and physician judgments. Health Serv Res 1976;11:508–515.

(6) Hunt SM, McEwen J. The development of a subjective health indicator. Sociol Health Illness 1980;2:231–246.

(7) McKenna SP, Hunt SM, McEwen J. Weighting the seriousness of perceived health problems using Thurstone's method of paired comparisons. Int J Epidemiol 1981;10:93–97.

(8) Martini CJM, McDowell I. Socio-medical measurements of health in primary care. London: Report submitted to Social Sciences Research Council, London, December, 1978.

(9) Hunt SM, McKenna SP, Williams J. Reliability of a population survey tool for measuring perceived health problems: a study of patients with osteoarthrosis. J Epidemiol Community Health 1981:35:297–300.

(10) Martini CJM, McDowell IW. Socio-medical measures of health in primary care. London: Report submitted to Social Sciences Research Council, September 1977.

(11) McKenna SP, McEwen J, Hunt SM, Papp E. Changes in the perceived health of patients recovering from fractures. Public Health 1984:98:97–102.

(12) McKenna SP, Hunt SM, McEwen J. Absence from work and perceived health among mine rescue workers. J Soc Occup Med 1981:31:151–157.

(13) McKenna SP, Hunt S, McEwen J, Williams J, Papp E. Looking at health from the consumers' point of view. Occup Health 1980:32:350-355.

THE SICKNESS IMPACT PROFILE
(Marilyn Bergner, Betty S. Gilson, Ruth A. Bobbitt and William B. Carter, 1976, Revised 1981)

Purpose

The Sickness Impact Profile (SIP) was conceived as a measurement of perceived health status that would provide a descriptive profile of the changes in a person's behavior due to sickness (1). "It was designed to be broadly applicable across types and severities of illness and across demographic and cultural subgroups." (2, p787). The SIP was intended for use in measuring the outcomes of care, in health surveys, in program planning and policy formation, and in monitoring patient progress (3).

Conceptual Basis

The conceptual development originated from the observation that the ultimate aim of most health care is to reduce sickness or modify its effect on everyday activities (4). "Sickness" denotes the individual's own experience of illness, perceived through its effect on daily activities, feelings, and attitudes. In this sense, sickness is contrasted to disease, which denotes a professional or a provider's definition of illness based on clinical observations (5).

The SIP measures health status by assessing the impact of sickness on changing daily activities and behavior. Its concentration on behavior holds several advantages over recording feelings or clinical reports. Feeling states are variable, hard to measure, and are not accessible to external validation because of their subjectivity. Clinical assessments are limited to patients under care, or require medical interpretation of symptoms reported by those under study. Behavioral reports, by contrast, can be verified by observation and they can be obtained whether or not a patient is receiving care; they may also be less subject to cultural bias than reports of feelings (1).

The items in the SIP all concentrate on changes in performance rather than capacity (4). The behaviors included in the profile are considered significant from the individual, social, and health care points of view. They are held to represent "universal patterns" of limitations that may be affected by sickness or disease, regardless of the specific conditions, treatment, individual characteristics, or prognosis concerned (1).

Description

Work on the SIP began in 1972; statements describing changes in behavior attributable to sickness were compiled from professionals, from interviews with healthy and ill lay persons, and from a literature review. Following a succession of field trials (total sample = 1,108), the prototype, containing 312 statements grouped into 14 categories of activities, was refined to a final version with 136 statements in 12 categories. The SIP is composed of statements such as "I have difficulty reasoning and solving problems" and "I do not walk at all," each of which considers a change in behavior and specifies the extent of limitation.

Respondents check only the items that describe them on a given day and are related to their health, although the medical condition is not a consideration (1). Scores may be calculated using item weights that indicate the relative severity of limitation implied by each statement. The weights were derived from equal-appearing interval scaling procedures involving more than 100 judges (2, 6).

> The scaling permits the calculation of an SIP percent score which is the sum of the scale values of items checked divided by the sum of the scale values for all items multiplied by 100. This SIP percent score may be calculated for the entire SIP (the SIP overall score) as well as for each of the categories. (7, p58).

The full instrument is too long to reproduce here; copies are available at cost (see "Address" below). Exhibit 8.5 indicates the scope of the SIP and illustrates the types of items used. As shown in the exhibit, 3 of the 12 activity categories may also be summed to form a physical score and 5 others form a psychosocial score (2). The remaining 5 sections are scored separately.

Exhibit 8.5 The Sickness Impact Profile: Categories and Selected Items

Dimension	Category	Items describing behavior related to	Selected items
Independent categories	SR	Sleep and Rest	I sit during much of the day I sleep or nap during the day
	E	Eating	I am eating no food at all, nutrition is taken through tubes or intravenous fluids I am eating special or different food
	W	Work	I am not working at all I often act irritable toward my work associates
	HM	Home management	I am not doing any of the maintenance or repair work around the house that I usually do I am not doing heavy work around the house
	RP	Recreation and pastimes	I am going out for entertainment less I am not doing any of my usual physical recreation or activities
I. Physical	A	Ambulation	I walk shorter distances or stop to rest often I do not walk at all
	M	Mobility	I stay within one room I stay away from home only for brief periods of time
	BCM	Body care and movement	I do not bathe myself at all, but am bathed by someone else I am very clumsy in body movements
II. Psychosocial	SI	Social interaction	I am doing fewer social activities with groups of people I isolate myself as much as I can from the rest of the family
	AB	Alertness behavior	I have difficulty reasoning and solving problems, for example, making plans, making decisions, learning new things I sometimes behave as if I were confused or disoriented in place or time, for example, where I am, who is around, directions, what day it is
	EB	Emotional behavior	I laugh or cry suddenly I act irritable and impatient with myself, for example,

Dimension	Category	Items describing behavior related to	Selected items
	C	Communication	talk badly about myself, swear at myself, blame myself for things that happen I am having trouble writing or typing I do not speak clearly when I am under stress

Reproduced from Bergner M, Bobbitt RA, Carter WB, Gilson BS. The Sickness Impact Profile: development and final revision of a health status measure. Med Care 1981;19:789,Table 1. With permission.

The profile can be administered by an interviewer in 20 to 30 minutes, or it can be self-administered. User's and trainer's manuals are available (4).

Reliability

In a comprehensive discussion of reliability, Pollard et al. reported the results of various tests of the 235-item and 146-item version of the SIP (8, 9) while reliability results for the final 136-item version were reported by Bergner et al. (2). Test-retest reliability in these various trials was consistently high (0.88 to 0.92) for the overall score. Reliability was higher for the interviewer-administered (0.97) than for the self-administered version (0.87). Reproducibility of the individual items averaged 0.50, while for the 12 category scores it was 0.82 (2, pp793, 796). The reliability of overall scores did not vary by type or level of sickness; the short form was as reliable as the long form (2, 8, 9). Deyo et al. applied the SIP in a study of 79 arthritics (mean age, 57 years). Test-retest reliability (Spearman correlation) was 0.91 for 23 patients (10, Table 6).

Internal consistency was examined within each category and for the instrument as a whole. Cronbach's coefficient alpha was 0.97 for the 235-item version and 0.94 for the final 136-item version, although mailed self-administered questionnaires had the lower internal consistency alpha of 0.81 (2, p793).

Validity

The validity trials compared the SIP with subjective ratings made by the respondents, with clinical assessments and with other functional assessment instruments. The results of field trials using the final version of the SIP showed higher correlations than were obtained using the preliminary versions: 0.69 with a self-assessment of limitation; 0.63 with a self-assessment of sickness; 0.50 with a clinician's assessment of limitation; and 0.40 with a clinician's assessment of sickness (2, Table 4).

The rank correlation between Katz's Index of Activities of Daily Living and SIP scores was 0.46 for 73 rehabilitation patients; the relatively low correlation derives from the broader scope of the SIP and perhaps also from the low validity of the Katz instrument (see Chapter 3). The combined score for the five SIP categories that most clearly reflect ADL behaviors correlated 0.64 (7, p65). The correlation between the SIP and the National Health Interview Survey questions on activity limitation was 0.55 (2, p795).

A comparison of the SIP responses and clinical indicators was made for patients in each of three diagnostic groups for which clinical tests could be expected to reflect patient functioning. For 15 hip replacement patients, the overall SIP score correlated 0.81 with an index of physical functioning. A similar comparison for 15 patients with rheumatoid arthritis yielded a correlation of 0.66. For hyperthyroid patients the overall SIP score correlated 0.41 with thyroid function measurements (2, Table 8).

Deyo et al. reported correlations between SIP overall physical and psychosocial scores and several indicators of disease severity for 79 arthritic patients. The results are shown in Table 8.3. (10). Correlations with a clinician's rating of the patient's functional classification were 0.36 for the physical dimension and 0.02 for the psychosocial dimension (10).

Alternative Forms

As described in the review of the Lambeth screening instrument in Chapter 3, the SIP was adapted for use in England and was called the Functional Limitations Profile (11, 12). Linguistic changes were made and scale weights were recalculated, although these agreed closely with the original weights for the United States. A Chicano-Spanish version has also been developed (13).

Commentary

The SIP has been developed with exemplary care and thoroughness. Like the OECD index, the SIP attempts to be universally applicable, capable of assessing any sickness and not restricted to particular types of medical condition. The reliability results are good, the validity findings promising, and this scale

Table 8.3 Correlations Between SIP Scores and Criterion Variables

| | SIP | | |
	Overall score	Physical dimension	Psychosocial dimension
Duration of RA	0.26*	0.36†	0.03
Morning stiffness	0.23*	0.15	0.32†
Hematocrit	−0.29*	−0.26*	−0.12
Sedimentation rate (ESR)	0.36*	0.44†	0.11
Anatomic stage	0.17	0.31†	−0.01
Evidence of mental health problems	0.11	−0.03	0.27†

*$p < 0.05$
†$p < 0.01$

Adapted from Deyo RA, Inui TS, Leininger JD, Overman SS. Measuring functional outcomes in chronic disease: a comparison of traditional scales and a self-administered health status questionnaire in patients with rheumatoid arthritis. Med Care 1983;21:187,Table 2.

is likely to become a standard against which to judge other methods. We have no hesitation in recommending its use in clinical and survey research.

Address

Marilyn Bergner, PhD, Professor, Health Policy and Management, School of Hygiene and Public Health, The Johns Hopkins University, 624 North Broadway, Baltimore, Maryland, USA 21205

References

(1) Bergner M, Bobbitt RA, Kressel S, Pollard WE, Gilson BS, Morris JR. The Sickness Impact Profile: conceptual formulation and methodology for the development of a health status measure. Int J Health Serv 1976;6:393–415.

(2) Bergner M, Bobbitt RA, Carter WB, Gilson BS. The Sickness Impact Profile: development and final revision of a health status measure. Med Care 1981;19:787–805.

(3) The Sickness Impact Profile: a brief summary of its purpose, uses and administration. Seattle, Washington: University of Washington, Department of Health Services, January 1978.

(4) Gilson BS, Bergner M, Bobbitt RA, Carter WB. The Sickness Impact Profile: final development and testing, 1975–1978. Seattle, Washington: University of Washington, Department of Health Services, 1979.

(5) Gilson BS, Gilson JS, Bergner M, Bobbitt RA, Kressel S, Pollard WE, Vesselago M. The Sickness Impact Profile: development of an outcome measure of health care. Am J Public Health 1975;65:1304–1310.

(6) Carter WB, Bobbitt RA, Bergner M, Gilson BS. Validation of an interval scaling: the Sickness Impact Profile. Health Serv Res 1976;11:516–528.

(7) Bergner M, Bobbitt RA, Pollard WE, Martin DP, Gilson BS. The Sickness Impact Profile: validation of a health status measure. Med Care 1976;14:57–67.

(8) Pollard WE, Bobbitt RA, Bergner M, Martin DP, Gilson BS. The Sickness Impact Profile: reliability of a health status measure. Med Care 1976;14:146–155.

(9) Pollard WE, Bobbitt RA, Bergner M. Examination of variable errors of measurement in a survey based social indicator. Soc Indicat Res 1978;5:279–301.

(10) Deyo RA, Inui TS, Leininger JD, Overman SS. Measuring functional outcomes in chronic disease: a comparison of traditional scales and a self-administered health status questionnaire in patients with rheumatoid arthritis. Med Care 1983;21:180–192.

(11) Patrick DL. Standardisation of comparative health status measures: using scales developed in America in an English speaking country. Paper presented at the Third Biennial Conference on Health Survey Research Methods, Reston VA, 17 May 1979.

(12) Patrick DL, ed. Health and care of the physically disabled in Lambeth. Report of Phase II of The Longitudinal Disability Interview Survey. London: St. Thomas's Hospital Medical School, Department of Community Medicine, 1982.

(13) Gilson BS, Erickson D, Chavez CT, Bobbitt RA, Bergner M, Carter WB. A Chicano version of the Sickness Impact Profile. Cult Med Psychiatry 1980;4:137–150.

THE MULTILEVEL ASSESSMENT INSTRUMENT
(M. Powell Lawton, 1982)

Purpose

The Multilevel Assessment Instrument (MAI) was designed to measure the overall well-being of elderly persons living in the community. It covers health problems, activities of daily living skills, psychological well-being, environmental quality and social interaction.

Conceptual Basis

Lawton argued that to assess the quality of life of an elderly person, ratings must be made on four dimensions: behavioral competence, psychological well-being, perceived quality of life and objective quality of the environment (1). Based on this conceptual framework, the MAI built on existing measurement instruments, notably the Multidimensional Functional Assessment Questionnaire. Lawton argued that the MAI incorporated, but went beyond, existing instruments by considering environmental factors, by separating social interaction from personal pursuits such as hobbies and by separating cognitive ability from psychological well-being (1). The functional abilities section of the MAI was based on the theme of "behavioral competence," which Lawton viewed in terms of a hierarchy of increasingly complex activities ranging from the basic biological functions required for life maintenance, through perception and cognition, followed by skills for physical self-maintenance, up to exploratory behavior and complex social interactions (2). The term "multilevel assessment" is used to imply assessment on each of the levels of this hierarchy.

Description

This is one of several measurement scales developed at the Philadelphia Geriatric Center. Others that are reviewed in this book include the Physical Self-Maintenance Scale and the Philadelphia Geriatric Center Morale Scale. The MAI comprises seven dimensions with 147 items; a further 81 items cover medical and demographic data, but these are not considered in this review. Items were taken from a wide variety of established indices (1), and the MAI incorporates the ADL and IADL questions from the MFAQ. The psychological domain includes questions on morale and psychiatric symptoms, and the environmental dimension covers housing quality and personal security (1). Space does not permit listing all the MAI questions, but the seven dimensions are shown in Exhibit 8.6 (note: this describes a revised questionnaire). Most of the dimensions are divided into subscales of which there are 14 in all (for example, perceived environment includes housing quality, neighborhood quality, and personal security). Each subscale contains between 3 and 24 items.

The instrument is administered in a home interview that takes an average of 50 minutes to complete. Some of the information must be obtained from

Exhibit 8.6 The Scope of the Multilevel Assessment Instrument, Showing Numbers of Items in Each Subscale

	Number of items
1. Physical health:	
Self-rated health	4
Use of health services	3
Health conditions	26
Mobility	3
Use of aids, prostheses, etc.	13
2. Cognition:	
Mental status	6
Cognitive symptoms	4
3. Activities of daily living:	
IADL Scale	10
Personal Self-Maintenance Activities	6
4. Time use:	
Social activities, sports, hobbies	18
5. Social relations and interactions:	
Family	12
Friends	5
6. Personal adjustment:	
Morale	9
Psychiatric symptoms	3
7. Perceived environment:	
Housing quality	9
Neighborhood quality	12
Personal security	4
	147

Adapted from Lawton MP, Moss M, Fulcomer M, Kleban MH. A research and service oriented Multilevel Assessment Intrument. J Gerontol 1982;37:96,Table 2.

the elderly person, but much can be obtained from the spouse or other informant. Scores are based on the numbers of items checked in each section; these may be added to give scores for each of the seven dimensions. Unweighted scores were found to correlate well with more complicated scoring methods (1).

Reliability

Lawton reported several studies of the agreement between two independent raters. Intraclass correlations between ratings on the seven dimensions ranged from 0.88 (for the IADL scale) to a low of 0.58 (for the social interaction scale (1, p95). Agreement between two interviewers lay within a one point discrepancy for 95% of the ratings on the summary scales for a sample of 484 (1). Alpha internal consistency results for 590 respondents ranged from 0.69 for the cognitive and psychiatric symptom scales to 0.93 for activities of daily living. Two coefficients, for health behavior and personal security, were lower at 0.39 and 0.57. Three-week test re-test reliabilities for 22 respondents ranged from 0.55 to 0.99 with the exception of ADL, which had a correlation of 0.35 (2, Table 2).

Validity

The MAI showed a weak ability to distinguish respondents living independently in the community from those in institutional care. Correlations for the seven dimension scores fell between 0.05 and 0.54 (1, Table 2).

Correlations with a psychologist's independent rating of 590 individuals was 0.23 for the cognition dimension of the MAI, although, curiously, agreement between the psychologist's rating of other dimensions and the MAI scores was higher, ranging from 0.56 to 0.69. Agreement with ratings made by a housing administrator on 180 respondents for the seven dimensions ranged from 0.12 (for social interaction) to 0.59 (for ADL). The interviewers who applied the MAI made their own summary ratings of each dimension, and these were correlated against scores on the MAI. Coefficients ranged from 0.36 to 0.87 (1, Table 2). Lawton and Brody reported correlations between the IADL section and the Physical Self-Maintenance Scale and a variety of other measurements. The correlations ranged from 0.36 to 0.62 (2, Table 6).

Commentary

This instrument is a good example of a scale based on a clearly enunciated conceptual framework and on existing measurements. The reliability findings are promising, and yet the scale will clearly benefit from further testing and refinement. The validity results show quite low correlations between the method and independent assessments. Those scales showing low validity coefficients also showed low reliability scores, and Lawton noted that the psychometric properties of the social interaction and time use scales require improvement. The developers of the MAI also experienced some problems in selecting the most appropriate questions for the environmental scales. The low validity agreement between the psychologist's rating of cognition and the corresponding MAI score is a cause for concern; it may be that the cognition measure discriminates only at very low levels of cognitive functioning. Lawton discussed the strengths and weaknesses of the MAI, and argued in favor of a simple scoring system and against abbreviating the scale. He noted that scale norms based on representative population samples are not yet available, and the social and environmental domains show particular need for further research and development. He concluded that the physical health, the cognition and the ADL dimensions of the MAI are the most robust.

This scale shows potential, but still lacks adequate documentation and validity analysis. Nonetheless, it seems that the MAI will continue to be refined, and we recommend that those who wish to assess the well-being of the elderly living in the community contact Dr. Lawton to find out whether a revised form has been developed.

Address

M. Powell Lawton, PhD, Philadelphia Geriatric Center, 5301 Old York Road, Philadelphia, Pennsylvania, USA 19141

References

(1) Lawton MP, Moss M, Fulcomer M, Kleban MH. A research and service oriented Multilevel Assessment Instrument. J Gerontol 1982;37:91–99.

(2) Lawton MP, Brody EM. Assessment of older people: Self-Maintaining and Instrumental Activities of Daily Living. Gerontologist 1969;9:179–186.

THE OARS MULTIDIMENSIONAL FUNCTIONAL ASSESSMENT QUESTIONNAIRE
(Older Americans Resources and Services, Duke University, 1975)

Purpose

The OARS Multidimensional Functional Assessment Questionnaire (MFAQ) was developed to give a comprehensive profile of the level of functioning and need for services of older persons who live at home but who have some degree of impairment (1). It can be used as a screening instrument, to evaluate outcomes and in modeling the cost-effectiveness of alternative approaches to providing care.

Conceptual Basis

The Older Americans Resources and Services (OARS) Program was the clinical facet of the Duke University Center for the Study of Aging and Human Development. The program was concerned with reducing inappropriate institutionalization and with evaluating alternatives to institutional care for the elderly (2). The MFAQ was intended to give a broad ranging patient assessment for integrating services tailored to the needs of the older person.

Description

The OARS questionnaire is divided into two parts: the Multidimensional Functional Assessment Questionnaire and the Services Assessment Questionnaire. The MFAQ includes five sections, covering social and economic resources, mental and physical health, and activities of daily living. Sixty-six questions are asked of the respondent and a further ten questions record judgments made by an informant. Many of the questions have subparts, making a total of 120 items, as reported in Table 8.2 at the beginning of this chapter. In addition, the interviewer makes five overall ratings, one for each of the sections, based on information collected in the interview. The Services Assessment Questionnaire covers services received and needed. The MFAQ evolved from revisions to an Intake Form, developed for an outpatient clinic population, that was later modified into a Community Survey Questionnaire for assessing people at home (3). While these instruments were designed for the elderly, items were later added to the MFAQ to make it suitable for people aged 18 years and over. Questions were drawn from existing instruments and the source of each is given in the manual.

Exhibit 8.7 Contents of the Multidimensional Functional Assessment Questionnaire

In addition to basic demographic and interview specific information, the MFAQ includes two sections: Part A, Assessment of Individual Functioning, and Part B, Assessment of Services Utilization.

Part A: Assessment of individual functioning

Part A is divided into seven major sections. These sections, in order, with a listing of the number of primary questions (some questions include several items) and a description of their content, are:

Section	No. of questions	Content
Basic demographic	11	Address; date; interviewer; informant; place of interview; duration; sex; race; age; education; telephone number.
Social resources	9	Marital status; resident companions; extent and type of contact with others; availability of confidante; perception of loneliness; availability, duration, and source of help.
Economic resources	15	Employment status; major occupation of self (and of spouse, if married); source and amount of income; number of dependents; home ownership or rental, and cost; source and adequacy of financial resources; health insurance; subjectively assessed adequacy of income.
Mental health	6	Short Portable Mental Status Questionnaire (SPMSQ), a ten-item test of organicity; extent of worry, satisfaction, and interest in life; assessment of present mental status and change in the past five years; fifteen-item Short Psychiatric Evaluation Schedule.
Physical health	16	Physician visits, days sick, in hospital and/or nursing home in past six months; medications in past month; current illnesses and their extent of interference; physical, visual, and hearing disabilities; alcoholism; participation in vigorous exercise; self-assessment of health.
Activities of daily living	15	Extent of capacity to: telephone, travel, shop, cook, do housework, take medicine, handle money, feed self, dress, groom, walk, transfer, bathe, and control bladder and bowels. Also, presence of another to help with ADL tasks.
Informant assessments	10	Information on the focal person's level of functioning on each of the five dimensions is sought from a knowledgeable informant. Specifically: Social: Capacity to get along with others; availability, duration, and source of help in time of need. Economic: Extent to which income meets basic self-maintenance requirements. Mental: Ability to make sound judgements,

300

Section	No. of questions	Content
		cope; interest in life; comparison with peers; change in past five years.
		Physical: Assessment of health; extent of interference of health problems.
Interviewer section		
(a) interview specific	4	Sources of information; reliability of responses.
(b) interview assessments	15	Social: Availability and duration of help when needed; adequacy of social relationships.
		Economic: Assessed adequacy of income; presence of reserves; extent to which basic needs are met.
		Mental: Ability to make sound judgements, cope; interest in life; behavior during interview.
		Physical: Whether obese or malnourished.
		Rating scales: Five six-point scales, one for each dimension.

Part B: Services assessment

For each of the twenty-four nonoverlapping services named below, enquiry is made into (a) utilization in the past six months, (b) intensity of present utilization (e.g., frequency), (c) service provider (e.g., self, family and friends, agency), and (d) perceived current need for service.

1. Transportation
2. Social/recreational
3. Employment
4. Sheltered employment
5. Educational services, employment related
6. Remedial training
7. Mental health
8. Psychotropic drugs
9. Personal care
10. Nursing care
11. Medical services
12. Supportive services and prostheses
13. Physical therapy
14. Continuous supervision
15. Checking
16. Relocation and placement
17. Homemaker-household
18. Meal preparation
19. Administrative, legal, and protective
20. Systematic multidimensional evaluation
21. Financial assistance
22. Food, groceries
23. Living quarters (housing)
24. Coordination, information, and referral

Reproduced from Multidimensional functional assessment: the OARS methodology. A manual. 2nd ed. Durham, North Carolina: Duke University, Center for the Study of Aging and Human Development, 1978:13–15. Copyright Duke University Center for the Study of Aging and Human Development. With permission. Permission required to use.

The MFAQ is administered by a trained interviewer. Two-day interviewer training courses are available from the Duke University Center for Aging ; further details on administering the scale are given in the manual (2, p133). The method was designed as a single interview schedule to be used in its entirety—the originators advise against extracting particular sections (1). It takes about 45 minutes to complete, the time required for Part A being about 30 minutes (2).

The entire scale is too long to present here; it is available in the OARS manuals (1, 2). The contents of the MFAQ are summarized in Exhibit 8.7; a rationale for the topics included is given by Pfeiffer. As an illustration of the actual questions, Exhibit 8.8 shows the ADL and IADL sections.

The five sections of the MFAQ are scored by a rater who reads the answers to each item and then summarizes the level of function for that section on a six-point scale: 1, outstanding functioning; 2, good functioning; 3, mild impairment; 4, moderate impairment; 5, severe impairment; and 6, complete impairment. This information can be handled in several ways: the five section ratings may be presented as a profile (2), or the five ratings may be added to form a Cumulative Impairment Score. Scores below 10 suggest excellent functioning, while those over 18 indicate significant impairment in several areas (2). Third, the number of sections on which a patient shows significant impairment (scores of 4 or more) may be counted. Finally, each of the five scores may be dichotomized into not impaired (ratings 1 to 3) and impaired (4 to 6). This produces 32 permutations, and the respondent is classified into one of these (2).

Reliability

Extensive reliability testing has been carried out on Part A of the MFAQ and on the Community Service Questionnaire from which the MFAQ was derived (1, 2). Because section scores on the MFAQ are typically assigned on the basis of judgments by raters who review the questionnaire responses, the assessment of inter-rater agreement is especially important. Fillenbaum and Smyer reported inter-rater agreement for the MFAQ for 11 raters who evaluated 30 patients. Intraclass correlations ranged from 0.66 for physical health to 0.87 for self-care (3, p432). Raters were in complete agreement for 74% of the ratings.

Other reliability data refer to the Community Service Questionnaire, giving inter-rater Kendall coefficients of concordance between 0.70 and 0.93, with 11 out of 25 coefficients being 0.85 or above (2, p32). Ratings of the same questionnaires made 12 to 18 months apart gave correlations between 0.47 and 1.00, with only 6 of 35 coefficients lying below 0.80 (2, p32).

Five week test-retest correlations for 30 elderly subjects were 0.82 for the physical ADL questions, 0.71 for the IADL questions, 0.79 for those on economic resources. The test-retest correlation for the objective questions on social resources was 0.71, and that for the subjective questions was 0.53. Coefficients for life satisfaction and mental health were lower: 0.42 and 0.32, respectively (2, p30).

Validity

Fillenbaum and Smyer presented criterion validity results for the MFAQ on 33 family medicine patients. Separate criterion ratings were established for each section in the questionnaire (3). Spearman correlations between the MFAQ and these ratings were 0.68 for the economic section, 0.67 for mental health, 0.82 for physical health, and 0.89 for self-care capacity (3, Table 3).

Several validity results are available for the Intake Form and the Commu-

Exhibit 8.8 The Multidimensional Functional Assessment Questionnaire: ADL and IADL Sections

Activities of daily living

Now I'd like to ask you about some of the activities of daily living, things that we all need to do as a part of our daily lives. I would like to know if you can do these activities without any help at all, or if you need some help to do them, or if you can't do them at all.

[Be sure to read all answer choices if applicable in questions 56 through 69 to respondent.]

Instrumental ADL

56. Can you use the telephone . . .
    2 without help, including looking up numbers and dialing,
    1 with some help (can answer phone or dial operator in an emergency, but need a special phone or help in getting the number or dialing),
    0 or are you completely unable to use the telephone?
    – Not answered

57. Can you get to places out of walking distance . . .
    2 without help (can travel alone on buses, taxis, or drive your own car),
    1 with some help (need someone to help you or go with you when traveling) or
    0 are you unable to travel unless emergency arrangements are made for a specialized vehicle like an ambulance?
    – Not answered

58. Can you go shopping for groceries or clothes [assuming subject has transportation] . . .
    2 without help (taking care of all shopping needs yourself, assuming you had transportation),
    1 with some help (need someone to go with you on all shopping trips),
    0 or are you completely unable to do any shopping?
    – Not answered

59. Can you prepare your own meals . . .
    2 without help (plan and cook full meals yourself),
    1 with some help (can prepare some things but unable to cook full meals yourself),
    0 or are you completely unable to prepare any meals?
    – Not answered

60. Can you do your housework . . .
    2 without help (can scrub floors, etc.),
    1 with some help (can do light housework but need help with heavy work),
    0 or are you completely unable to do any housework?
    – Not answered

61. Can you take your own medicine . . .
    2 without help (in the right doses at the right time),
    1 with some help (able to take medicine if someone prepares it for you and/or reminds you to take it),
    0 or are you completely unable to take your medicines?
    – Not answered

62. Can you handle your own money . . .
    2 without help (write checks, pay bills, etc.),
    1 with some help (manage day-to-day buying but need help with managing your checkbook and paying your bills),
    0 or are you completely unable to handle money?
    – Not answered

EXHIBIT 8.8 (*continued*)

Physical ADL

63. Can you eat . . .
    2 without help (able to feed yourself completely),
    1 with some help (need help with cutting, etc.),
    0 or are you completely unable to feed yourself?
    – Not answered

64. Can you dress and undress yourself . . .
    2 without help (able to pick out clothes, dress and undress yourself),
    1 with some help,
    0 or are you completely unable to dress and undress yourself?
    – Not answered

65. Can you take care of your own appearance, for example combing your hair and (for men) shaving . . .
    2 without help,
    1 with some help,
    0 or are you completely unable to maintain your appearance yourself?
    – Not answered

66. Can you walk . . .
    2 without help (except from a cane),
    1 with some help from a person or with the use of a walker, or crutches, etc.,
    0 or are you completely unable to walk?
    – Not answered

67. Can you get in and out of bed . . .
    2 without any help or aids,
    1 with some help (either from a person or with the aid of some device),
    0 or are you totally dependent on someone else to lift you?
    – Not answered

68. Can you take a bath or shower . . .
    2 without help,
    1 with some help (need help getting in and out of the tub, or need special attachments on the tub),
    0 or are you completely unable to bathe yourself?
    – Not answered

69. Do you ever have trouble getting to the bathroom on time?
    2 No
    0 Yes
    1 Have a catheter or colostomy
    – Not answered
    [*If "Yes" ask* a.]
    a. How often do you wet or soil yourself (either day or night)?

        1 Once or twice a week
        0 Three times a week or more
        – Not answered

70. Is there someone who helps you with such things as shopping, housework, bathing, dressing, and getting around?
    1 Yes
    0 No
    – Not answered

[*If "Yes" ask* a. *and* b.]
a. Who is your major helper?
   Name _____ Relationship _____
b. Who else helps you?
   Name _____ Relationship _____

Reproduced from Multidimensional functional assessment: the OARS methodology. A manual. 2nd ed. Durham, North Carolina: Duke University, Center for the Study of Aging and Human Development, 1978:68. Copyright Duke University Center for the Study of Aging and Human Development. With permission. Permission required to use.

nity Survey Questionnaire, the earlier versions of the MFAQ. Scores on physical and mental health from the questionnaire were compared with ratings made by psychiatrists and physicians' assistants for 82 patients. The Spearman correlation for mental health was 0.62 and for physical health it was 0.70 ($p <$ 0.001) (2, p27). A comparison of MFAQ scores with health care expenditures was made by Laurie, showing a steep rise in expenditures (by a factor of 13) as the MFAQ scores rose from the lowest to the highest level of impairment (2). Scores from three contrasting populations—985 community residents, 78 patients, and 76 institutionalized elderly—showed clearly differing profiles on the instrument (5, Figure 1).

Commentary

The OARS work has been cited as influential in the design of several subsequent scales, including the CARE of Gurland et al. The development work has been carefully carried out over a long period of time by a large team. The questionnaire is being used in a number of settings, reflecting the emphasis on developing a multi-purpose instrument (4). This flexibility is reflected in the alternative approaches to scoring the questionnaire: "the same basic set of data can be analyzed in several different ways to meet the needs of its many different users" (2).

Much of the reliability testing refers to previous versions of the instrument, although the results suggest that the method can be applied and scored in a consistent manner. The manuals provide clear details of the development, administration and quality of the instrument. The ADL and IADL sections show especially good validity and reliability, making them apparently superior to many of the purpose-built ADL instruments reviewed in Chapter 3. The OARS team counsels against applying these separately, but it appears likely that these two sections will be tested as separate scales in their own right. We have little hesitation in recommending the MFAQ as a valuable instrument for providing a very detailed and comprehensive patient profile.

Address

George L. Maddox, PhD, Chairman, University Council on Aging and Human Development, Center for the Study of Aging and Human Development, Duke University Medical Center, Durham, North Carolina, USA 27710

References

(1) Pfeiffer E, ed. Multidimensional functional assessment: the OARS methodology. A manual. Durham, North Carolina: Duke University, Center for the Study of Aging and Human Development, 1975.

(2) Multidimensional functional assessment: the OARS methodology. A manual. 2nd ed. Durham, North Carolina: Duke University, Center for the Study of Aging and Human Development, 1978.

(3) Fillenbaum GG, Smyer MA. The development, validity, and reliability of the OARS Multidimensional Functional Assessment Questionnaire. J Gerontol 1981;36:428–434.

(4) George LK, Fillenbaum GG. OARS methodology: a decade of experience in geriatric assessment. J Am Geriatr Soc 1985;33:607–615.

(5) Maddox GL. Assessment of functional status in a programme evaluation and resource allocation model. In: Holland WW, Ipsen J, Kostrzewski J, eds. Measurement of levels of health. Copenhagen: World Health Organization, 1979:353–366. (WHO Regional Publications European Series No. 7).

THE COMPREHENSIVE ASSESSMENT AND REFERRAL EVALUATION
(Barry Gurland, 1977, Revised 1983)

Purpose

The Comprehensive Assessment and Referral Evaluation (CARE) is a semi-structured interview that evaluates the health and social problems of people aged 65 years and over living in the community (1, 2). It covers psychiatric, medical, nutritional, economic and social problems and was intended to assess the individual's need for care and preventive services and to indicate the likely prognosis.

Conceptual Basis

The main feature of the CARE is its unusually broad scope. There are several reasons for this. In assessing people living in the community, the interpretation of symptoms may be more complex than among hospitalized patients:

> The situation is very different with regard to persons who have been randomly selected from the community based population. It cannot be assumed that their symptoms (if any) have clinical significance, nor, if they do have significance, to which disciplinary domain they might pertain. For example, weight loss which may indicate depression in a hospitalized psychiatric patient may, in a community resident, just as well be normal (e.g., the person is on a reducing diet), due to a medical condition (e.g., a wasting disease), or due to a social condition (e.g., poverty, or lack of help in preparing food). (1, p18).

Gurland et al. also noted that most elderly people suffer from more than one health or social problem, and each must be distinguished in order to determine appropriate treatment (2). Treatment will depend on the combination of problems encountered and may require continual monitoring of all of them.

The conceptual model on which the CARE is based identifies a causal sequence of health problems in the elderly. The sequence begins with age, race and social circumstances; these influence medical condition and cognitive states, and thereby influence functional capacity. Functional capacity in turn may cause the person to seek care and may also lead to demoralization and family inconvenience (3).

Description

Gurland described the CARE as follows:

> The CARE is a new assessment technique which is intended to reliably elicit, record, grade and classify information on the health and social problems of the older person. The CARE is basically a semi-structured interview guide and an inventory of defined ratings. It is designated *comprehensive* because it covers psychiatric, medical, nutritional, economic and social problems rather than the interests of only one professional discipline. The style, scope and scoring of the CARE makes it suitable for use with both patients and non-patients, and a potentially useful aid in determining whether an elderly person should be *referred,* and to whom, for a health or social service. The CARE can also be employed in *evaluating* the effectiveness of that service if given. (1, p10).

The items included in the CARE were drawn from existing instruments, including Wing's Present State Examination, Gurland's SSIAM, the MFAQ and various ADL scales (1). Developmental tests of the CARE were carried out in London and in New York.

The original version of the CARE contained 1,500 items and was administered in an interview lasting about 90 minutes (2). Shortened version have subsequently been derived (2): the CORE-CARE (329 items; see Exhibit 8.9) and the SHORT-CARE (143 items).

Original versions of the CARE required extensive training to administer, but later versions may be applied by interviewers with standard training (2). The interview is not completely standard, permitting the interviewer to alter the order of questions to suit each respondent. A manual gives questions that the interviewer is trained to partly memorize to enhance the flow of the interview (1). To clarify the meaning of questions to a respondent who does not understand, the guide contains standard alternative question phrasings.

Scores for the CORE-CARE are provided for 22 "indicator scales" covering psychiatric and medical problems, service needs and social conditions. These scales were formed by selecting items from the original interview schedule on the basis of face validity, expert judgments of importance and internal consistency (4). Item selection was based on data collected from 445 randomly selected elderly residents in New York and 396 in London. Exhibit 8.9 summarizes the 22 indicator scales while Exhibit 8.10 gives an example of one of the scales. Copies of the questionnaire are available from the author; scoring instructions may be obtained from the National Technical Information Service, US Department of Commerce, Springfield, Virginia, USA 22151.

The SHORT-CARE is intended as a simpler instrument focusing on psychiatric impairment and physical disability. It contains 143 items drawn from six

Exhibit 8.9 22 Indicator Scales of the CORE-CARE

	Number of items	
Psychiatric problems		
1. Cognitive impairment	10	
2. Depression/demoralization	29	
3. Subjective memory problems	9	
		48
Physical problems		
4. Somatic symptoms	34	
5. Heart disorder	15	
6. Stroke effects	9	
7. Cancer	6	
8. Respiratory symptoms	6	
9. Arthritis	9	
10. Leg problems	9	
11. Sleep disorder	8	
12. Hearing disorder	14	
13. Vision disorder	11	
14. Hypertension	4	
15. Ambulation problems	27	
16. Activity limitation	3⁰	
		191
Service needs		
17. Service utilization	15	
		15
Environmental social problems		
18. Financial hardship	8	
19. Dissatisfaction with neighborhood	8	
20. Fear of crime	18	
21. Social isolation	34	
22. Retirement dissatisfaction	7	
		75
		329

Adapted from Golden RR, Teresi JA, Gurland BJ. Development of indicator scales for the Comprehensive Assessment and Referral Evaluation (CARE) interview schedule. J Gerontol 1984;39:141–145,Tables 1, 2.

Exhibit 8.10 An Example of an Indicator Scale from the CORE-CARE

Cognitive impairment
1. Doesn't know his age
2. Doesn't know the year of his birth
3. Doesn't know the number of years in neighborhood
4. Doesn't know his address
5. Doesn't know the rater's name, first try
6. Can't recall the President's name, current or previous
7. Doesn't know the month
8. Doesn't know the year
9. Doesn't know the rater's name, second try
10. Failed knee-hand-ear test

Adapted from Golden RR, Teresi JA, Gurland BJ. Development of indicator scales for the Comprehensive Assessment and Referral Evaluation (CARE) interview schedule. J Gerontol 1984;39:141–144,Table 1.

of the CORE-CARE scales: depression/demoralization, dementia, memory problems, sleep, somatic symptoms and activity limitation. The interview is in two parts. The first, taking about 30 minutes to complete, contains 143 items; the second part contains additional items on depression and dementia that are used to identify the need for clinical intervention (5).

Reliability

Alpha internal consistency scores for the 22 CORE-CARE indicator scales were high, ranging from 0.72 for retirement dissatisfaction to 0.95 for activity limitation (3, Tables 1–5; 1, Table 2). Intercorrelations among the indicator scales were reported by Golden (4).

The agreement between two raters for 30 interviews on the CORE-CARE gave kappas ranging from 0.70 to 0.80 (4, p145). For the original CARE instrument, the intraclass correlation was used to measure agreement among four raters in applying the scale to videotaped interviews with eight older women subjects. Agreement was close for the psychiatric dimensions with correlations between 0.82 and 0.97 (1, Table 3). Agreement was lower for the medical and physical dimensions, and ranged widely, reflecting the specialty of the rater (1). Correlations ranged from 0.01 to 0.83. Agreement for the social dimensions was intermediate, with correlations ranging from 0.48 to 0.92 (1, Table 3).

Inter-rater reliability for the SHORT-CARE was 0.76 for dementia, 0.94 for depression, and 0.91 for disability (5, p167). Coefficient alphas for the same scales, calculated on a population sample of 283 elderly people, were 0.64, 0.75 and 0.84.

Validity

Validity of the SHORT-CARE was reported by Gurland et al. (5). The convergent validity was 0.33 for the depression scale, 0.51 for cognitive impairment and 0.70 for disability (3, Table 5). For 26 respondents, classified as psychiatric cases or normal by psychiatrists, the sensitivity of the combined SHORT-CARE psychiatric scales was 100%, the specificity 71%. Predictive validity results were impressive, in that the "diagnosed pervasive dementias had one year outcomes consistent with that expected of dementia (e.g., death, institutional admission, deterioration) in all cases . . ." (5, p167). Those diagnosed as demented at initial interview had a mortality of 27% compared with 6% for an age-matched sample drawn from the remaining interviewees. Those who were diagnosed as depressed at initial interview had a higher use of psychotropic medication than others.

The extensive validity results for the complete CARE instrument are presented under three headings: construct, criterion and predictive validity.

Construct Validity. Teresi et al. reported the construct validity of the CARE, using multitrait-multimethod matrices and path analyses. They provided extensive details of the correlations between the CARE scales and data provided by family informants and from global diagnostic ratings (3). The results provided strong evidence for the validity of the measures of functional capacity (correlations ranging from 0.51 to 0.70). The validity coefficients for the medical scales ranged from 0.47 to 0.59. Validity of the service utilization scale was somewhat lower, although adequate, with correlations falling between 0.40 and 0.75. The correlations for service needs were lower, ranging from 0.29 to 0.54 (3, p150). Correlations between CARE scales and the judgments made by other informants were highest for the scales that assess behavior or are more objective (activity limitation, medical conditions, service use), with correlations falling in the range 0.47 to 0.70 (3, Table 5). Agreement over the more subjective ratings (depression, service needs) ranged from 0.30 to 0.60.

Criterion Validity. The CARE depression and cognitive impairment scales were compared with clinicians' ratings of 26 cases, 16 of whom had some form of psychiatric impairment. Kappa coefficients were 0.76 and 0.78 for the two CARE scales, giving sensitivity results of 93% and 67% (3, p154). The CARE was compared with two criterion scales that assessed family inconvenience and the extent to which the family had made plans to institutionalize the elderly relative. Sensitivity and specificity analyses yielded overall correct classification rates for the CARE activity limitation scale ranging from 60% to 89% (6, Tables 1, 2). Equivalent figures for the cognitive impairment scale ranged from 0.44 to 0.85, according to the cutting point used (6, Table 3).

Predictive Validity. The predictive ability of 21 of the indicator scales to identify people who subsequently died was examined; discrimination was significant for seven scales ($p < 0.01$), with odds ratios as high as 3.1 (6, Table 5). Logistic regression was used to test the ability of several CARE scales to predict death, a diagnosis of dementia or depression, activity restriction and service utilization. The results, presented in terms of odds ratios attaching to each indicator scale, suggest that the likelihood of the outcomes, given a high score on the CARE, are as much as five to ten times greater than for those with low scores.

Alternative Forms

Other abbreviated forms of the CARE include: MERGE-CARE, IN-CARE, and GLOBAL-CARE (2).

Commentary

Gurland et al. have shown that the validity of the SHORT-CARE is such that it can be used by psychiatrists or non-psychiatrists to provide reliable diagnoses of depression and dementia. It appears to represent a useful screening tool. The CARE scales are in the process of being further developed and refined at the time of writing.

The validity testing of the CARE is extensive, and the available results are impressive. Later versions do not require the detailed training of interviewers needed for earlier versions, and Gurland and his colleagues report that the

CARE has been used in other settings with reliable results. This broad-ranging assessment shows great potential in evaluating elderly people living in the community. The purpose of the CARE instruments is similar to that of the MAI and MFAQ scales also reviewed in this chapter. All give comprehensive assessments for elderly people living in the community. Of the three, the MAI is perhaps the least fully tested. The other two scales show similar levels of reliability and validity; the MFAQ has the advantage of an extensive user's manual and documentation, while the CARE has the advantage of being available in several shortened versions.

Address

Barry J. Gurland, MRCP (London), FRC Psych, Columbia University Center for Geriatrics, 100 Haven Avenue, Tower 3-29F, New York, New York, USA 10032

References

(1) Gurland B, Kuriansky J, Sharpe L, Simon R, Stiller P, Birkett P. The Comprehensive Assessment and Referral Evaluation (CARE)—rationale, development and reliability. Int J Aging Hum Dev 1977;8:9–42.

(2) Gurland BJ, Wilder DE. The CARE interview revisited: development of an efficient, systematic clinical assessment. J Gerontol 1984;39:129–137.

(3) Teresi JA, Golden RR, Gurland BJ, Wilder DE, Bennett RG. Construct validity of indicator-scales developed from the Comprehensive Assessment and Referral Evaluation interview schedule. J Gerontol 1984;39:147–157.

(4) Golden RR, Teresi JA, Gurland BJ. Development of indicator scales for the Comprehensive Assessment and Referral Evaluation (CARE) interview schedule. J Gerontol 1984;39:138–146.

(5) Gurland B, Golden RR, Teresi JA, Challop J. The SHORT-CARE: an efficient instrument for the assessment of depression, dementia and disability. J Gerontol 1984;39:166–169.

(6) Teresi JA, Golden RR, Gurland BJ. Concurrent and predictive validity of indicator scales developed for the Comprehensive Assessment and Referral Evaluation interview schedule. J Gerontol 1984;39:158–165.

THE QUALITY OF WELL-BEING SCALE (Formerly the Index of Well-Being) (J.W. Bush, J.P. Anderson, R.M. Kaplan and Others, 1973, Revised 1976)

Purpose

The Quality of Well-Being Scale (QWB) is an indicator of disability and of need for care that can be applied to individuals and to populations and can be used with any type of disease. The QWB summarizes current well-being in a single number that represents an assessment of the social undesirability of the patient's problem; this value can be adjusted to indicate the likely prognoses of any medical condition that is present. This enables the QWB to be used in indicating the present and future need for health services (1, 2).

Conceptual Basis

In order to compare the success of different therapies for different types of disease, the QWB scale was developed as one component of an approach to quantifying health status. It was developed initially to operationalize "wellness" for a General Health Policy Model, a long-term effort to develop an alternative to economic cost-benefit analysis for resource allocation in the health field. To provide a complete evaluation of a health care program, it is necessary to have an index that combines mortality with estimates of the quality of life among survivors. The QWB does this. The scale

> quantifies the health output of any treatment in terms of the years of life, adjusted for their diminished quality, that it produces or saves. Thus, a "Well-Year" can be defined conceptually as the equivalent of a year of completely well life, . . . A disease that reduces the health-related quality of life by one-half, for example, will take away .500 Well-Years over the course of one year. If it affects two people, it will take away 1.0 Well-Year (= 2 × .500). . . . Dividing the cost of a program by the number of Well-Years gives its relative efficiency or "cost-effectiveness." (3, p64).

The QWB scale is based on a three-component model of health. First, the assessment of health begins with an objective appraisal of current functional status, based on the individual's performance, classifying this into one of

> the universe of all possible situations between optimum function and death . . . From an extensive specialty-by-specialty review of medical reference works, we listed all the ways, however minor, that diseases and injuries can affect a person's behavior and role performance, regardless of etiology. (4, p485).

Second, a value reflecting relative desirability or utility is associated with each functional level (1, 5). The QWB includes death, thus making possible a ratio rather than an interval scale. This avoids the problem inherent in other indices that, where death is ignored, the death of a disabled patient will appear to improve the population estimate of health status (4). Third, health implies a consideration not only of present state, but also of future changes (prognoses). This would permit a distinction to be drawn between two people with equal present functional ability, but one of whom has a fatal disease: information crucial in assessing future need for health care.

Description

The QWB was originally called the Health Status Index (1); the title was subsequently changed to the Index of Well-Being (4) and then to Quality of Well-Being to indicate its emphasis on the quality of life or "Well-Life Expectancy" (3). An unweighted version used by Reynolds, Rushing and Miles is called the Function Status Index (6).

The procedure for classifying an individual may be described in three stages, corresponding to the three components of the concept of health noted above.

Assessing Functional Status. A structured interview is used to classify the respondent's function level and to record any symptoms or medical problems experienced during the previous eight days. The data on symptoms are used in a later stage of the rating procedure (see below). The questions are phrased in terms of performance and not capacity; self-reports are used rather than observation. Four aspects of function are considered: mobility or confinement (e.g., does the individual leave the house, is he confined to a hospital or institution?); physical activity, especially ambulation or confinement to bed; social activity (e.g., work, housekeeping) and self-care. The categories on each scale are mutually exclusive and exhaustive and range from full independence to death (7). Apart from death (which is scored as zero), the physical ability scale has four categories and the others have five, as we show in Exhibit 8.11, which summarizes the information contained in Exhibit 8.12.

Questions in the interview schedule were drawn mainly from the Health Interview Survey and from the Social Security Administration Survey of the disabled but have been extensively revised. Copies of the questionnaire, which is too long to reproduce here, and the 30-page interviewer manual can be ordered at cost from Dr. Kaplan. The questionnaire is structured so that general screening questions lead to more extensive investigations of problems raised. At least 18 questions are asked of all respondents. The questionnaire requires 10 to 15 minutes to administer (8).

Of 101 possible combinations* of function levels, not all are observed to occur. The authors have identified 43 function levels (originally 31), that are logically possible and that have been observed empirically (4, 7). Descriptions of the 43 levels are shown in Exhibit 8.12. As an example, someone in a wheel-

Exhibit 8.11 Dimensions and Function Levels of the Quality of Well-Being Scale

Function level	Mobility	Physical activity	Social activity
1.	In special care unit	In bed or chair	Had help with self-care
2.	In hospital	Moved own wheelchair without help	Performed self-care but not work, school or housework
3.	In house	Walked with physical limitations	Limited in amount or kind of work, school, or housework
4.	Did not drive, or had help to use bus or train	Walked without physical limitations	Did work, school, or housework, but other activities were limited
5.	Drove car and used bus or train without help		Did work, school, or housework and other activities

*Calculated as death (code 0 on each scale) plus 5 × 4 × 5 other steps on the three scales.

Exhibit 8.12 The Quality of Well-Being Scale, Showing the Combinations of Mobility, Physical Activity and Social Activity Items and Associated Social Preference Weights

Function level number (i)	Mobility	Physical activity	Social activity	Level of well-being (W_j)
		Scale		
		NO SYMPTOM/PROBLEM COMPLEX		
L 43	Drove car and used bus or train without help (5)	Walked without physical problems (4)	Did work, school, or housework, and other activities (5)	1.000
		SYMPTOM/PROBLEM COMPLEX PRESENT		
L 42	Drove car and used bus or train without help (5)	Walked without physical problems (4)	Did work, school, or housework, and other activities (5)	0.7433
L 41	Drove car and used bus or train without help (5)	Walked without physical problems (4)	Did work, school, or housework, but other activities limited (4)	0.6855
L 40	Drove car and used bus or train without help (5)	Walked without physical problems (4)	Limited in amount or kind of work, school, or housework (3)	0.6683
L 39	Drove car and used bus or train without help (5)	Walked without physical problems (4)	Performed self-care, but not work, school, or housework (2)	0.6955
L 38	Drove car and used bus or train without help (5)	Walked without physical problems (4)	Had help with self-care activities (1)	0.6370
L 37	Drove car and used bus or train without help (5)	Walked with physical limitations (3)	Did work, school, or housework, and other activities (5)	0.6769
L 36	Drove car and used bus or train without help (5)	Walked with physical limitations (3)	Did work, school, or housework, but other activities limited (4)	0.6172
L 35	Drove car and used bus or train without help (5)	Walked with physical limitations (3)	Limited in amount or kind of work, school, or housework (3)	0.6020
L 34	Drove car and used bus or train without help (5)	Walked with physical limitations (3)	Performed self-care, but not work, school, or housework (2)	0.6292
L 33	Drove car and used bus or train without help (5)	Walked with physical limitations (3)	Had help with self-care activities (1)	0.5707
L 32	Did not drive, or had help to use bus or train (4)	Walked without physical problems (4)	Did work, school, or housework, but other activities limited (4)	0.6065

314

Function level number (i)	Scale			Level of well-being (W_j)
	Mobility	Physical activity	Social activity	
L 31	Did not drive, or had help to use bus or train (4)	Walked without physical problems (4)	Limited in amount or kind of work, school, or housework (3)	0.5913
L 30	Did not drive, or had help to use bus or train (4)	Walked without physical problems (4)	Performed self-care, but not work, school, or housework (2)	0.6185
L 29	Did not drive, or had help to use bus or train (4)	Walked without physical problems (4)	Had help with self-care activities (1)	0.5600
L 28	Did not drive, or had help to use bus or train (4)	Walked with physical limitations (3)	Did work, school, or housework, but other activities limited (4)	0.5402
L 27	Did not drive, or had help to use bus or train (4)	Walked with physical limitations (3)	Limited in amount or kind of work, school, or housework (3)	0.5250
L 26	Did not drive, or had help to use bus or train (4)	Walked with physical limitations (3)	Performed self-care, but not work, school, or housework (2)	0.5523
L 25	Did not drive, or had help to use bus or train (4)	Moved own wheelchair without help (2)	Limited in amount or kind of work, school, or housework (3)	0.5376
L 24	Did not drive, or had help to use bus or train (4)	Moved own wheelchair without help (2)	Performed self-care, but not work, school, or housework (2)	0.5649
L 23	In house (3)	Walked without physical problems (4)	Performed self-care, but not work, school, or housework (2)	0.6488
L 22	In house (3)	Walked without physical problems (4)	Had help with self-care activities (1)	0.5902
L 21	In house (3)	Walked with physical limitations (3)	Did work, school, or housework, but other activities limited (4)	0.5704
L 20	In house (3)	Walked with physical limitations (3)	Limited in amount or kind of work, school, or housework (3)	0.5552
L 19	In house (3)	Walked with physical limitations (3)	Performed self-care, but not work, school, or housework (2)	0.5824
L 18	In house (3)	Walked with physical limitations (3)	Had help with self-care activities (1)	0.5239
L 17	In house (3)	Moved own wheelchair without help (2)	Performed self-care, but not work, school, or housework (2)	0.5950

Table 9.12 (continued)

Function level number (i)	Mobility	Scale Physical activity	Social activity	Level of well-being (W_j)
L 16	In house (3)	Moved own wheelchair without help (2)	Had help with self-care activities (1)	0.5364
L 15	In house (3)	In bed or chair (1)	Performed self-care, but not work, school, or housework (2)	0.5715
L 14	In house (3)	In bed or chair (1)	Had help with self-care activities (1)	0.5129
L 13	In hospital (2)	Walked without physical problems (4)	Performed self-care, but not work, school, or housework (2)	0.6057
L 12	In hospital (2)	Walked without physical problems (4)	Had help with self-care activities (1)	0.5471
L 11	In hospital (2)	Walked with physical limitations (3)	Performed self-care, but not work, school, or housework (2)	0.5394
L 10	In hospital (2)	Walked with physical limitations (3)	Had help with self-care activities (1)	0.4808
L 9	In hospital (2)	Moved own wheelchair without help (2)	Performed self-care, but not work, school, or housework (2)	0.5520
L 8	In hospital (2)	Moved own wheelchair without help (2)	Had help with self-care activities (1)	0.4934
L 7	In hospital (2)	In bed or chair (1)	Performed self-care, but not work, school, or housework (2)	0.5284
L 6	In hospital (2)	In bed or chair (1)	Had help with self-care activities (1)	0.4699
L 5	In special care unit (1)	Walked without physical problems (4)	Performed self-care, but not work, school, or housework (2)	0.5732
L 4	In special care unit (1)	Walked without physical problems (4)	Had help with self-care activities (1)	0.5147
L 3	In special care unit (1)	Walked with physical limitations (3)	Performed self-care, but not work, school, or housework (2)	0.5070
L 2	In special care unit (1)	Walked with physical limitations (3)	Had help with self-care activities (1)	0.4483
L 1	In special care unit (1)	In bed or chair (1)	Had help with self-care activities (1)	0.4374
L 0	Dead (0)	Dead (0)	Dead (0)	0.0000

Reproduced from Kaplan RM, Bush JW, Berry CC. Health status: types of validity and the Index of Well-Being. Health Serv Res 1976;11:486–488.Table 1. With permission.

chair who remains indoors, and who can care for himself but not work would be coded 3, 2, 2.

Scaling the Responses. For each of the 43 function levels a "preference weight" has been established empirically, ranging from 1 (complete well-being) to 0 (death). The appropriate preference weight is assigned to the respondent's function level, and the resulting score is known as the Quality of Well-Being score, or W (see Exhibit 8.12). Thus, in the example of the individual rated 3, 2, 2, the corresponding function level is L17 and W is 0.595. Although death was scored as the lowest state in the QWB, the authors noted that it is possible to provide a score below zero to represent a state "worse than death," such as a prolonged vegetative existence (3).

The weights reflect social preferences or judgments of the relative importance that members of society associate with each function level (4, 9). The preference weights do not take into consideration the patient's diagnosis. Bush emphasized that preference ratings should be collected empirically rather than be based on the assumptions or clinical experience of the researchers as the two types of estimate have been shown to vary (10). The weights were derived from an equal-appearing interval scaling task using a population sample in which 867 subjects rated approximately 500 items (4). Kaplan, Bush and Berry compared different approaches to deriving such weights, and concluded that category weighting was more appropriate than magnitude estimation (9). Further validation of the scaling procedure has been reported by Kaplan and Ernst (11). To express the well-being of a population, a simple formula is used to calculate the average W (4, p493).

Indicating Prognosis. To reflect the concept of health status as a combination of present state and prognosis, the third stage of rating a respondent involves adjusting W to reflect prognoses for any condition(s) the individual may have. This gives the "Well-Life Expectancy" *(E)* and the relevant equation is given by Kaplan (4, p484). Prognoses are expressed in terms of the probabilities of future transitions to other levels of function and well-being (worse or better) after a fixed lapse of time (1, 9). Estimates of transition probabilities may be obtained from empirical studies of patient's progress. Currently, Kaplan et al. do not propose to estimate transition probabilities for every disease; probabilities are available for the likelihood of developing mental retardation following various forms of phenylketonuria (12).

The indices W and E may be further refined by adjusting for the presence or absence of 36 symptoms or problems that "might limit function" (3) in which case the indices are designated W^* and E^* (9, p506). This involves adding a weight ranging from -0.0027 to 0.2567, with lower values representing more undesirable problems (4). When a respondent has multiple problems the one considered "most undesirable" is taken as dominant (9). The methods used to obtain the weights were described by Patrick et al. (7, 13) and by Bush et al. (9, 14). By recording symptoms, even where these are not sufficient to cause a restriction in activity levels, the index is held to be sensitive to minor deviations from complete well-being.

The 36 symptoms and problems are said to cover the "full array of the symptoms and problems, except those of mental health, that occur in people's daily lives" (4). The authors note that if the definition and measurement of physical health is successful, applications to mental and social conditions will be possible (7).

Reliability

Considerable attention has been paid to the reliability of estimating preference weights. The reliability coefficient obtained when judges reassessed scale values for 29 function levels was 0.90 (3, 13). The preference weights obtained from different judges at different times showed systematic but small variations (8).

Kaplan and Bush noted that in applying the instrument in assessing over 50,000 person days, the classification accuracy exceeded 96% (3, p70). Test-retest reliability of the W statistic was studied by correlating the rating of the first day with the mean of those made on eight subsequent days. Correlations in excess of 0.93 were obtained (8).

Validity

Arguments for the content validity of the index are given by Kaplan et al. (4) and by Reynolds et al. (6). The QWB is the only instrument that considers mortality, symptoms, and problems as well as functional levels—all of which are central components of the concept of health.

Kaplan et al. reported correlations of -0.75 between the score of the QWB scale and the number of reported symptoms and of -0.96 between the score and the number of chronic health problems (4, pp498, 497). The correlation with the number of physician contacts in the preceding eight days was -0.55.

Alternative Forms

Reynolds, Rushing and Miles have suggested a simplified scoring procedure for their version of the index called the Function Status Index (FSI) (6). They also recorded behavior on the previous day rather than the previous eight days, and separated the social activity scale and self-care scales (6). From a sample of 8,036 respondents in Alabama, a correlation of -0.61 was obtained between the FSI and the number of chronic health problems reported (6, Table 2). A gamma coefficient of -0.53 was obtained with the number of physician contacts (6, Table 3). Reynolds et al. also reported a correlation of -0.48 with a health worry scale (6, pp279, 281). Harkey et al. applied the FSI in a study (N = 16,569) of the relationship between social class and functional status (15).

Commentary

The QWB seems a suitable health index with which to close our book. It has been influential in the design of other scales, such as the Arthritis Impact Measurement Scale and the Rand Functional Limitations Battery. The QWB also represents a bridge between the subjective indices that predominate in the field of sociomedical measurement and purely mathematical population indices such as that of Chiang (16). It is one of the most complex instruments we have reviewed (similar, perhaps, to some of the pain measurements) and represents a radical and innovative approach to the whole field. No other scale has confronted the issues of placing health, disability and death on a single scale and, although it is possible to criticize such an attempt, it is a theme widely considered as important by those working in health planning. The thoroughness of the conceptual formulation of the method is impressive, especially in that it incorporates an estimate of prognosis. Obviously, the practical task of deriving the required transition probabilities for all diseases would be daunting (17) but it is possible to use follow-up studies to estimate these for particular conditions.

The QWB has, of course, been criticized. Apparent inconsistencies were noted in the weights for a few of the 43 health states where a more disabled state is preferred to a less disabled one (18). Bush et al. responded to this criticism, reporting extensive justifications for their scaling procedures, and pointing out that desirability may differ for acute and chronic conditions. For acute conditions, for example, " . . . being in a wheelchair is sometimes more comfortable (and therefore more desirable) than struggling to walk with limitations (e.g., with crutches) . . ." (10). The prognostic dimension permits the QWB to be applied equally to acute and chronic states, whereas other scales (such as the OECD instrument) have kept acute and chronic causes of functional limitation separate because of their different implications for the need for care.

The index has been used in evaluating screening programs for phenylketonuria (12), thyroid conditions and hypertension (19) as well as programs for tuberculin testing (1, 5), estrogen therapy (20) and pneumonia (21). Kaplan and Bush summarized these studies in a table that compares the cost-effectiveness of each screening program per well-year gained (3). However, it seems doubtful that the QWB will ever see routine use as an evaluative tool. Many of the other scales in this book are more practical and have the virtue of being widely used. The importance of the QWB lies in its conceptual approach and in its very existence: it serves to illustrate a wholly different approach that could be made to the process of measuring health status and planning care.

Address

R.M. Kaplan, PhD, Professor, Department of Psychology, San Diego State University, San Diego, California, USA 92182

References

(1) Fanshel S, Bush JW. A Health-Status Index and its application to health-services outcomes. Operations Res 1970;18:1021–1065.

(2) Chen MM, Bush JW, Patrick DL. Social indicators for health planning and policy analysis. Policy Sci 1975;6:71–89.

(3) Kaplan RM, Bush JW. Health-related quality of life measurement for evaluation research and policy analysis. Health Psychol 1982;1:61–80.

(4) Kaplan RM, Bush JW, Berry CC. Health status: types of validity and the Index of Well-Being. Health Serv Res 1976;11:478–507.

(5) Bush JW, Fanshel S, Chen MM. Analysis of a tuberculin testing program using a Health Status Index. Socio-Econ Plan Sci 1972;6:49–68.

(6) Reynolds WJ, Rushing WA, Miles DL. The validation of a Function Status Index. J Health Soc Behav 1974;15:271–288.

(7) Patrick DL, Bush JW, Chen MM. Toward an operational definition of health. J Health Soc Behav 1973;14:6–23.

(8) Kaplan RM, Bush JW, Berry CC. The reliability, stability, and generalizability of a Health Status Index. American Statistical Association, Proceedings of the Social Statistics Section, 1978:704–709.

(9) Kaplan RM, Bush JW, Berry CC. Health Status Index: category rating versus magnitude estimation for measuring levels of well-being. Med Care 1979;17:501–523.

(10) Bush JW, Anderson JP, Kaplan RM, Blischke WR. "Counterintuitive" preferences in health-related quality-of-life measurement. Med Care 1982;20:516–525.

(11) Kaplan RM, Ernst JA. Do category rating scales produce biased preference weights for a health index? Med Care 1983;21:193–207.

(12) Bush JW, Chen MM, Patrick DL. Health Status Index in cost effectiveness: analysis of PKU program. In: Berg RL, ed. Health status indexes. Chicago: Hospital Research and Educational Trust, 1973:172–209.

(13) Patrick DL, Bush JW, Chen MM. Methods for measuring levels of well-being for a Health Status Index. Health Serv Res 1973;8:228–245.

(14) Blischke WR, Bush JW, Kaplan RM. Successive intervals analysis of preference measures in a Health Status Index. Health Serv Res 1975;10:181–198.

(15) Harkey J, Miles DL, Rushing WA. The relation between social class and functional status: a new look at the drift hypothesis. J Health Soc Behav 1976;17:194–204.

(16) Chiang CL. An index of health: mathematical models. Washington, DC: National Center for Health Statistics, 1965. (Vital Health Statistics Series 2).

(17) Chen MM, Bush JW, Zaremba J. Effectiveness measures. In: Shuman L, Speas R, Young J, eds. Operations research in health care—a critical analysis. Baltimore: Johns Hopkins University Press, 1975:276–301.

(18) Anderson GM. A comment on the Index of Well-Being. Med Care 1982;20:513–515.

(19) Weinstein MC, Stason WB. Foundations of cost-effectiveness analysis for health and medical practices. N Engl J Med 1977;296:716–721.

(20) Weinstein MC. Estrogen use in post-menopausal women—costs, risks & benefits. N Engl J Med 1980;303:308–316.

(21) Willems JS, Sanders CR, Riddiough MA, Bell JC. Cost-effectiveness of vaccination against pneumococcal pneumonia. N Engl J Med 1980;303:553–559.

CONCLUSION

This chapter reviews some of the most recently developed measurement methods that are in many ways the showpiece of current health measurement technology. Few of the methods we have described here suffer from the criticisms that were raised of the other instruments reviewed in the book: lack of conceptual formulation, poor reliability and validity, and a tendency toward the development of alternative versions that are not strictly comparable. They also represent the major research instruments, as opposed to strictly clinical scales, that are now being used in evaluative studies to measure physical well-being: frequently one of these techniques is selected in preference to those reviewed in Chapter 3. We should stress, of course, that we have had to be selective and have excluded several instruments that could be relevant to certain users. An example is the ESCROW profile, used with the Barthel and PULSES scales as part of an assessment of needs for care—a field close to that of the Functional Assessment Inventory of Crewe and Athelstan. The ESCROW profile covers the social and economic resources available to a person that will affect his ability to live independently in the community. Despite its relevance, we did not include the scale because of the apparently low levels of validity and reliability obtained in the early trials of the method.

Looking to the future, we would like to see fuller testing of sections taken from these instruments as alternatives to some of the established, but apparently inferior, scales that were reviewed in Chapter 3. For example, can the ADL and IADL scales from the MFAQ be used independently as separate instruments? It is desirable that the gap between the research instruments described here and the scales familiar to clinicians be bridged to improve the quality of routine clinical assessments. This was an emphasis in the development of the Nottingham profile, that sought to emulate the psychometric qualities of the research instruments, but was designed to be brief and simple enough to be applied in routine clinical settings.

9

Recommendations and Conclusions

THE CURRENT STATUS OF HEALTH MEASUREMENT

The experience of preparing a broad-ranging review such as this book has been valuable in revealing several facts about the current status of health measurements. It has also fostered in us certain attitudes concerning how we would like to see the field develop in the future. Accordingly, in concluding we wish to draw together some of the themes introduced previously.

The reader will have been struck by the considerable variation in the quality and sophistication of the health measurements presented. This may reflect the relative newness of the field: the development of health indices is a recent endeavor compared with measuring intelligence or public opinion. Certainly, health measurement has benefited from the theoretical and technical advances in test construction already achieved in the social sciences, but the application of this knowledge to health measurements has been uneven. Pain scales seem to have been most successful in exploiting the more sophisticated scaling techniques, while measurements of psychological well-being have devoted the greatest attention to validity testing. Meanwhile, the field of functional disability shows a different picture: the profusion of measurement scales is rivaled only by their lack of technical sophistication. The doubtful quality of many of these scales appears to have fostered the reaction of developing yet more scales, whose superiority is more often assumed then demonstrated. We should now pay closer attention to refining and testing existing instruments than to developing new methods, and when a new method is clearly required its design should be based on a careful analysis of the strengths and weaknesses of previous scales. Each new scale should then be exhaustively compared with existing methods—an activity all too rarely undertaken in the field of functional disability measurements. We hope (perhaps credulously) that the contrast between the quality of the different types of measurement reviewed here will encourage those who develop physical rating scales to carry out more thorough validation studies in future.

On the theme of building on prior experience, we have repeatedly mentioned the desirability of a conceptual definition of the topic being measured. This is intended to stress the role of measurement in scientific discovery: as science ultimately tests theories we must know what theoretical orientation each health index represents. This goal has been quite well achieved in the fields of pain measurement and emotional well-being, and to a certain extent in quality of life measures. Many of the measurements of functional disability, however, pay little more than lip service to the idea of a conceptual approach to the topic: the WHO definition may be mentioned, or passing reference may be made to the distinction between disability and handicap. Although a useful start, this could be refined to indicate more closely what questions should be included and why.

While we may complain about the weakness and lack of coordinated development work in certain areas of health measurement, we must also acknowledge that the universal, perfect index will never exist and that it is impossible to select one set of questions applicable to all diseases and all individuals. Nevertheless, the approach followed in developing health indices can be universally applicable. It should also be noted that our measurement problems are not unique, and we are reminded of the lack of agreement over how to measure far simpler topics such as occupational status or smoking behavior. Given some successes and some areas of weakness, what should be done to strengthen this field?

GUIDELINES FOR DEVELOPING HEALTH MEASUREMENTS

Many of the following comments may be seen as preliminary steps towards fostering a science of health measurement, equivalent to psychometrics or econometrics. Important decisions affecting the welfare of patients or the expenditure of public funds are based on the results of health measurements, so we argue in the strongest terms for a responsible attitude towards ensuring the quality of these measurements. An ethic of quality control in the development of health measurement methods is often lacking. Although various recommendations have been made on how to develop, test and present a health measurement (1–5), these have not yet been assembled in a central or authoritative source equivalent to the American Psychological Association's handbook (1). We believe it is in the interests of this field to formulate guidelines on the development and presentation of health measurement techniques. Formalized guidelines could, perhaps, be published under the aegis of a body such as the International Epidemiological Association.

Guidelines must tackle two common shortcomings in health indices: inadequate development and testing of the instrument itself, and a lack of clarity in the published descriptions of it. It is always hard to describe a measurement in sufficient detail within the constraints of a standard journal article, a problem that emphasizes the desirability of producing a manual describing the method and its administration. If a measurement has been adequately tested, it is certainly worth the additional effort of preparing a manual to describe it fully. This has been done for several of the indices we describe in this book, although most manuals exhibit significant weaknesses. Several pertinent suggestions on preparing manuals are included in the APA Standards (1), which guided the following comments.

1. Published articles or a manual should provide a full description of the purpose of the method, specifying the population for which it is designed, the populations on which it has been tested, and the intended use for the data collected. The method must be made readily available to the user, perhaps by having it formally printed and distributing it at cost; a copy should be included in the manual. The otherwise excellent manual for the General Health Questionnaire can be faulted for its omission of a copy of the scale itself (curious, since it had already been published in previous reports). Each method should be given a name that accurately describes its content; some published ADL scales have not been named, making it difficult for subsequent users to explain which scale they have used. The description of the method should also outline pitfalls in its administration and interpretation, and should show how high and low scores are to be interpreted (see the "Commentary" on the Health Opinion Survey in Chapter 4).

2. A rationale should be given for the design of the instrument; what conceptual definition of the topic of measurement does it reflect? As an example, the presentation of an anxiety measurement should discuss alternative theoretical approaches to the concept, and the approach taken by the measurement should be clearly specified. Specification in this detail has been achieved for relatively few of the indices that we review; the scales of Bradburn, of Bush and of Melzack provide examples of adequate conceptual formulations.

3. The way in which questions were selected should be indicated: where did they come from and how were they sampled? The manual should describe the general development of the instrument; good illustrations of this are contained in descriptions of the General Health Questionnaire and of the Sickness Impact Profile.

4. Revisions to the method should be clearly explained and data on the reliability and validity of the latest version should be presented. It is unfortunate that academic pressure to publish encourages the presentation of preliminary versions; this runs the danger that users become confused and continue to use outdated versions of a measurement. The worst case of this was seen in the Health Opinion Survey, in which many validation studies have been wasted as they do not test comparable versions of the method; the Life Satisfaction Index has also suffered in this way. Many users have a tendency to abbreviate and alter the published measurement and the tactic used by Goldberg, when he recommended various abbreviations to the General Health Questionnaire, appears to be successful in forestalling this problem. Correlations between the alternative versions should be given.

5. Instructions must be clear enough to ensure standard administration and scoring of the method. Even for self-administered questionnaires there is a need to indicate the precise instructions given to the respondent. The answer scale must be shown, and the setting in which the method was administered during the validation studies described. A good example of attention to detail of this type is given in the Structured and Scaled Interview to Assess Maladjustment described in Chapter 5. Details on scoring are at times unclear in

published reports; how, for example, should missing data be handled? How should change scores be calculated—as absolute changes or as a percentage of the initial score? When there are alternative scoring methods, the advantages of each need to be given and their intercorrelation should be stated; Melzack has done this for his pain scale. Wherever possible, reference scores from large population studies should be provided to indicate percentile values against which a given score may be compared. Various measurements have been applied in major population studies that would permit the derivation of reference standards, although these have frequently not been published. Dupuy's General Well-Being Schedule, for example, was used in national surveys and reference standards by age and sex would be simple to produce and would provide a useful addition to our knowledge about how to interpret results obtained using the measurement. Secondary analyses of this type might provide material for student theses.

6. The validity and reliability testing should examine both the internal structure of the method (its internal consistency and factor structure) and also its relation to alternative measurements of the same concept. In criterion validation, the rationale for the selection of the criterion scores must be given, and attention paid to *their* validity. Validation studies should specify the level of correlation to be considered as adequate: all too often authors present a list of coefficients that may range anywhere from 0.15 to 0.45 and then conclude that the results demonstrate the construct validity of the method, an approach that seems to preclude refutation of validity. More formal approaches that help to avoid capricious interpretation of construct validity results include the multi-trait-multimethod matrix approach. At the very least, a formal declaration should be made of the levels of validity coefficients that are being taken as indicative of validity. In general, remarkably little information is yet available on the comparison between rival measurement methods in the health field: few studies have tested concurrent validity. The use of statistical techniques in the validation studies should be appropriate and sample sizes should be adequate. This is especially true of factor analytic studies—the majority we reviewed were applied incorrectly, due either to small sample sizes or to the use of inappropriate response scales.

7. Ideally, each measurement method should be tested by users other than the original authors, indicating that it holds a wide appeal and that it can be used successfully by others to provide consistent results.

FINAL REMARKS

We repeat our awareness that these guidelines are exacting and represent an ideal that few scales have achieved. And yet the difficulty of the task should not encourage us to condone inferior work. Why should health be measured any less accurately than other fields such as educational attainment?

There are several possible avenues for the development of the area of health measurement. First, many methodological advances simply have not been applied here, making health indices less good than they could potentially be.

Our tabular summaries of the strengths and weaknesses of existing measurements before the reviews are intended to give an initial stimulus to further work in consolidating the field, and the guidelines above suggest how this may be done. Second, we require more formal channels of recognition of the field: the development of a journal of health measurement analogous to *Psychometrika* would help to avoid the continuing diversity of sources for publishing such articles. Methodological conferences on health indices are becoming more common, and university courses in measurement and evaluation indicate the depth of interest. A recognized body such as the Society for Epidemiological Research could be asked to take on a coordinating role in formalizing guidelines, making recommendations on choices among rival methods, and possibly developing a journal.

As authors we may look forward to the time when a new edition of this book is required, for this would imply an advance in the field and the establishment of new methods that are superior to many of the ones we have included. At such a time we would also attempt to expand the work to include some of the other topics such as patient satisfaction scales and measurements of sensory problems that were originally planned, but for which space in this book proved insufficient.

References

(1) American Psychological Association. Standards for educational and psychological tests. Washington, DC: American Psychological Association, 1974.
(2) Sullivan DF. Disability components for an index of health. Washington, DC: U.S. Department of Health, Education, and Welfare, National Center for Health Statistics, 1971. (Data Evaluation and Methods Research Series 2, No. 42. Public Health Service Publication No. 1000).
(3) Moriyama IM. Problems in the measurement of health status. In: Sheldon EB, Moore W, eds. Indicators of social change: concepts and measurements. New York: Russell Sage, 1968:573–599.
(4) Sackett DL, Chambers LW, MacPherson AS, Goldsmith CH, Mcauley RG. The development and application of indices of health: general methods and a summary of results. Am J Public Health 1977;67:423–427.
(5) Miller JE. Guidelines for selecting a health status index: suggested criteria. In: Berg RL, ed. Health Status Indexes. Chicago: Hospital Research and Education Trust, 1973:243–247.

Glossary of Technical Terms

Alpha Cronbach's alpha is a generalized formula for expressing the internal consistency reliability of a test.

Category Scaling See Scaling.

Coefficient of Concordance While a rank order correlation shows the agreement between two sets of rankings, Kendall's coefficient of concordance provides a measure of the relationship among several rankings of objects or individuals. It is the nonparametric equivalent of the intraclass correlation.

Correlation A measure of association that indicates the degree to which two or more sets of observations fit a linear relationship. There exist various formulae for estimating the strength of the correlation; in each case the range lies between -1 and $+1$. A correlation close to zero indicates no association between the observations; as correlations rise, it becomes more possible to predict the value of the second observation from a knowledge of the first. The formula most commonly encountered is Pearson's r, suited to data measured at the interval or ratio scale level. Kendall's tau and Spearman's rho correlations may be used to indicate the association between variables measured at the ordinal level, and are termed "rank order correlations."

Discriminant Analysis A multivariate statistical procedure that indicates how adequately a set of variables (here, typically, the replies to questions in a health index) differentiate between two or more groups of people who are known to differ on some characteristic (here, typically being sick or well). The analysis selects the set of questions that show the most marked contrast in pattern of replies between the groups, i.e., the most discriminative questions.

Equal-Appearing Interval Scales See Scaling.

Factor Analysis Factor (or principal component) analysis is a mathematical technique that permits the reduction of a large number of interrelated observations to a smaller number of common dimensions or factors. As an example, a factor analysis of questions asked to assess intelligence might indicate discrete groups of questions that assess verbal ability, numerical ability and visual-spatial judgments. The factors are composed of observations that intercorrelate; observations on one factor are distinct from those on other factors.

Goal Attainment Scaling An evaluation method that assesses the efficacy of a program in attaining predetermined goals.

Guttman Scaling See Scalogram Analysis.

Intraclass Correlation In testing the reliability of a measurement, correlation coefficients such as Pearson's r may be used to compare the ratings of a number of patients made by two raters. The intraclass correlation generalizes this procedure and expresses the agreement among more than two raters.

Internal Consistency See Reliability.

Inter-Rater Reliability The extent to which results obtained by different raters or interviewers using the same measurement method will agree. The agreement is calculated using a correlation coefficient, appropriately the intraclass correlation when several raters are involved.

Interval Scale See Scales of Measurement.

Item The term "item" is used to refer to individual questions or response phrases in any health measurement. It replaces the more obvious term "question" simply because not all response categories are actually phrased as questions: some use rating scales, others use agree/disagree statements.

Item-Total Correlation The correlation of each question in a health index with the total score is used as an indication of the internal consistency or homogeneity of the scale, suggesting how far each question contributes to the overall theme being measured.

Kappa As a coefficient of agreement between two raters, kappa expresses the level of agreement that is observed beyond the level that would be expected by chance alone. A typical formula is

$$K = (p_o - p_c)/(1 - p_c),$$

where p_o is the observed proportion of agreement, and p_c is the proportion of agreement expected by chance alone. Chance agreement occurs because the rating given by rater 1 happens to coincide with that given by rater 2. The p_c is assessed as follows:

$$p_c = p_1 p_2 + (1 - p_1)(1 - p_2),$$

where p_1 is the probability of rater 1 diagnosing a case, and p_2 is the equivalent probability for the second rater. Although in theory the range of kappa is from 0 to 1, in practice its upper value is limited by the sensitivity and specificity of the test (see Grave WM, et al. Arch Gen Psychiatry 1981;38:408–413).

Kendall's Tau See Correlation.

Likelihood Ratio This is an approach to summarizing the results of sensitivity and specificity analyses for various cutting points on diagnostic or screening tests. Each cutting point produces a value for the true positive ratio (i.e., sensitivity) and the false positive ratio (i.e., specificity). The ratio of true to false positives is the likelihood ratio for each cutting point. These values are plotted on a graph whose axes show true and false positive values; the curve that results is known as a receiver operating characteristic (ROC) curve. This way of presenting validity data may aid in selecting the optimal cutting point, as described by McNeil BJ, et al. N Engl J Med 1975;293:211–215. See also Sensitivity, Specificity.

Magnitude Estimation See Scaling.

Multitrait-Multimethod Matrix A format for presenting validity and reliability correlations in which the agreement among several measurement methods (multimethod) as applied to several traits (multitrait) is shown in a manner that simplifies the interpretation of construct validity. It is assumed, for example, that the correlations between different measurement methods will be higher when applied to the same topic of measurement than when applied to different topics. (A clear example of the approach and the underlying assumptions is given by Campbell DT, Fiske DW. Covergent and discriminant validation by the multitrait-multimethod matrix. Psychol Bull 1959;56:81–105).

Ordinal Scale See Scales of Measurement.

Path Analysis A procedure for testing causal hypotheses that indicates the extent to which a hypothesized causal pattern fits empirical data. Path analysis could, for example, be used in analyzing a set of data to calculate the relative strength of the causal influence exerted by smoking, obesity, sedentary living and cholesterol levels in predicting cardiovascular disease. The strength of the causal influence is indicated by path coefficients.

Pearson Correlation See Correlation.

Positive Predictive Value The proportion of all people who were identified by a measurement or screening test as apparently having the disease who actually do have it.

Predictive Validity The accuracy with which a measurement predicts some future event, such as mortality (see Chapter 2, page 28).

Rank Order Correlation See Correlation.

Reliability The proportion of variance in a measurement that is not error variance (see page 32). In practice, reliability refers to the stability of a measurement: how far it will give the same results on separate occasions. This is closely related to the internal consistency of the method: how far the questions it contains all measure the same theme.

Rho See Correlation.

Ridit Used in presenting the results of several health indices, a ridit is a way of expressing the observed score relative to an identified population (hence "ridit"). The average ridit calculated for the group of interest shows the probability that a member of that group is "worse off" than someone in the identified, reference population distribution. As an example, if the average ridit for a subgroup is .625, then 62.5% of the people in the reference population have a better score (e.g., are less sick) than the average individual in the subgroup.

Scalability Coefficient See Scalogram Analysis.

Scales of Measurement The mathematical qualities of numerical measurement scales vary and are of four main types.

1. Nominal scales. Numbers are assigned arbitrarily with no implication of an inherent order to their categories, as in telephone numbers. Such scales may only be used as classifications; no statistical analyses may be carried out that use the numerical characteristics of the scale.
2. Ordinal scales. Classification into a scale that implies a distinct order among the categories (such as house numbers on a street), but where there is no natural assumption concerning the relative distance between adjacent values. Statistical methods such as rank order correlations may be used.
3. Interval scales. Interval scales are so named because the distance between numbers in one region of the scale is assumed to be equal to the distance between numbers at another region of the scale (as in Fahrenheit or Celsius scales). Addi-

tion and subtraction are permissible, but not multiplication or division of such scales; statistical analyses such as the Pearson correlation, factor analysis or discriminant analysis may be used with interval scales.

4. Ratio scales. A ratio scale is an interval scale with a true zero point, so that ratios between values are meaningfully defined. Examples include weight, height, and income, as in each case it is meaningful to speak of one value being so many times greater or less than another value. All arithmetical operations, including multiplication and division, may be applied, and all types of statistical analysis may be used.

Scaling A set of procedures used to assign numerical weights to replies to health questions to reflect the severity of disability implied. Scaling methods are of two broad types—category scaling (such as Thurstone's "equal-appearing interval" procedure), which produces weights at an interval scale level, and magnitude estimation, which provides a ratio scale. An index that uses category scaling is the Sickness Impact Profile (Chapter 8); the Pain Perception Profile is an example of a scale using magnitude estimation (Chapter 7). By no means do all health indices use any form of scaling to derive numerical weights for response categories. Several scales described in this book have shown similar results with weighted and unweighted scoring systems (see the PAMIE scale, the Multilevel Assessment Instrument or the Health Opinion Survey).

Scalogram Analysis This method of analysis is used to select questions that lie in a hierarchical order such that agreeing to an item at one end of the scale implies a positive answer to all other items on the scale. For example, a scale of functional ability may ask about walking ability using items like "I can walk a block or more," "I can walk 100 yards," "I can walk outside my house," and "I can move around in my room." Statistical techniques developed by Guttman and others analyze the pattern of responses to such items and show how closely they lie in a consistent hierarchy of severity: are there respondents who said "I can walk a block or more" but said they could not walk 100 yards? If so, the intention of the scale to measure varying levels of mobility may not have been met, perhaps because some respondents do not understand 100 yards, or because they feel that a "block or more" may be less than 100 yards. Whatever the reason, the items may be reworded during the test development process. The hierarchical consistency is evaluated by coefficients of scalability and of reproducibility that range from 0.0 to 1.0. The coefficient of scalability indicates how far the questions form a cumulative scale, and should exceed 0.6 if the scale is truly unidimensional. The coefficient of reproducibility shows how accurately the scale score indicates a person's entire pattern of responses. In a valid scale the coefficient of reproducibility will fall above 0.9.

Sensitivity The ability of a measurement method or screening test to identify those who have a condition, calculated as the percentage of all cases with the condition who were judged by the test to have the condition: the "true positive" rate.

Spearman Correlation See Correlation.

Specificity The ability of a measurement to correctly identify those who do *not* have the condition in question.

Tau See Correlation.

Test-Retest Reliability The stability, or repeatability of a measurement is evaluated in terms of the correlation between a measurement applied to a sample of people and the same measurement applied at a later time (typically one or two weeks later).

Validity The extent to which a measurement method measures what it is intended to. A fuller discussion of validity is given on pages 26–31.

Visual Analogue Scale A broadly applicable format for a measurement scale in which the respondent places a mark at a point on a 10 cm line that indicates the intensity of his response. Phrases are printed at the ends of the line (e.g., "no pain" and "pain as bad as you can imagine") to indicate the scope of the scale (see page 236).

Yule's Q A correlation formula used for estimating the association between two binary variables.

Index